Abdominal Obesity and the Endocannabinoid System

Abdominal Obesity and the Endocannabinoid System

From Basic Aspects to Clinical Management of Related Cardiometabolic Risk

Edited by

Jean-Pierre Després
Université Laval
Quebec, Canada

Vincenzo Di Marzo
Consiglio Nazionale delle Ricerche
Pozzuoli, Napoli, Italy

informa
healthcare

New York London

Informa Healthcare USA, Inc.
52 Vanderbilt Avenue
New York, NY 10017

Printed in the United States of America on acid-free paper
10 9 8 7 6 5 4 3 2 1

International Standard Book Number ISBN-13: 978-1-4200-6084-3
International Standard Book Number ISBN-10: 1-4200-6084-8

Library of Congress Cataloging-in-Publication Data

Abdominal obesity and the endocannabinoid system : from basic aspects to clinical management of related cardiometabolic risk / edited by Jean-Pierre Despres,Vincenzo Di Marzo.
p. ; cm.
Includes bibliographical references and index.
ISBN-13: 978-1-4200-6084-3 (hardcover : alk. paper)
ISBN-10: 1-4200-6084-8 (hardcover : alk. paper) 1. Obesity–Molecular aspects.
2. Abdomen. 3. Cannabinoids. I. Després, Jean-Pierre. II. Di Marzo, Vincenzo.
[DNLM: 1. Obesity–complications. 2. Abdominal Fat. 3. Cardiovascular Diseases. 4. Endocannabinoids–physiology. 5. Metabolic Syndrome X. WD 210 A1355 2008]
RC628.A233 2008
362.196'398–dc22

2008042736

For Corporate Sales and Reprint Permissions call 212–520-2700 or write to: Sales Department, 52 Vanderbilt Avenue, 16th floor, New York, NY 10017.

Visit the Informa Web site at
www.informa.com

and the Informa Healthcare Web site at
www.informahealthcare.com

Foreword

The worldwide development of an obesity epidemic with associated diabetes and cardiovascular disease represents one of the major challenges of the 21st century. Both the biomedical research investigator as well as the clinician are being challenged to advance our present understanding of the etiology and pathophysiology of obesity as well as to develop new therapeutic approaches to control the epidemic. During the last several years major new insights have been made in our understanding of the clinical importance of the adipocyte. The role of the adipocyte has evolved from that of an uninteresting storage organ for lipids to that of a dynamic endocrine organ which secretes hormones and cytokines which play a pivotal role in regulating metabolism, inflammation, and cardiovascular disease. Of particular importance has been the realization that there are marked differences in the metabolism of visceral and peripheral adiposity. Current evidence indicates that visceral obesity accompanied by ectopic fat in the liver and muscle is associated with insulin resistance and an increased risk of the development of diabetes and vascular disease. The frequent combination of visceral obesity and insulin resistance with increased triglycerides, low HDL, increased blood pressure and elevated blood glucose has led to the codification of this multiplex risk factor as the insulin resistance syndrome or metabolic syndrome. Although the academic community has struggled with the selection of the most effective nosology to deal with this constellation of risk factors, the underlying evidence that patients with the metabolic syndrome are at risk for the future development of diabetes and cardiovascular events continues to accrue. The addition of risk factors associated with the metabolic syndrome to the classical risk factors for cardiovascular disease has resulted in the concept of global cardiometabolic risk. The ultimate clarification of whether the metabolic risk factors associated with visceral adiposity and ectopic fat will predict cardiovascular events beyond or independently from the classical risk factors awaits further clinical studies. An additional advancement in the clinical assessment of high risk patients will be the delineation of individual risk factors as a continuum of severity rather than a dichotomized classification system. For the practicing physician a clinical clue for the identification of the high risk obese patient with insulin resistance and the metabolic syndrome from the low risk equally obese individual is an increased waist circumference and elevated triglycerides.

A major breakthrough in our understanding of the pathophysiological basis of obesity and the metabolic syndrome has been the elucidation of the role of the endocannabinoid system in the regulation of caloric intake and metabolism. The identification of the CB1 receptor and the metabolic effects of regulation of the endocannabinoid pathways in the brain as well as peripheral organs have provided major new insights into lipid and glucose metabolism as well as obesity. Although a definitive understanding of the endocannabinoid system is being actively pursued in laboratories around the world, the ability to modulate a potentially dysfunctional endocannabinoid system in obesity and the metabolic syndrome has arrived. Clinical experience with CB1 antagonists, in conjunction with aggressive lifestyle changes, is currently underway and the evaluation of side effects as well as the selection of the appropriate patient for treatment will be ascertained.

The chapters in this book provide an up to date unique compendium of basic research and clinical information from investigators with expertise in both obesity and the endocannabinoid system. A comprehensive analysis of the topics presented in the individual chapters will provide the reader with an exceptional in-depth knowledge of this exciting and explosive area of medicine

Bryan Brewer, Jr.
Cardiovascular Research Institute
Washington Hospital Center
Washington, D.C., U.S.A.

Preface

Why a book on abdominal obesity and the endocannabinoid system? This work summarizes about 20 years of exciting developments and conceptual advances in our understanding of the form of overweight/obesity carrying the highest risk for chronic disease: visceral obesity. Indeed, we now better understand that many complications of obesity are more related to the distribution of body fat than to excess total fat per se. On the other hand, studies conducted over the last decade have documented the importance of the endocannabinoid system in the control of regional fat deposition and in the regulation of carbohydrate and lipid metabolism. Thus, it is only recently that we have begun to recognize the interplay between a dysfunctional endocannabinoid system and visceral obesity and its complications. These notions have tremendously important clinical implications on how to target the endocannabinoid system in order to reduce abdominal obesity. Unfortunately, the pharmaceutical industry and regulatory agencies have used the old "overall obesity" paradigm to evaluate "anti-obesity" drugs under development, including the antagonists of endocannabinoid action. This traditional view of obesity, assessed in the old fashioned way on the basis of indices of relative weight such as the body mass index, have led to a very difficult and uncertain path for drug developers and for physicians and their patients who are still expecting a "miracle drug".

This book is currently the most comprehensive effort at describing the endocannabinoid system as a whole and its role in the regulation of body fat distribution and of abdominal obesity-related metabolic complications that increase the risk of type 2 diabetes and cardiovascular disease. Whether pharmaceutical companies and regulatory bodies will agree on better experimental designs and more carefully selected patient populations for the evaluation of drugs targeting the endocannabinoid system is, at this stage, unclear. We hope that this comprehensive effort will help shed light on these issues.

Jean-Pierre Després
Vincenzo Di Marzo

Contents

Contributors

Martin Adiels Wallenberg Laboratory, Sahlgrenska University Hospital, Göteborg, Sweden

Marie-Christine Alessi Laboratoire d'Hématologie, Faculté de Médecine, Université de la Méditerranée, Inserm, Marseille, France

Asem Ali Mayo Clinic, Rochester, Minnesota, U.S.A.

Robert M. Anthenelli Department of Psychiatry, Tri-State Tobacco and Alcohol Research Center, University of Cincinnati College of Medicine, Cincinnati, Ohio, U.S.A.

Nir Barzilai Albert Einstein College of Medicine of Yeshiva University, Jack and Pearl Resnick Campus, Bronx, New York, U.S.A.

Luigi Bellocchio Endocrinology Unit and Center of Applied Biomedical Research (CRBA), Department of Internal Medicine and Gastroenterology, S. Orsola-Malpighi Hospital, University of Bologna, Bologna, Italy

Alvin Berger Metabolon, Inc., Durham, North Carolina, U.S.A. Department of Nutrition, University of North Carolina, Chapel Hill, North Carolina, U.S.A.

Richard N. Bergman Department of Physiology and Biophysics, University of Southern California, Los Angeles, California, U.S.A.

Jan Borén Wallenberg Laboratory, Sahlgrenska University Hospital, Göteborg, Sweden

Galina Burdyga School of Biomedical Sciences, University of Liverpool, Liverpool, U.K.

Karyn Catalano Department of Physiology and Biophysics, University of Southern California, Los Angeles, California, U.S.A.

Cristina Cervino Endocrinology Unit and Center of Applied Biomedical Research (CRBA), Department of Internal Medicine and Gastroenterology, S. Orsola-Malpighi Hospital, University of Bologna, Bologna, Italy

Jenny D. Chiu Department of Physiology and Biophysics, University of Southern California, Los Angeles, California, U.S.A.

Daniela Cota INSERM U862, Université Bordeaux 2, Bordeaux, France

Jean-Pierre Després Québec Heart Institute, Hôpital Laval Research Centre and Division of Kinesiology, Department of Social and Preventive Medicine, Université Laval, Québec City, QC, Canada

Vincenzo Di Marzo Endocannabinoid Research Group, Institute of Biomolecular Chemistry, National Research Council, Pozzuoli, Naples, Italy

Graham J. Dockray School of Biomedical Sciences, University of Liverpool, Liverpool, U.K.

Ester Fride Departments of Behavioral Sciences and Molecular Biology, Ariel University Center, Ariel, Israel

Luc F. Van Gaal Department of Endocrinology, Diabetology and Metabolism, Antwerp University Hospital, Antwerp, Belgium

Hertzel C. Gerstein Department of Medicine and Population Health Research Institute, McMaster University and Hamilton Health Sciences, Hamilton, Ontario, Canada

Nikolai Gobshtis Departments of Behavioral Sciences and Molecular Biology, Ariel University Center, Ariel, Israel

Lisa N. Harrison Department of Physiology and Biophysics, University of Southern California, Los Angeles, California, U.S.A.

Jaimee L. Heffner Department of Psychiatry, Tri-State Tobacco and Alcohol Research Center, University of Cincinnati College of Medicine, Cincinnati, Ohio, U.S.A.

Isabel Hsu Department of Physiology and Biophysics, University of Southern California, Los Angeles, California, U.S.A.

Derek M. Huffman Albert Einstein College of Medicine of Yeshiva University, Jack and Pearl Resnick Campus, Bronx, New York, U.S.A.

Viorica Ionut Department of Physiology and Biophysics, University of Southern California, Los Angeles, California, U.S.A.

Angelo A. Izzo Endocannabinoid Research Group, Department of Experimental Pharmacology, University of Naples Federico II, Naples, Italy

Peter M. Janiszewski School of Kinesiology and Health Studies, Queen's University, Kingston, Ontario, Canada

Michael D. Jensen Mayo Clinic, Rochester, Minnesota, U.S.A.

Richard Jones Division of Gastroenterology, Hope Hospital, University of Manchester, Manchester, U.K.

Irène Juhan-Vague Laboratoire d'Hématologie, Faculté de Médecine, Université de la Méditerranée, Inserm, Marseille, France

Morvarid Kabir Department of Physiology and Biophysics, University of Southern California, Los Angeles, California, U.S.A.

Stella P. Kim Department of Physiology and Biophysics, University of Southern California, Los Angeles, California, U.S.A.

Tim C. Kirkham School of Psychology, University of Liverpool, Eleanor Rathbone Building, Bedford Street South, Liverpool, England, U.K.

Thomas W. Klein Department of Molecular Medicine, School of Basic Biomedical Sciences, College of Medicine, University of South Florida, Tampa, Florida, U.S.A.

Cathryn Kolka Department of Physiology and Biophysics, University of Southern California, Los Angeles, California, U.S.A.

George Kunos Section on Neuroendocrinology, Laboratory of Physiological Studies, NIAAA, National Institutes of Health, Bethesda, Maryland, U.S.A.

Max Lafontan Unité Inserm 858, Institut de Médecine Moléculaire de Rangueil, Hôpital Rangueil and Université Paul Sabatier, Toulouse Cedex, France

Benoît Lamarche Institute of Nutraceuticals and Functional Foods, Laval University, Québec, Canada

Isabelle Lemieux Québec Heart Institute, Hôpital Laval Research Centre, Québec City, Canada

Jaana Lindström Department of Public Health, University of Helsinki and Diabetes Unit, Department of Health Promotion and Chronic Disease Prevention, National Public Health Institute, Helsinki, Finland

Sophie Lotersztajn INSERM U 841, Université Paris XII-Val de Marne, AP-HP, Groupe hospitalier Henri Mondor-Albert Chenevier, Service d'Hépatologie et de Gastroentérologie, Creteil, France

Maya Lottati Department of Physiology and Biophysics, University of Southern California, Los Angeles, California, U.S.A.

Ariane Mallat INSERM U 841, Université Paris XII-Val de Marne, AP-HP, Groupe hospitalier Henri Mondor-Albert Chenevier, Service d'Hépatologie et de Gastroentérologie, Creteil, France

Isabel Matias U862 Centre de Recherche INSERM François Magendie, Université de Bordeaux 2, Bordeaux, France

Pál Pacher Section on Oxidative Stress Tissue Injury, Laboratory of Physiological Studies, NIAAA, National Institutes of Health, Bethesda, Maryland, U.S.A.

Uberto Pagotto Endocrinology Unit and Center of Applied Biomedical Research (CRBA), Department of Internal Medicine and Gastroenterology, S. Orsola-Malpighi Hospital, University of Bologna, Bologna, Italy

Renato Pasquali Endocrinology Unit and Center of Applied Biomedical Research (CRBA), Department of Internal Medicine and Gastroenterology, S. Orsola-Malpighi Hospital, University of Bologna, Bologna, Italy

Paul Poirier Department of Cardiology, Faculty of Pharmacy, Institut Universitaire de Cardiologie et de Pneumologie Hôpital Laval, Québec, Canada

Zubin Punthakee Department of Medicine, McMaster University and Hamilton Health Sciences, Hamilton, Ontario, Canada

Shimon Rabichev Departments of Behavioral Sciences and Molecular Biology, Ariel University Center, Ariel, Israel

Caroline Rhéaume Department of Medicine, Faculty of Medicine, Institut Universitaire de Cardiologie et de Pneumologie Hôpital Laval, Québec, Canada

Caroline Richard Institute of Nutraceuticals and Functional Foods, Laval University, Québec, Canada

Joyce M. Richey Department of Physiology and Biophysics, University of Southern California, Los Angeles, California, U.S.A.

Robert Ross School of Kinesiology and Health Studies, Department of Medicine, Division of Endocrinology and Metabolism, Queen's University, Kingston, Ontario, Canada

Luis M. Ruilope Hypertension Unit, Hospital 12 de Octubre, Madrid, Spain

André J. Scheen Division of Diabetes, Nutrition and Metabolic Disorders, CHU Sart Tilman, University of Liege, Liege, Belgium

Tracy A. Sherwood Department of Molecular Medicine, School of Basic Biomedical Sciences, College of Medicine, University of South Florida, Tampa, Florida, U.S.A

Ulf Smith The Lundberg Laboratory for Diabetes Research, Center of Excellence for Cardiovascular and Metabolic Research, Department of Molecular and Clinical Medicine, The Sahlgrenska Academy, University of Gothenburg, Gothenburg, Sweden

Darko Stefanovski Department of Physiology and Biophysics, University of Southern California, Los Angeles, California, U.S.A.

Marja-Riitta Taskinen Department of Medicine, Helsinki University Central Hospital, Helsinki, Finland

André Tchernof Molecular Endocrinology and Oncology Research Center & Department of Nutrition, Laval University Medical Research Center and Laval University, Québec, Canada

David G. Thompson Division of Gastroenterology, Hope Hospital, University of Manchester, Manchester, U.K.

Jaakko Tuomilehto Department of Public Health, University of Helsinki and Diabetes Unit, Department of Health Promotion and Chronic Disease Prevention, National Public Health Institute, Helsinki, Finland and South Ostrobothnia Central Hospital, Seinäjoki, Finland

Alain Veilleux Molecular Endocrinology and Oncology Research Center & Department of Nutrition, Laval University Medical Research Center and Laval University, Québec, Canada

Valentina Vicennati Endocrinology Unit and Center of Applied Biomedical Research (CRBA), Department of Internal Medicine and Gastroenterology, S. Orsola-Malpighi Hospital, University of Bologna, Bologna, Italy

Orison O. Woolcott Department of Physiology and Biophysics, University of Southern California, Los Angeles, California, U.S.A.

Dan Zheng Department of Physiology and Biophysics, University of Southern California, Los Angeles, California, U.S.A.

1 Abdominal Obesity, Metabolic Syndrome, and Risk of Cardiovascular Disease

Jean-Pierre Després

Québec Heart Institute, Hôpital Laval Research Centre and Division of Kinesiology, Department of Social and Preventive Medicine, Université Laval, Québec City, QC, Canada

Vincenzo Di Marzo

Endocannabinoid Research Group, Institute of Biomolecular Chemistry, National Research Council, Pozzuoli, Naples, Italy

INTRODUCTION

Although it is well accepted that obesity is a health hazard and a risk factor for cardiovascular disease (CVD) and type 2 diabetes (1–4), physicians have been perplexed by the remarkable heterogeneity noticed among equally obese individuals. For instance, some obese patients are not characterized by any CVD risk factors, whereas others have type 2 diabetes and/or clinical signs of coronary heart disease (CHD) (5–10). Thus, although we recognize that obesity causes prejudice to health, why is this condition so heterogeneous in terms of its clinical manifestations?

Epidemiological and experimental studies published over the last three decades have contributed to establish the notion that it is the subgroup of overweight or obese patients characterized by an excess of abdominal fat, especially by a selective deposition of intra-abdominal or visceral adipose tissue, who is at the highest risk of developing type 2 diabetes and CVD (11–13).

OBESITY: MORE THAN EXCESS BODY WEIGHT

The relationship between body weight and mortality, CHD, or diabetes has been documented in many epidemiological studies (1,2,14). Thus, when populations are studied, there is a clear linear or curvilinear relationship between relative weight (the most common index used being the body mass index or BMI expressed in kg/m^2) and the presence of comorbidities such as type 2 diabetes and CVD. However, in clinical practice, physicians are constantly confronted to the problem that some equally obese individuals may or may not be characterized by the expected comorbidities of obesity. Because of this apparently weak relationship with comorbidities, obesity has for a long time not been considered among the "heavyweights" of modifiable CVD risk factors, which have traditionally included smoking, diabetes, a dyslipidemic state and hypertension.

More than half a century ago, Jean Vague from the University of Marseille had recognized that the complications of obesity were not dependent upon excess body fat mass per se but were rather the consequence of the regional distribution of body fat (15,16). Vague coined the term android or male-type obesity to characterize the form of overweight/obesity observed among his patients with diabetes or clinical signs of CVD, whereas he proposed that the lower body form of obesity frequently found in premenopausal obese women was rather benign (Fig. 1) (15,16). These remarkable clinical observations did not receive a lot of attention from the medical community, and it took more than 35 years before Vague's hypothesis received further support from "modern" prospective epidemiological studies.

Björntorp and colleagues from the University of Gothenburg in Sweden and Kissebah and his group in Milwaukee (U.S.A.) almost simultaneously published results showing highly significant relationships between regional body fat distribution and the comorbidities of obesity (17–20).

More recently, the international case-control INTERHEART study has provided robust evidence that among the 27,000 individuals stratified on the basis of their BMI values, subjects in the top quintiles of waist-to-hip ratio (WHR) were characterized by an increased odds ratio

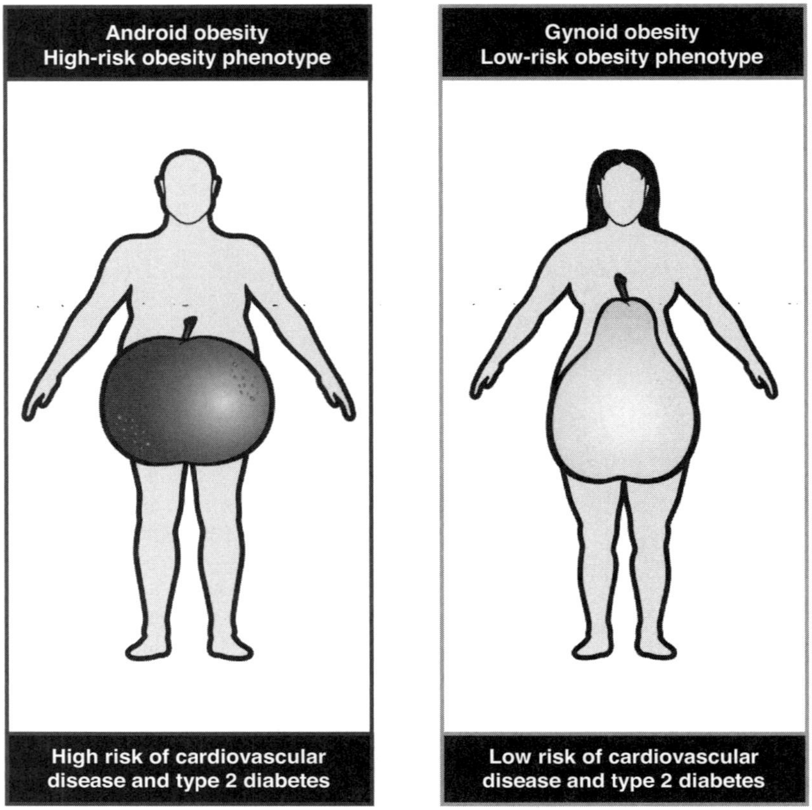

Figure 1 Android and gynoid obesity phenotype as first defined by Vague with preferential accumulation of adipose tissue in the abdominal and gluteo-femoral regions, respectively. The android pattern of adipose tissue distribution is closely associated with the metabolic complications of obesity, whereas the gynoid pattern is seldom associated with an altered metabolic profile.

of myocardial infarction (MI) (21). Therefore, this case-control study found that the proportion of abdominal fat is much more important to consider in the identification of individuals with clinical signs of CHD than the BMI. Additional evidence from other prospective studies has, however, indicated that both the BMI and the proportion of abdominal fat contribute to the risk of diabetes and CVD. For instance, data from large epidemiological studies including the IDEA and EPIC-Norfolk studies have further provided robust evidence that measuring waist circumference adds to the information provided by the BMI, as it helps physicians identify the subgroup of overweight/obese patients likely to be characterized by a greater accumulation of abdominal fat and at greater risk of diabetes and CVD (22,23).

ABDOMINAL OBESITY: A DEEPER LOOK AT THE CULPRIT ADIPOSE DEPOT

However, an increased waist circumference could be the result of an increased accumulation of subcutaneous fat or of visceral fat. Figure 2 shows two cross-sectional images of the abdomen which are obtained by computed tomography. The image is usually obtained by scanning the abdomen at the level of L4–L5. Computed tomography was a specialized equipment found in academic centres 2 or 3 decades ago. It has now become available even in regional hospitals making the measurement of visceral adiposity fairly simple for the patient and the physician. Because of the differences in the attenuation values of adipose, muscle, and bone tissues, it is very easy when studying the image to distinguish fat from muscle and bone. In the present figure, the intra-abdominal or visceral adipose tissue is highlighted in white. This Figure shows abdominal scans of two male subjects who have the same age, same BMI, same amount of total body fat but with a high or low accumulation of visceral adipose tissue determined by computed tomography. It is quite obvious that the subject on the right panel (subject B) had a

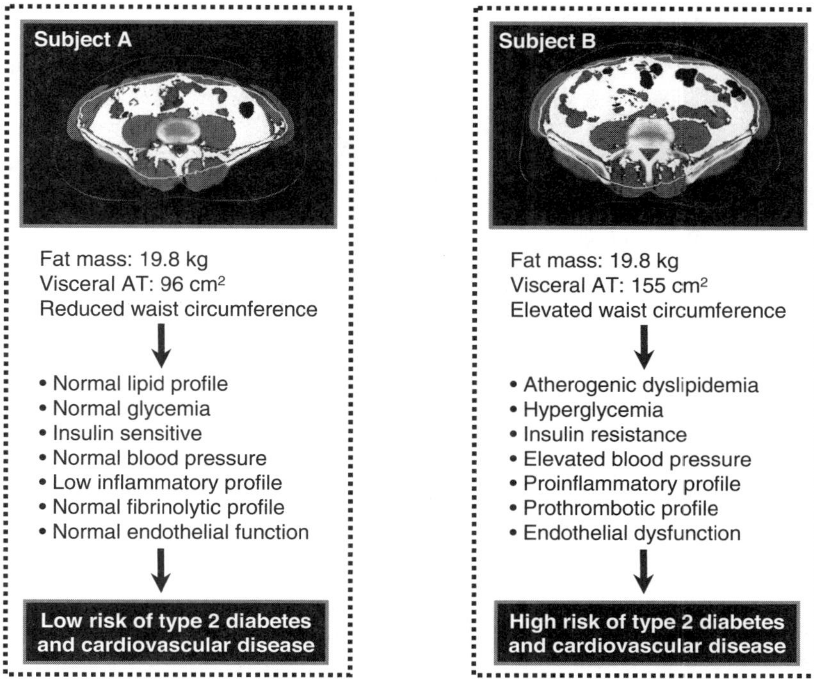

Figure 2 Marked differences in visceral adipose tissue accumulation measured by computed tomography in two subjects having the same amount of total body fat (19.8 kg) quantified by underwater weighing. Despite similar amount of total body fat, subject B has a greater cross-sectional accumulation of visceral adipose tissue (155 cm^2) than subject A (96 cm^2). This higher accumulation of visceral adipose tissue is associated with a diabetogenic and atherogenic metabolic risk profile.

greater accumulation of visceral fat than the subject on the left panel (subject A), despite the fact that both men had exactly the same amount of total body fat.

When we studied plasma glucose and insulin responses to a 75-g oral glucose load among subgroups of obese patients with the same level of obesity but with high versus low levels of visceral fat, we found trivial differences in glucose tolerance and in the insulin response between obese subjects with little visceral fat and lean controls (10). However, viscerally obese patients were characterized by a greater glycemic response observed in the presence of marked hyperinsulinemia, suggesting a greater level of insulin resistance in subjects with high levels of visceral adipose tissue compared to equally obese individuals with a low accumulation of visceral fat. Thus, viscerally obese patients represent a subgroup at much greater risk of developing type 2 diabetes.

When simple indices of the lipid profile were examined among the same three groups of subjects, only the viscerally obese patients were characterized by marked hypertriglyceridemia and by reduced HDL-cholesterol levels (10). Thus, visceral obesity in both men and women is associated with insulin resistance and with the high triglyceride–low HDL-cholesterol dyslipidemic state. Similar results were reported in both men and women (6,10).

Additional metabolic studies conducted in several laboratories around the world have shown that among equally obese patients, subjects with an excess of visceral adipose tissue have the most deteriorated metabolic risk profile (24–27). These individuals show insulin resistance and compensatory hyperinsulinemia as a sign of insulin resistance. Among genetically susceptible subjects, this condition favors the development of glucose intolerance and eventually leads to type 2 diabetes when the insulin-resistant state is accompanied by a relative deficit in insulin secretion (28). It is, however, important to point out that even in the absence of glucose intolerance and of marked hyperglycemia, visceral obesity and insulin resistance have been associated with a very typical dyslipidemic profile which includes hypertriglyceridemia, low HDL-cholesterol concentration, elevated apolipoprotein B as a marker of an increased concentration of atherogenic lipoproteins, and an increased concentration of small, dense LDL particles (7,29–31). In addition to the dyslipidemic insulin resistant profile of viscerally obese patients, these individuals are characterized by an impaired fibrinolysis, an increased susceptibility to thrombosis, endothelial dysfunction (as an early sign of endothelial damage) and an inflammatory profile (Fig. 2) (8,32–35).

The cardiovascular risk associated with some of the features of visceral obesity has not been examined extensively as markers of insulin resistance, and related abnormalities have not been commonly measured in large prospective studies. In the Québec Cardiovascular Study, a prospective study conducted in a sample of initially asymptomatic middle-aged men, there was an opportunity to test the hypothesis that fasting hyperinsulinemia, as a crude marker of insulin resistance, could be a relevant marker of CHD risk (36). Furthermore, as hyperinsulinemic men are also often characterized by elevated apolipoprotein B and small LDL particles, we tested the hypothesis that this triad of abnormalities (hyperinsulinemia, elevated apolipoprotein B, small LDL particles), which is commonly found in viscerally obese individuals, could increase the risk of CHD (37).

For comparison purposes, men of the Québec Cardiovascular Study who had none of the features of the atherogenic metabolic triad at baseline were considered as the reference group to whom a CHD odds ratio of 1.0 was attributed. Men characterized by the three abnormalities had a substantially increased risk of CHD (20.8-fold increase in CHD risk over a 5-year follow-up). Adjustment of this odds ratio for traditional risk factors and lipid variables such as LDL-cholesterol, triglycerides, and HDL-cholesterol failed to substantially alter the odds ratio associated with the presence of hyperinsulinemia, elevated apolipoprotein B, and small LDL particles; such ratio remaining elevated by 18-fold among men characterized by the atherogenic metabolic triad compared to men having none of these abnormalities. In comparison, the presence of the traditional lipid triad (elevated triglycerides, LDL-cholesterol, and reduced HDL-cholesterol) increased CHD risk by 4.4-fold. These results from the Québec Cardiovascular Study provided evidence that more refined markers of the metabolic consequences of visceral obesity could improve our ability to assess CHD risk beyond traditional risk factors and lipid variables. Further work is clearly warranted to examine this question.

Thus, some of the complications of abdominal obesity associated with an excess of visceral fat appear to increase the risk of CHD beyond what could be predicted from the presence of traditional risk factors. As an atherogenic dyslipidemia and a state of insulin resistance are conditions frequently observed among patients with abdominal obesity and excess visceral adipose tissue accumulation in clinical practice, it has been suggested that the most prevalent form of the metabolic syndrome was found among patients with an elevated waistline and an excess of visceral adipose tissue (31). In addition to these complications, inflammation has also been examined in the context of abdominal obesity and studies have shown that it is associated with abdominal fat accumulation (8,38). For instance, we had previously reported that high C-reactive protein (CRP) concentrations were associated with an elevated waist circumference and with a greater accumulation of visceral adipose tissue (8). Multivariate analyses revealed that waist circumference was by far the best predictor of individual differences in CRP concentration found in our sample.

ADIPOSE TISSUE: A REMARKABLE ENDOCRINE ORGAN

The reason for this close relationship between the expanded waistline and the elevated CRP could result from the fact that there is evidence of macrophage infiltration in adipose tissue of abdominally obese patients (39). These macrophages could become a production site of inflammatory cytokines such as tumor necrosis factor (TNF)-α and interleukin (IL)-6 that could have a local impact on adipose tissue metabolism as well as on systemic effects exacerbating the dysmetabolic profile noted among patients with an excess of visceral adipose tissue (40–44). For instance, the TNF-α could make the adipose tissue insulin resistant (45) and also has an inhibitory effect on the production of adiponectin (46) (an important adipose tissue–derived cytokine which has been suggested to have anti-atherogenic and antidiabetic properties) (47). In addition, the release of IL-6 by fat cells is known to stimulate the production of CRP through the liver (48).

Therefore, although the so-called "portal free fatty acid hypothesis" has been suggested to explain some of the metabolic abnormalities associated with excess adipose tissue accumulation, the hyperlipolytic state of the expanded visceral depot cannot, by itself, explain all the metabolic abnormalities observed in viscerally obese patients (49). However, if we consider the exciting new findings indicating that adipose tissue is an important endocrine organ (50) and a site of production of inflammatory cytokines such as IL-6 and TNF-α and of a potentially protective cytokine such as adiponectin (the production of the latter being reduced in visceral obesity), one can now better understand why marked alterations are observed in the metabolic profile of viscerally obese patients (8,38,42,51). Therefore, the hyperlipolytic state and proinflammatory profile of the expanded visceral fat depot could explain the constellation of metabolic abnormalities found in viscerally obese patients.

METABOLIC SYNDROME: CLEARING THE CONFUSION BETWEEN THE DEFINITION AND SCREENING TOOLS

Thus, abdominal obesity characterized by excess visceral fat accumulation is the form of overweight/obesity associated with a constellation of abnormalities increasing the risk of diabetes and CVD. In this context, the introduction of the metabolic syndrome as a concept by the National Cholesterol Education Program—Adult Treatment Panel III (NCEP-ATP III) in 2001 and the identification of simple criteria to identify in clinical practice individuals likely to be characterized by the features of the metabolic syndrome were important milestones in preventive medicine (52). Furthermore, NCEP-ATP III has recommended the measurement of waist circumference rather than BMI to put further emphasis on the important role played by abdominal obesity as the most prevalent form of the athero-thrombotic, inflammatory abnormalities of the metabolic syndrome (53). It is, however, important to point out that the NCEP-ATP III criteria do not represent the definition of the metabolic syndrome. Indeed, the metabolic syndrome was defined by NCEP-ATP III as a cluster of athero-thrombotic, inflammatory abnormalities increasing the risk of type 2 diabetes and CVD, its most prevalent form being found in patients with abdominal obesity and insulin resistance (53). This definition of a constellation of risk factors has unfortunately too often been confused with the five clinical criteria proposed by NCEP-ATP III to identify individuals likely to be characterized by the metabolic syndrome.

Furthermore, in the American Diabetes Association (ADA)/European Association for the Study of Diabetes (EASD) document, the relevance of the diagnosis of the metabolic syndrome has been questioned (54). It was suggested, for instance, that the metabolic syndrome cannot by itself appropriately assess global cardiovascular risk and this criticism is certainly justified. Whether the diagnosis of the metabolic syndrome adds to global CVD risk assessed on the basis of traditional risk factors has not been properly examined in the literature. Furthermore, not all patients with the metabolic syndrome are characterized by the same clustering abnormalities, and once a diagnosis is established, traditional risk factors have to be treated following guidelines. Whether the presence/absence of the metabolic syndrome will modify the therapeutic pharmacological approaches remains an open question for the moment.

It is very important to emphasize the notion that although there are other causes of insulin resistance and of the metabolic syndrome, this constellation of metabolic abnormalities is most frequently found among patients with abdominal obesity and with an excess visceral adipose tissue accumulation. This is the most prevalent form of the metabolic syndrome as recognized by NCEP-ATP III and by the recent International Diabetes Federation (IDF) guidelines (52,55). This prevalent form of the metabolic syndrome should not be confused with the various clinical tools, criteria that have been proposed by several organizations to identify individuals who are likely to have the constellation of metabolic abnormalities. Therefore, the various criteria from different organizations do not represent different definitions of the metabolic syndrome but rather tools which can be used in clinical practice to identify patients likely to be characterized by the clustering abnormalities of the syndrome. In addition, there is a very lively debate as to whether visceral adiposity or insulin resistance is the key core culprit. Clearly, insulin resistance is an essential component of the clustering abnormalities of the metabolic syndrome. However, in clinical practice, it is important to emphasize to the primary care physician that abdominal obesity, especially when accompanied by an excessive visceral fat accumulation, is by far the most prevalent form of insulin resistance. Therefore, while additional studies are needed to better understand the pathophysiological aspects of the metabolic syndrome, it is clear that the prevalent form of the metabolic syndrome is accompanied by visceral adiposity and insulin resistance and that these are core features which are predictive of additional metabolic abnormalities increasing the risk of complications.

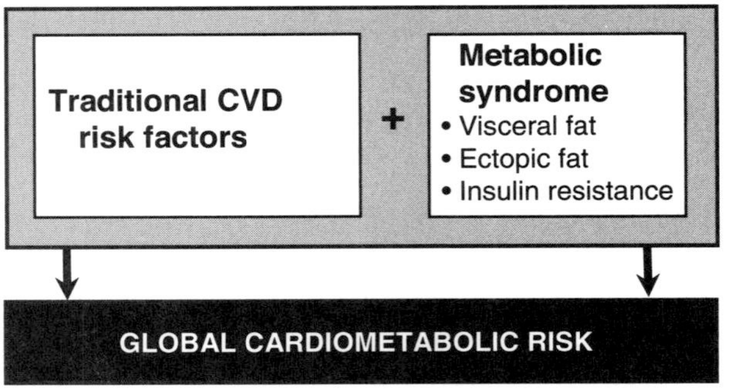

Figure 3 The concept of global cardiometabolic risk. It is now established that the metabolic syndrome is associated with an increased relative risk of cardiovascular disease (CVD). Under this model, the metabolic syndrome constitutes a novel modifiable risk factor for CVD. In clinical practice, the metabolic syndrome is often accompanied by an insulin-resistance state, visceral obesity, and ectopic fat, which reflect the presence of a dysfunctional adipose tissue. As a classical approach, the clinician interested by the evaluation of global CVD risk will consider traditional risk factors and calculate a global risk score using algorithms. However, because of the high prevalence of the metabolic syndrome and of its associated risk, it is also important to take into account the cardiovascular risk associated with the metabolic syndrome along with the risk associated with traditional risk factors (age, sex, genetic susceptibility, lipid profile, blood pressure, smoking habits), this risk being described as global cardiometabolic risk. There is currently a debate as to whether the metabolic syndrome adds to global CVD risk assessed by traditional risk factors and further work in this area is clearly warranted.

Thus, one should distinguish the conceptual definition of the metabolic syndrome from tools which can be used by physicians to identify individuals most likely to have the features of metabolic syndrome. Among those tools and clinical criteria, it has been suggested that waist circumference and fasting triglyceride levels are probably the two early key markers of an increased probability of being characterized by the features of the metabolic syndrome (29).

FROM ABDOMINAL OBESITY TO METABOLIC SYNDROME AND GLOBAL CARDIOMETABOLIC RISK

Therefore, physicians should keep in mind that it is important to first assess global CVD risk on the basis of the traditional risk factors. Clearly, smoking, hypertension, a dyslipidemic state, and the presence of diabetes are key modifiable CVD risk factors. Global risk engines do exist such as the Framingham (56) or the PROCAM (57) algorithms, and modifiable traditional risk factors are playing a very important role in driving the patient's absolute risk of CVD in addition to factors such as age and gender. However, the presence of the metabolic syndrome has been shown to increase the relative risk of CVD by approximately 2-fold (58,59). However, increasing the risk of CVD by 2-fold does not necessarily put the patient at high absolute risk of CVD. Figure 3 illustrates the notion that one has to pay attention to both the traditional risk factors and the metabolic syndrome. Clearly, we need more results from prospective studies to address the question whether the presence of the metabolic syndrome has an impact on the global CVD risk assessed on the sole basis of traditional risk factors.

For the time being, it is proposed that the global CVD risk resulting from the presence of traditional risk factors and from the features of the metabolic syndrome defines global cardiometabolic risk (60,61). Additional prospective studies with measurements of traditional risk factors and of various features of the metabolic syndrome are urgently needed to provide physicians with better risk assessment algorithms. This is particularly important considering the very high prevalence of patients with type 2 diabetes, with abdominal obesity, and with the features of the metabolic syndrome in clinical practice.

CONCLUSION

We need to pay attention to the abdominally obese patient with a large waistline and with clinical features of the metabolic syndrome, and we need to target a root cause of their additional cardiometabolic risk, which is abdominal obesity resulting from their sedentary/affluent lifestyle. Unfortunately, until we reshape our urban and living environment to promote physical activity and healthy nutrition, physicians will have a hard time improving the lifestyle of their patients because the medical system is currently ill equipped to handle this huge wave of sedentary patients with abdominal obesity, metabolic syndrome, and type 2 diabetes. To have a true impact on this epidemic of abdominal obesity and type 2 diabetes, a multidisciplinary approach will be required involving all relevant stakeholders. Meanwhile, it is hoped that we will work on improving our clinical approach aiming at the optimal assessment and management of high-risk abdominally obese patients.

ACKNOWLEDGMENTS

The work of the author has been supported by research grants from the Canadian Institutes of Health Research, the Canadian Diabetes Association, the Heart and Stroke Foundation, and by the Foundation of the Québec Heart Institute. Dr. Després is the Scientific Director of the International Chair on Cardiometabolic Risk, which is supported by an unrestricted grant from Sanofi-Aventis awarded to Université Laval.

REFERENCES

1. Willett WC, Manson JE, Stampfer MJ, et al. Weight, weight change, and coronary heart disease in women. Risk within the 'normal' weight range. JAMA 1995; 273(6):461–465.
2. Colditz GA, Willett WC, Rotnitzky A, et al. Weight gain as a risk factor for clinical diabetes mellitus in women. Ann Intern Med 1995; 122(7):481–486.
3. Kissebah AH, Freedman DS, Peiris AN. Health risk of obesity. Med Clin North Am 1989; 73:111–138.
4. Bray GA. Complications of obesity. Ann Intern Med 1985; 103:1052–1062.
5. Pascot A, Lemieux I, Prud'homme D, et al. Reduced HDL particle size as an additional feature of the atherogenic dyslipidemia of abdominal obesity. J Lipid Res 2001; 42(12):2007–2014.
6. Pouliot MC, Després JP, Nadeau A, et al. Visceral obesity in men. Associations with glucose tolerance, plasma insulin, and lipoprotein levels. Diabetes 1992; 41(7):826–834.
7. Tchernof A, Lamarche B, Prud'homme D, et al. The dense LDL phenotype. Association with plasma lipoprotein levels, visceral obesity, and hyperinsulinemia in men. Diabetes Care 1996; 19(6):629–637.
8. Lemieux I, Pascot A, Prud'homme D, et al. Elevated C-reactive protein: Another component of the atherothrombotic profile of abdominal obesity. Arterioscler Thromb Vasc Biol 2001; 21(6):961–967.
9. Couillard C, Bergeron N, Prud'homme D, et al. Postprandial triglyceride response in visceral obesity in men. Diabetes 1998; 47:953–960.
10. Després JP, Moorjani S, Lupien PJ, et al. Regional distribution of body fat, plasma lipoproteins, and cardiovascular disease. Arteriosclerosis 1990; 10(4):497–511.
11. Nicklas BJ, Penninx BW, Cesari M, et al. Association of visceral adipose tissue with incident myocardial infarction in older men and women: The health, aging and body composition study. Am J Epidemiol 2004; 160(8):741–749.
12. Kuk JL, Katzmarzyk PT, Nichaman MZ, et al. Visceral fat is an independent predictor of all-cause mortality in men. Obes Res 2006; 14(2):336–341.
13. Boyko EJ, Fujimoto WY, Leonetti DL, et al. Visceral adiposity and risk of type 2 diabetes: A prospective study among Japanese Americans. Diabetes Care 2000; 23(4):465–0471.
14. Manson JE, Willett WC, Stampfer MJ, et al. Body weight and mortality among women. N Engl J Med 1995; 333(11):677–685.
15. Vague J. Sexual differentiation, a factor affecting the forms of obesity. Presse Méd 1947; 30:339–340.
16. Vague J. The degree of masculine differentiation of obesities: A factor determining predisposition to diabetes, atherosclerosis, gout and ulric calculous disease. Am J Clin Nutr 1956; 4:20–34.
17. Ohlson LO, Larsson B, Svardsudd K, et al. The influence of body fat distribution on the incidence of diabetes mellitus: 13.5 years of follow-up of the participants in the study of men born in 1913. Diabetes 1985; 34:1055–1058.
18. Krotkiewski M, Björntorp P, Sjöström L, et al. Impact of obesity on metabolism in men and women. Importance of regional adipose tissue distribution. J Clin Invest 1983; 72:1150–1162.
19. Kissebah AH, Vydelingum N, Murray R, et al. Relation of body fat distribution to metabolic complications of obesity. J Clin Endocrinol Metab 1982; 54(2):254–260.

20. Larsson B, Svardsudd K, Welin L, et al. Abdominal adipose tissue distribution, obesity, and risk of cardiovascular disease and death: 13 year follow-up of participants in the study of men born in 1913. Br Med J 1984; 288:1401–1404.
21. Yusuf S, Hawken S, Ounpuu S, et al. Obesity and the risk of myocardial infarction in 27,000 participants from 52 countries: A case-control study. Lancet 2005; 366(9497):1640–1649.
22. Balkau B, Deanfield JE, Després JP, et al. International Day for the Evaluation of Abdominal Obesity (IDEA): A study of waist circumference, cardiovascular disease, and diabetes mellitus in 168,000 primary care patients in 63 countries. Circulation 2007; 116(17):1942–1951.
23. Canoy D, Boekholdt SM, Wareham N, et al. Body fat distribution and risk of coronary heart disease in men and women in the European prospective investigation into cancer and nutrition in Norfolk cohort: A population-based prospective study. Circulation 2007; 116(25):2933–2943.
24. Bacha F, Saad R, Gungor N, et al. Obesity, regional fat distribution, and syndrome X in obese black versus white adolescents: Race differential in diabetogenic and atherogenic risk factors. J Clin Endocrinol Metab 2003; 88(6):2534–2540.
25. Ross R, Aru J, Freeman J, et al. Abdominal adiposity and insulin resistance in obese men. Am J Physiol Endocrinol Metab 2002; 282(3):E657-E663.
26. Ross R, Freeman J, Hudson R, et al. Abdominal obesity, muscle composition, and insulin resistance in premenopausal women. J Clin Endocrinol Metab 2002; 87(11):5044–5051.
27. Cnop M, Landchild MJ, Vidal J, et al. The concurrent accumulation of intra-abdominal and subcutaneous fat explains the association between insulin resistance and plasma leptin concentrations: Distinct metabolic effects of two fat compartments. Diabetes 2002; 51(4):1005–1015.
28. Prentki M, Nolan CJ. Islet beta cell failure in type 2 diabetes. J Clin Invest 2006; 116(7):1802–1812.
29. Lemieux I, Pascot A, Couillard C, et al. Hypertriglyceridemic waist. A marker of the atherogenic metabolic triad (hyperinsulinemia, hyperapolipoprotein B, small, dense LDL) in men? Circulation 2000; 102:179–184.
30. Després JP, Lemieux I, Prud'homme D. Treatment of obesity: need to focus on high risk abdominally obese patients. BMJ 2001; 322(7288):716–720.
31. Després JP. Is visceral obesity the cause of the metabolic syndrome? Ann Med 2006; 38(1):52–63.
32. Juhan-Vague I, Morange P, Renucci JF, et al. Fibrinogen, obesity and insulin resistance. Blood Coagul Fibrinolysis 1999; 10(Suppl. 1):S25-S28.
33. Juhan-Vague I, Alessi MC. PAI-1, obesity, insulin resistance and risk of cardiovascular events. Thromb Haemost 1997; 78(1):656–660.
34. Mertens I, Van Der Planken M, Corthouts B, et al. Is visceral adipose tissue a determinant of von Willebrand factor in overweight and obese premenopausal women? Metabolism 2006; 55(5):650–655.
35. Couillard C, Ruel G, Archer WR, et al. Circulating levels of oxidative stress markers and endothelial adhesion molecules in men with abdominal obesity. J Clin Endocrinol Metab 2005; 90(12):6454–6459.
36. Després JP, Lamarche B, Mauriège P, et al. Hyperinsulinemia as an independent risk factor for ischemic heart disease. N Engl J Med 1996; 334:952–957.
37. Lamarche B, Tchernof A, Mauriège P, et al. Fasting insulin and apolipoprotein B levels and low-density lipoprotein particle size as risk factors for ischemic heart disease. JAMA 1998; 279(24):1955–1961.
38. Hak AE, Stehouwer CD, Bots ML, et al. Associations of C-reactive protein with measures of obesity, insulin resistance, and subclinical atherosclerosis in healthy, middle-aged women. Arterioscler Thromb Vasc Biol 1999; 19(8):1986–1991.
39. Weisberg SP, McCann D, Desai M, et al. Obesity is associated with macrophage accumulation in adipose tissue. J Clin Invest 2003; 112(12):1796–1808.
40. Després JP. Inflammation and cardiovascular disease: Is abdominal obesity the missing link? Int J Obes Relat Metab Disord 2003; 27(Suppl. 3):S22-S24.
41. Berg AH, Scherer PE. Adipose tissue, inflammation, and cardiovascular disease. Circ Res 2005; 96(9):939–949.
42. Côté M, Mauriège P, Bergeron J, et al. Adiponectinemia in visceral obesity: Impact on glucose tolerance and plasma lipoprotein and lipid levels in men. J Clin Endocrinol Metab 2005; 90(3):1434–1439.
43. Matsuzawa Y. Therapy Insight: Adipocytokines in metabolic syndrome and related cardiovascular disease. Nat Clin Pract Cardiovasc Med 2006; 3(1):35–42.
44. Hotamisligil GS. Molecular mechanisms of insulin resistance and the role of the adipocyte. Int J Obes Relat Metab Disord 2000; 24(Suppl. 4):S23-S27.
45. Hotamisligil GS, Spiegelman BM. Tumor necrosis factor alpha: A key component of the obesity-diabetes link. Diabetes 1994; 43(11):1271–1278.
46. Bruun JM, Lihn AS, Verdich C, et al. Regulation of adiponectin by adipose tissue-derived cytokines: In vivo and in vitro investigations in humans. Am J Physiol Endocrinol Metab 2003; 285(3):E527-E533.
47. Nedvidkova J, Smitka K, Kopsky V, et al. Adiponectin, an adipocyte-derived protein. Physiol Res 2005; 54(2):133–140.
48. Gabay C, Kushner I. Acute-phase proteins and other systemic responses to inflammation. N Engl J Med 1999; 340(6):448–454.

49. Jensen MD. Is visceral fat involved in the pathogenesis of the metabolic syndrome? Human model. Obesity (Silver Spring) 2006; 14(Suppl. 1):20S–24S.
50. Flier JS. The adipocyte: Storage depot or node on the energy information superhighway? Cell 1995; 80(1):15–18.
51. Yudkin JS, Stehouwer CD, Emeis JJ, et al. C-reactive protein in healthy subjects: Associations with obesity, insulin resistance, and endothelial dysfunction: A potential role for cytokines originating from adipose tissue? Arterioscler Thromb Vasc Biol 1999; 19(4):972–978.
52. Expert Panel on Detection, Evaluation, and Treatment of High Blood Cholesterol in Adults. Executive Summary of the Third Report of the National Cholesterol Education Program (NCEP) Expert Panel on Detection, Evaluation, and Treatment of High Blood Cholesterol in Adults (Adult Treatment Panel III). JAMA 2001; 285(19):2486–2497.
53. Grundy SM, Brewer HB Jr., Cleeman JI, et al. Definition of metabolic syndrome: Report of the National Heart, Lung, and Blood Institute/American Heart Association conference on scientific issues related to definition. Circulation 2004; 109(3):433–438.
54. Kahn R, Buse J, Ferrannini E, et al. The metabolic syndrome: Time for a critical appraisal: Joint statement from the American Diabetes Association and the European Association for the Study of Diabetes. Diabetes Care 2005; 28(9):2289–2304.
55. Alberti KG, Zimmet P, Shaw J. The metabolic syndrome—A new worldwide definition. Lancet 2005; 366(9491):1059–1062.
56. Wilson PW, D'Agostino RB, Levy D, et al. Prediction of coronary heart disease using risk factor categories. Circulation 1998; 97(18):1837–1847.
57. Assmann G, Cullen P, Schulte H. Simple scoring scheme for calculating the risk of acute coronary events based on the 10-year follow-up of the prospective cardiovascular Munster (PROCAM) study. Circulation 2002; 105(3):310–315.
58. Galassi A, Reynolds K, He J. Metabolic syndrome and risk of cardiovascular disease: A meta-analysis. Am J Med 2006; 119(10):812–819.
59. Gami AS, Witt BJ, Howard DE, et al. Metabolic syndrome and risk of incident cardiovascular events and death: A systematic review and meta-analysis of longitudinal studies. J Am Coll Cardiol 2007; 49(4):403–414.
60. Després JP, Lemieux I. Abdominal obesity and metabolic syndrome. Nature 2006; 444(7121):881–887.
61. Després JP, Lemieux I, Bergeron J, et al. Abdominal obesity and the metabolic syndrome: Contribution to global cardiometabolic risk. Arterioscler Thromb Vasc Biol 2008; 28(6):1039–1049.

2 Abdominal Obesity in Type 2 Diabetes

Isabelle Lemieux
Québec Heart Institute, Hôpital Laval Research Centre, Québec City, Canada

Jean-Pierre Després
Québec Heart Institute, Hôpital Laval Research Centre and
Division of Kinesiology, Department of Social and Preventive Medicine, Université Laval, Québec City, Canada

INTRODUCTION

There is a worldwide increase in the prevalence of obesity (1,2), which contributes to the increasing incidence of type 2 diabetes. This phenomenon represents a challenge to control cardiovascular disease (CVD), as more than 75% of patients with type 2 diabetes will die from cardiovascular complications (Fig. 1) (3,4). Type 2 diabetes has therefore reached epidemic proportions (5,6), and the International Diabetes Federation estimates that almost 333 millions of individuals will be affected by type 2 diabetes by 2025 (7). As the parallel rapid growth of overweight/obesity and of type 2 diabetes is striking (2), some investigators have coined the term "diabesity" (6,8) to stress the link between these two conditions; excess body weight (fat) being the major cause of type 2 diabetes.

In this regard, a strong positive relationship between excess adiposity and the risk of type 2 diabetes has been reported in epidemiological studies, since many years (9–11). More recently, results of the Nurses' Health Study, which enrolled almost 12,000 women followed for 14 years, have highlighted the fact that the risk of type 2 diabetes was increased even in women whose body mass index (BMI; a marker of total adiposity) was in the range of 23.0 to 25.0 kg/m^2 (considered as "normal" weight) compared with women whose BMI was less than 22.0 kg/m^2 (10). This study also reported that an increase in body weight (from 7.0 to 10.9 kg) was associated with a 2-fold increase in the risk of developing type 2 diabetes over the 14-year follow-up (10). Moreover, middle-aged women who lost more than 5.0 kg had a significantly reduced risk of type 2 diabetes compared to women with stable body weight. However, despite this well-established contribution of obesity to the risk of type 2 diabetes, it is also recognized that not all obese individuals will develop this metabolic disease. Some factors have been identified which can contribute to explain the heterogeneity associated with the obesity state. In this regard, numerous studies have shown that the regional distribution of body fat plays a significant role in the modulation of the obesity health hazard. In the present chapter, we will specially focus on the importance of paying attention to body fat distribution, particularly to visceral adiposity as the hazardous form of obesity in the evaluation of type 2 diabetes risk.

REGIONAL BODY FAT DISTRIBUTION: DOES IT REALLY MATTER? REVIEW OF THE EVIDENCE

Early pioneering work from Dr. Jean Vague from the University of Marseille has allowed for the first time to recognize that the distribution of body fat could influence disease risk beyond overall obesity (12,13). Vague made the early observation that diabetes and CVD were the diseases that were more often observed among overweight/obese patients characterized by a preferential accumulation of fat in the upper body region (he referred to it as android obesity) than among those who preferentially accumulated adipose tissue in the lower part of their body, that is, around their hips and thighs (a condition that he described as gynoid obesity) (12,13). Since these remarkable landmark observations, many cross-sectional and prospective studies have tied type 2 diabetes to body fat distribution. As early as in 1969, it was reported that type 2 diabetic patients were characterized by more total body fat than nondiabetic subjects, and that this fat surplus was preferentially distributed in the trunk as determined by skinfold

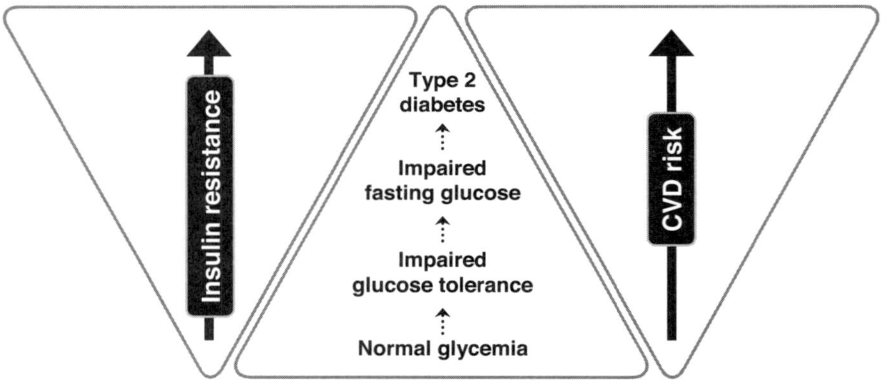

Figure 1 The risk of type 2 diabetes increases as a function of increasing glycemia. This phenomenon, in whole or in part, is the consequence of an insulin-resistant state. On the other hand, the risk of cardiovascular disease (CVD) also increases in a stepwise manner across the glycemia continuum, and the majority of patients with type 2 diabetes (>75%) will die from CVD.

measurements (14). Moreover, a greater proportion of obese women with upper body fat had glucose values in the diabetes range compared to equally obese women characterized by fat localized principally in the gluteo-femoral area (15). In a large sample size of more than 15,000 women, the predominance of fat in the upper body region was associated with a relative risk of diabetes which was as high as among women with severe obesity (16). In this study, the simultaneous presence of severe obesity and of upper body fat yielded a 10.3-fold increased risk of diabetes.

The risk of developing diabetes over a 13.5-year follow-up period has also been investigated in the sample of middle-aged men from the Gothenburg Prospective Study (17). When men were stratified into tertiles of BMI and of waist-to-hip ratio (as an index of the proportion of abdominal fat), it was evident that even among lean individuals (men in the first BMI tertiles), those in the top tertile for the waist-to-hip ratio had a 6-fold increase in the risk of developing diabetes (from 0.5% incidence to 2.9%). On the other hand, being in the top BMI tertile in the absence of an elevated waist-to-hip ratio was not associated with an increased risk of developing diabetes. Finally, among equally overweight/obese individuals (the three subgroups of men in the top BMI tertile), the proportion of abdominal fat as estimated by the waist-to-hip ratio had a huge impact on the risk of developing diabetes; the risk being increased by 30-fold among overweight individuals from the lowest to the top waist-to-hip ratio tertile. The role played by obesity and body fat distribution in type 2 diabetes risk was also examined in women of the Gothenburg prospective study (18). Similar conclusions were reached with body fat distribution in the abdominal region (as determined by the waist-to-hip ratio) as well as the total amount of fat, which were both important risk factors for diabetes (18). Therefore, results of the Gothenburg Prospective Study were one of the key results of early findings, which provided the evidence that we had to go beyond measuring the BMI to better appreciate the risk of diabetes associated with overweight and obesity.

More recently, several large prospective studies have confirmed the role played by abdominal obesity in the modulation of the risk of type 2 diabetes (19–21). The Nurses' Health Study followed for 8 years a cohort of over 43,000 women free of diabetes and other major chronic diseases at baseline (20). Women in the study who were characterized by an elevated waist circumference ($>90^{th}$ percentile), as an indicator of the absolute amount of abdominal fat, had a 5.1-fold increased risk of developing type 2 diabetes compared to women with a low waist circumference ($<10^{th}$ percentile). Furthermore, a consistent increase in type 2 diabetes risk was observed as waist circumference increased within each BMI category. The Health Professionals Follow-Up Study conducted in 27,270 men, examined the predictive risk of type 2 diabetes according to BMI, waist circumference or waist-to-hip ratio subgroups (21). Age-adjusted relative risks during the 13-year follow-up across quintiles of waist circumference were 1.0, 2.0, 2.7, 5.0, and 12.0; those for quintiles of waist-to-hip ratio were 1.0, 2.1, 2.7, 3.6, and 6.9; whereas those for quintiles of BMI were 1.0, 1.1, 1.8, 2.9, and 7.9. Additional analyses revealed that waist circumference and BMI were similar and better than waist-to-hip ratio in predicting type 2 diabetes risk. Finally, robust evidence from the International Day for the Evaluation of Abdominal Obesity (IDEA) was made available in 2008 (19). Briefly, the IDEA study is an epidemiological cross-sectional study conducted in 63 countries and involved more than 6400 primary care physicians who were instructed on how to properly measure the waist circumference of their patients evaluated on two separate half days. At the end of the study, data on waist circumference and BMI were obtained in about 100,000 women and 70,000 men and the relationship with the prevalence of type 2 diabetes and CVD was examined. There was a continuous relationship between waist circumference and the prevalence of diabetes and CVD in both men and women. Moreover, the BMI and waist circumference were both associated with diabetes and CVD. Of utmost importance, at any BMI value, an elevated waist circumference was predictive of a greater risk of diabetes or CVD.

Based on the results of the above-mentioned studies, measuring abdominal obesity, especially with waist circumference, allows to further refine the risk associated with total adiposity.

VISCERAL ADIPOSITY AND TYPE 2 DIABETES RISK: A HIGH-RISK OBESITY PHENOTYPE

Visceral Obesity and Metabolic Disturbances Predictive of Type 2 Diabetes

Although waist-to-hip ratio and waist circumference have been widely used to characterize abdominal obesity, they do not distinguish subcutaneous from visceral (intra-abdominal) adipose tissue. Only imaging techniques such as computed tomography or magnetic resonance imaging have allowed to precisely measure the size of these two metabolically distinct abdominal fat depots (22). Measurements performed with these techniques have shown that individuals with a greater proportion of visceral adipose tissue are at substantially higher risk of being insulin resistant and of developing atherogenic and diabetogenic complications. In this regard, in 1987, Fujioka and colleagues (23) were among the first to report that among individuals with similar BMI values, those with a preferential accumulation of visceral adipose tissue were characterized by higher glucose responses following an oral glucose tolerance test as well as by higher triglyceride concentrations than individuals who accumulated their excess fat in the subcutaneous depot. Following the publication of these results, several studies have reported similar associations between the accumulation of visceral fat and deteriorations of indices of glucose–insulin homeostasis (24–34). In a study performed more than 20 years ago, Sparrow et al. (28) reported that type 2 diabetic patients were characterized by a significantly greater amount of visceral adipose tissue than subjects with normal glucose tolerance after adjusting for age and BMI. In a sample of healthy nonobese (mean BMI = 24.7 kg/m^2) young men, a high visceral fat accumulation was associated with a decreased insulin sensitivity measured by the euglycemic–hyperinsulinemic glucose clamp (31). These findings suggest that even in nondiabetic, nonobese young men, an excess of visceral adipose tissue is associated with impairments in the metabolism of glucose and insulin.

Additional results have confirmed that visceral obesity, measured by imaging techniques, is the dangerous form of obesity which is correlated to substantial disturbances in indices of plasma glucose–insulin homeostasis (27,33–36). For instance, individuals carefully matched for total adiposity or subcutaneous fat, with either a low or a high accumulation of visceral adipose tissue, have been shown to be markedly different in their levels of insulin resistance and glucose tolerance (27,33–36). However, after being matched for visceral adiposity, individuals with low or high levels of subcutaneous fat were not found to differ in insulin sensitivity (33,34). These findings reinforce the notion that visceral adipose tissue is a robust marker of insulin resistance in abdominally obese individuals, independent of overall adiposity.

Visceral Obesity and Development of Type 2 Diabetes

Although many cross-sectional studies have demonstrated relationships between the high-risk form of obesity, visceral fat, and metabolic complications, only a few prospective studies have examined the contribution of high levels of visceral fat as a predictor of the onset of type 2 diabetes (37,38). Nevertheless, a study performed in Japanese-American men have clearly shown that subjects who developed type 2 diabetes during the course of the study had higher levels of visceral fat at baseline than subjects who did not develop type 2 diabetes, but this association disappeared after adjusting for glycemia (37). However, this study included only

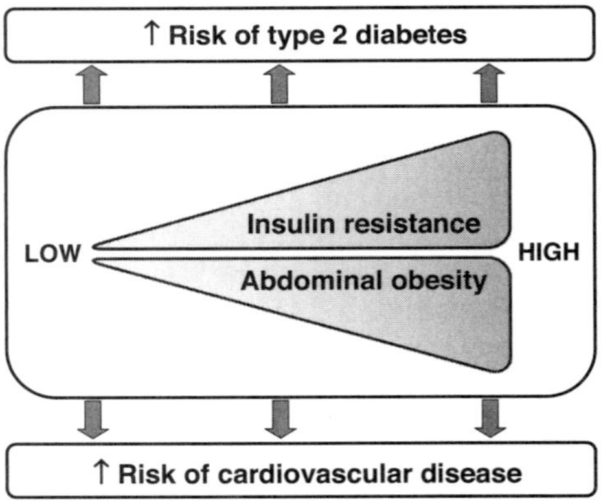

Figure 2 Abdominal obesity, especially visceral obesity, is closely interrelated to the development of an insulin-resistant state, being predictive of a greater risk of type 2 diabetes and cardiovascular disease.

men and a limited number of patients developed type 2 diabetes. In a larger sample size with a longer follow-up, further results were reported from the same cohort (38). Boyko and colleagues (38) have found that excess visceral fat at baseline preceded the development of type 2 diabetes over 6 to 10 years in this sample of Japanese Americans. This relationship remained significant even after controlling for fasting insulin, insulin secretion, glycemia, total and regional adiposity, and family history of diabetes.

This study confirms the notion that high levels of visceral adipose tissue play a critical role in the development of type 2 diabetes. Nevertheless, additional prospective studies on the associations between visceral adiposity and associated metabolic disturbances are clearly warranted in order to better understand and elucidate the role of visceral adiposity in the progression of metabolic complications linked with a deterioration of insulin action potentially leading to the onset of type 2 diabetes (Fig. 2).

TYPE 2 DIABETES IS NOT A HOMOGENEOUS CONDITION: IMPORTANCE OF ABDOMINAL OBESITY AND RELATED FEATURES

Although patients with type 2 diabetes are, as a group, at greater risk of coronary heart disease (CHD) than individuals with normal fasting glucose levels, studies recently conducted have shown that type 2 diabetes is a heterogeneous entity (39,40). Among patients with type 2 diabetes, only those characterized by abdominal obesity and therefore by the likely presence of features of the metabolic syndrome appear to be at increased CHD risk. For instance, Alexander and colleagues (39) examined the prevalence of CHD across subgroups of subjects with/without metabolic syndrome and type 2 diabetes. They found that the presence of the metabolic syndrome increased the risk of CHD even in nondiabetic individuals. However, among patients with type 2 diabetes, only individuals with the simultaneous presence of features of the metabolic syndrome were at greater risk of CHD. For instance, the prevalence of CHD in the small group of diabetic patients without the metabolic syndrome was similar to nondiabetic individuals without the metabolic syndrome.

Furthermore, we have recently published results which support the concept put forward by Alexander that type 2 diabetes is not a homogeneous condition regarding CHD risk (40). Indeed, in a cohort of women who underwent coronary angiography for the investigation of retrosternal pain, Blackburn and colleagues (40) reported that the odds ratio (OR) of being diagnosed with coronary artery disease (CAD) was significantly increased among type 2 diabetic women compared with nondiabetic women. However, CAD risk in women with type 2 diabetes was only significantly increased among those showing some features of the metabolic syndrome, such as fasting hyperinsulinemia, increased apolipoprotein B levels, and small LDL particles, a triad of metabolic abnormalities that we had reported to be predictive of a substantially increased CHD risk (41). Thus, diabetes per se was not predictive of CAD in the absence of the concomitant presence of features of the metabolic syndrome.

Although it is still debated whether diabetes observed in isolation (in the absence of the metabolic syndrome) increases CHD risk considerably, results of these studies emphasize the

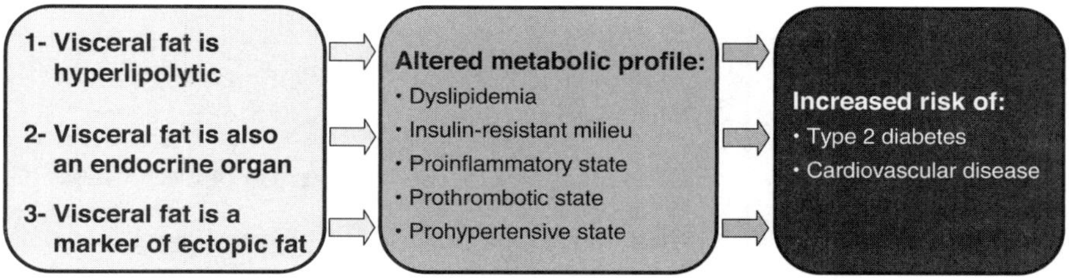

Figure 3 Several mechanisms by which visceral obesity, as the high-risk form of obesity, could be associated with an altered metabolic profile increasing the risk of type 2 diabetes and cardiovascular disease.

need to pay attention to other factors than glycemia to optimally assess and manage CHD risk among patients with type 2 diabetes.

PATHOPHYSIOLOGY OF EXCESS VISCERAL ADIPOSITY

The literature available on potential pathophysiological mechanisms linking excess visceral fat with an atherogenic and diabetogenic risk profile has been recently discussed and its review is beyond the scope of the present chapter (22,42). Figure 3 illustrates three scenarios that have been proposed to explain the link between visceral adiposity and related metabolic complications: (1) The hyperlipolytic state of the omental adipose tissue, which shows resistance to the action of insulin, contributes to expose the liver to increased levels of free fatty acids via the portal circulation. This situation generates several impairments in hepatic metabolic processes leading to hyperinsulinemia, glucose intolerance, and hypertriglyceridemia. (2) The adipose tissue, which is not only designed for fat storage and mobilization, but is also an endocrine organ releasing adipokines (e.g., adiponectin) including inflammatory cytokines (e.g., interleukin-6 and tumor necrosis factor-α), which contribute to the insulin resistant, inflammatory, prothrombotic, and hypertensive state of visceral obesity. (3) Excess visceral adipose tissue is in whole or in part an indicator of the relative incapacity of subcutaneous adipose tissue to play its role as a protective "metabolic sink." Therefore, individuals who cannot accumulate their energy surplus in the subcutaneous fat depot would display accumulation of fat at unwanted sites, such as the liver, the heart, the skeletal muscle and the pancreas, a phenomenon that has been described as ectopic fat. However, it is likely that all the above mechanisms are involved in the relationship of visceral obesity and metabolic complications.

CONCLUSION

It is clear that we are facing a diabetes epidemic worldwide which will not end until we properly prevent or at least assess and manage its underlying cause: abdominal obesity and more specifically visceral obesity. We must now urgently reshape our obesogenic and diabetogenic environments and this will imply the participation of all health care professionals, governments, and stakeholders in our fight against this "toxic" environment. In our current health care model, we legitimately treat the consequences of abdominal obesity in order to prevent, delay or at least treat the cardiovascular complications of patients with type 2 diabetes. However, because of the huge cardiovascular burden of type 2 diabetes, more focus should be placed on the prevention of this metabolic disease so closely related to abdominal obesity.

ACKNOWLEDGMENTS

The work of the authors has been supported by research grants from the Canadian Institutes of Health Research, the Canadian Diabetes Association, the Heart and Stroke Foundation and by the Foundation of the Québec Heart Institute. Dr. Després is the Scientific Director of the International Chair on Cardiometabolic Risk, which is supported by an unrestricted grant from Sanofi-Aventis awarded to Université Laval.

REFERENCES

1. Katzmarzyk PT. The Canadian obesity epidemic,1985–1998. CMAJ 2002; 166(8):1039–1040.
2. Mokdad AH, Ford ES, Bowman BA, et al. Prevalence of obesity, diabetes, and obesity-related health risk factors, 2001. JAMA 2003; 289(1):76–79.
3. Kannel WB, McGee DL. Diabetes and cardiovascular disease. The Framingham Study. JAMA 1979; 241(19):2035–2038.
4. Stamler J, Vaccaro O, Neaton JD, et al. Diabetes, other risk factors, and 12-yr cardiovascular mortality for men screened in the Multiple Risk Factor Intervention Trial. Diabetes Care 1993; 16(2):434–444.
5. Wild S, Roglic G, Green A, et al. Global prevalence of diabetes: Estimates for the year 2000 and projections for 2030. Diabetes Care 2004; 27(5):1047–1053.
6. Zimmet P, Alberti KGMM, Shaw J. Global and societal implications of the diabetes epidemic. Nature 2001; 414:782–787.
7. http://www.eatlas.idf.org/Prevalence/, accessed 22 April 2008.
8. Astrup A, Finer N. Redefining type 2 diabetes: 'Diabesity' or 'obesity dependent diabetes mellitus'? Obesity Rev 2000; 1:57–59.
9. Colditz GA, Willett WC, Stampfer MJ, et al. Weight as a risk factor for clinical diabetes in women. Am J Epidemiol 1990; 132:501–513.
10. Colditz GA, Willett WC, Rotnitzky A, et al. Weight gain as a risk factor for clinical diabetes mellitus in women. Ann Intern Med 1995; 122(7):481–486.
11. West KM, Kalbfleisch JM. Influence of nutritional factors on prevalence of diabetes. Diabetes 1971; 20:99–108.
12. Vague J. Sexual differentiation, a factor affecting the forms of obesity. Presse Méd 1947; 30:339–340.
13. Vague J. The degree of masculine differentiation of obesities: A factor determining predisposition to diabetes, atherosclerosis, gout and ulric calculous disease. Am J Clin Nutr 1956; 4:20–34.
14. Feldman R, Sender AJ, Siegelaub AB. Difference in diabetic and nondiabetic fat distribution patterns by skinfold measurements. Diabetes 1969; 18(7):478–486.
15. Kissebah AH, Vydelingum N, Murray R, et al. Relation of body fat distribution to metabolic complications of obesity. J Clin Endocrinol Metab 1982; 54(2):254–260.
16. Hartz AJ, Rupley DC, Jr., Kalkhoff RD,et al. Relationship of obesity to diabetes: Influence of obesity level and body fat distribution. Prev Med 1983; 12(2):351–357.
17. Ohlson LO, Larsson B, Svardsudd K, et al. The influence of body fat distribution on the incidence of diabetes mellitus: 13.5 years of follow-up of the participants in the study of men born in 1913. Diabetes 1985; 34:1055–1058.
18. Lundgren H, Bengtsson C, Blohme G, et al. Adiposity and adipose tissue distribution in relation to incidence of diabetes in women: Results from a prospective population study in Gothenburg, Sweden. Int J Obes 1989; 13(4):413–423.
19. Balkau B, Deanfield JE, Després JP, et al. International Day for the Evaluation of Abdominal Obesity (IDEA): A study of waist circumference, cardiovascular disease, and diabetes mellitus in 168,000 primary care patients in 63 countries. Circulation 2007; 116(17):1942–1951.
20. Carey VJ, Walters EE, Colditz GA, et al. Body fat distribution and risk of non-insulin-dependent diabetes mellitus in women. The Nurses' Health Study. Am J Epidemiol 1997; 145(7):614–619.
21. Wang Y, Rimm EB, Stampfer MJ, et al. Comparison of abdominal adiposity and overall obesity in predicting risk of type 2 diabetes among men. Am J Clin Nutr 2005; 81(3):555–563.
22. Després JP, Lemieux I. Abdominal obesity and metabolic syndrome. Nature 2006; 444(7121):881–887.
23. Fujioka S, Matsuzawa Y, Tokunaga K, et al. Contribution of intra-abdominal fat accumulation to the impairment of glucose and lipid metabolism in human obesity. Metabolism 1987; 36(1):54–59.
24. Kissebah AH. Insulin resistance in visceral obesity. Int J Obes 1991; 15(Suppl. 2):109–115.
25. Peiris AN, Sothmann MS, Hennes MI, et al. Relative contribution of obesity and body fat distribution to alterations in glucose insulin homeostasis: Predictive values of selected indices in premenopausal women. Am J Clin Nutr 1989; 49(5):758–764.
26. Pouliot MC, Després JP, Nadeau A, et al. Associations between regional body fat distribution, fasting plasma free fatty acid levels and glucose tolerance in premenopausal women. Int J Obes 1990; 14(4):293–302.
27. Pouliot MC, Després JP, Nadeau A, et al. Visceral obesity in men. Associations with glucose tolerance, plasma insulin, and lipoprotein levels. Diabetes 1992; 41(7):826–834.
28. Sparrow D, Borkan GA, Gerzof SG, et al. Relationship of fat distribution to glucose tolerance. Results of computed tomography in male participants of the Normative Aging Study. Diabetes 1986; 35(4):411–415.
29. Fujimoto WY, Newell-Morris LL, Grote M, et al. Visceral fat obesity and morbidity: NIDDM and atherogenic risk in Japanese American men and women. Int J Obes 1991; 15(Suppl. 2):41–44.

30. Després JP, Nadeau A, Tremblay A, et al. Role of deep abdominal fat in the association between regional adipose tissue distribution and glucose tolerance in obese women. Diabetes 1989; 38(3):304–309.
31. Park KS, Rhee BD, Lee KU, et al. Intra-abdominal fat is associated with decreased insulin sensitivity in healthy young men. Metabolism 1991; 40(6):600–603.
32. Peiris AN, Sothmann MS, Hoffmann RG, et al. Adiposity, fat distribution, and cardiovascular risk. Ann Intern Med 1989; 110(11):867–872.
33. Ross R, Aru J, Freeman J, et al. Abdominal adiposity and insulin resistance in obese men. Am J Physiol Endocrinol Metab 2002; 282(3):E657–E663.
34. Ross R, Freeman J, Hudson R, et al. Abdominal obesity, muscle composition, and insulin resistance in premenopausal women. J Clin Endocrinol Metab 2002; 87(11):5044–5051.
35. Després JP, Moorjani S, Lupien PJ, et al. Regional distribution of body fat, plasma lipoproteins, and cardiovascular disease. Arteriosclerosis 1990; 10(4):497–511.
36. Bacha F, Saad R, Gungor N, et al. Obesity, regional fat distribution, and syndrome X in obese black versus white adolescents: Race differential in diabetogenic and atherogenic risk factors. J Clin Endocrinol Metab 2003; 88(6):2534–2540.
37. Bergstrom RW, Newell-Morris LL, Leonetti DL, et al. Association of elevated fasting C-peptide level and increased intra-abdominal fat distribution with development of NIDDM in Japanese-American men. Diabetes 1990; 39(1):104–111.
38. Boyko EJ, Fujimoto WY, Leonetti DL, et al. Visceral adiposity and risk of type 2 diabetes: A prospective study among Japanese Americans. Diabetes Care 2000; 23(4):465–471.
39. Alexander CM, Landsman PB, Teutsch SM, et al. NCEP-defined metabolic syndrome, diabetes, and prevalence of coronary heart disease among NHANES III participants age 50 years and older. Diabetes 2003; 52:1210–1214.
40. Blackburn P, Lemieux I, Lamarche B, et al. Type 2 diabetes without the atherogenic metabolic triad does not predict angiographically assessed coronary artery disease in women. Diabetes Care 2008; 31(1):170–172.
41. Lamarche B, Tchernof A, Mauriège P, et al. Fasting insulin and apolipoprotein B levels and low-density lipoprotein particle size as risk factors for ischemic heart disease. JAMA 1998; 279(24):1955–1961.
42. Després JP, Lemieux I, Bergeron J, et al. Abdominal obesity and the metabolic syndrome: Contribution to global cardiometabolic risk. Arterioscler Thromb Vasc Biol 2008; 28(6):1039–1049.

3 Obesity and Hypertension

Paul Poirier

Department of Cardiology, Faculty of Pharmacy, Institut Universitaire de Cardiologie et de Pneumologie Hôpital Laval, Québec, Canada

Caroline Rhéaume

Department of Medicine, Faculty of Medicine, Institut Universitaire de Cardiologie et de Pneumologie Hôpital Laval, Québec, Canada

INTRODUCTION

Obesity, insulin resistance, and dysglycemia are common features in patients with systemic hypertension. Even if the relationship between these leading factors of cardiovascular disease is well known, the pathophysiology linking these features is not clear. Review of evidence from epidemiological and experimental studies, emphasizing a link between these three determinants of cardio-metabolic abnormalities, suggests that obesity (particularly abdominal obesity) may play a "central" role in the association between insulin resistance and systemic hypertension.

EXCESS WEIGHT AND BLOOD PRESSURE

The majority of patients with high blood pressure are overweight (1). Systemic hypertension is about six times more frequent in obese subjects than in lean men and women (1). Not only is systemic hypertension more frequent in obese subjects than in normal weight controls, but also weight gain in young people is a potent risk factor for subsequent development of systemic hypertension. A 10-kg higher body weight is associated with a 3.0-mmHg higher systolic and 2.3-mmHg higher diastolic blood pressure. These increases translate into an estimated 12% increased risk for CHD and 24% increased risk for stroke (2). In the vast majority of hypertensive patients, the occurrence of major events is the result of long-term exposure to multiple risk factors, and is usually preceded by the development of asymptomatic structural and functional abnormalities at the vascular and cardiac levels (3). Nevertheless, not every obese individual is hypertensive indicating that obesity is a heterogeneous condition. Also, it is well recognized that technical difficulties exist in the indirect measurement of blood pressure in the obese patient that may result in an overestimation of the level of blood pressure (4) or underestimation of the presence of left ventricular hypertrophy (Table 1).

Factors to be considered in linking obesity to an increase in blood pressure are related to changes in cardiac output and peripheral vascular resistance since BP = CO × SVR, where BP is blood pressure, CO is cardiac output, and SVR is systemic vascular resistance. These factors include: (1) direct impacts of obesity on hemodynamics and (2) mechanisms linking obesity and an increase in peripheral vascular resistance, for example, insulin resistance, sympathetic nervous system, and adipokines released from adipocytes, as well as the presence of sleep apnea. It is important that the physician who evaluates a referred patient for hypertension should be very suspicious of obese patients who admit habitual snoring, nocturnal gasping or choking, witnessed episodes of apnea, and daytime sleepiness, and should also consider sleep-disordered breathing (4). Obesity might be a confounding factor given the strong association of obesity with sleep-disordered breathing, and sleep apnea might be one of the intermediary mechanisms by which overweight is causally related to systemic hypertension.

Obesity per se is associated with alterations in hemodynamics (4). An increase in oxygen demand produced by excess adipose tissue (~1.5 mL/kg/min) requires an increase in cardiac output as well as a parallel increase in blood volume. Thus, obese individuals have increased in blood volume, stroke volume, and cardiac output. This high-output state is associated with a reduction in peripheral vascular resistance in individuals with normal blood pressure as would be predicted from Poiseuille's formula: $R = \Delta P/F = (8/\pi) \times (\eta) \times (l/r^4)$, where R is resistance,

Table 1 Detection of Left Ventricular Hypertrophy by QRS Voltage in Obesity

	Sensibility in obesity (%)	Specificity in obesity (%)	Accuracy in obesity (%)
Sokolow-Lyon	20	93	65
Romhilt-Estes point score $\geq$4	31	83	63
Cornell	49	93	76

Sokolow-Lyon voltage criteria: R in V_5 or V_6 + S in V_1 >35 mm.
Romhilt-Estes point score; Am Heart J 1968, 75: 752–758.
Cornell voltage criteria: R in aVL + S in V_3 >28 mm in men, >20 mm in women
Source: Adapted from Casale et al., J Am Coll Cardiol 1985, 6: 572–580.

$8/\pi$ is a numerical factor, η is blood viscosity, and l/r^4 is a geometric factor. Because of the marked influence of the geometric factor (to the fourth power) in the equation, vascular resistance is decreased. Thus, obese persons with an increase in blood pressure greater than optimal, that is, systemic hypertension, have a peripheral vascular resistance that is either inappropriately "normal," or increased. Therefore, while an increase in cardiac output may add to the increase in blood pressure, in the obese individual, an abnormal increase in blood pressure is primarily dependent on an increase in peripheral vascular resistance.

PATHOPHYSIOLOGICAL PROCESSES LINKING INSULIN TO HYPERTENSION

Since the first description of hyperinsulinemia in hypertensive patients (5), numerous investigations have been performed to clarify the link between insulin resistance and hypertension (6–8). Despite apparently conflicting results reported in the literature, a meta-analysis supported the role of hyperinsulinemia in the pathogenesis of essential hypertension (9). Since then, this role was corroborate by results from the San Antonio Heart study in which it was reported that elevated fasting insulin was among metabolic changes that may precede the development of hypertension (10). Insulin concentrations have also been associated with the incidence of hypertension in other large cohort such as the Atherosclerosis Risk in Communities (ARIC) study (11), the Coronary Artery Risk Development in (Young) Adults (CARDIA) study (12), as well as in the eastern Finland cohort (13). Recently, insulin resistance was also prospectively linked to incident hypertension. Interestingly, the Insulin Resistance Atherosclerosis Study (IRAS), observed an inverse association between insulin sensitivity (SI) and incident hypertension (10% decrease for every increase of SI unit) (14). A large cross-sectional study in the healthy population (normotensive without diabetes) has shown that each increase of 10 unit of insulin resistance corresponded to an increment of 1.7 mmHg of systolic and 2.3 mmHg of diastolic blood pressure (15). In young normotensive Americans, Falkner and coworkers reported a similar association (16). Finally, these results were recently confirmed in individuals without diabetes (7) as well as in individuals with diabetes (17). The pathogenesis through which insulin potentially induces hypertension is not clearly identified since there are most certainly numerous mechanisms involved. Except for a mild vasodilator effect encountered in insulin sensitive individual, it has been shown that insulin stimulates numerous processes (Table 1). All of the potential pathophysiological mechanisms linking insulin to hypertension have been investigated in experimental studies which were exhaustively summarized in a recent review (18). Nevertheless, the link between insulin resistance and blood pressure suffers from a lack of consistency from one study to another. Ferrannini et al. commented on the large differences in the strength of the association reported in several studies and suggested that confounders and sample size are primarily responsible for this discrepancy (15). Adding to this concept, one could add ethnicity as an important potential confounder. Indeed, the strength of the relationship between insulinemia, insulin resistance, and hypertension varies widely according to ethnic groups (1) showing no racial difference in the IRAS study (14), (2) weak associations in African-Americans as compared to white Americans in the ARIC (11) and the CARDIA studies (12), and (3) a strong relationship observed in European individuals (15). Thus, ethnicity is probably an important factor in the relationship between insulin and hypertension (19).

Small cross-sectional studies also showed that hypertensive subjects have a higher risk of insulin resistance compared to normotensive subjects (20,21) but not in all study (22). Metabolic pathways through which elevated blood pressure induces insulin resistance are not clearly understood. Hemodynamic basis (23,24), resistance to insulin-mediated glucose disposal (6), the renin–angiotensin system (RAS) (25,26), or the stimulation of nitric oxide (NO) synthesis (27) have all been implicated, but is still a topic of debate. Nevertheless, the link between insulin abnormalities and blood pressure has now been more accepted. But, the controversy of the direction of the link still remains. This is mainly due to the etiological heterogeneity of hypertension (6). Consequently, insulin may be viewed as an etiologic component of hypertension. Within this multifactorial framework of the etiology of hypertension, one must consider obesity as another major determinant.

In a population of hypertensive subjects without diabetes, it has been recently shown that obesity and insulin resistance have an additive effect which explains a significant variance of the model (38%) (28). In other words, obesity, insulin resistance, and hypertension are highly interrelated and there is collinearity among these parameters (25). Indeed, the Baltimore Longitudinal Study of Aging reported, in a Caucasian population of 649 patients, that the simple correlation between fasting insulin and blood pressure was secondary to the confounding effects of age and obesity (29). The correlation of blood pressure was considerably stronger, in both sexes, with body mass index (BMI), percent body fat, and waist/hip ratio than that of insulin levels (29). The strength of the relationship between insulin resistance, obesity, and hypertension triad was largely described in adult, as well as in childhood and adolescence 10 years ago (30).

Obesity is recognized as a major cause of hypertension in humans (31), and is also strongly associated with insulin resistance (32). For both associations, mechanisms are not fully understood. Many pathways are suspected, such as an activation of the RAS, increment in sympathetic nervous system activity, which mediates an increase in leptin secretion as well as an involvement of microvascular dysfunction (33). These mechanisms may contribute to the increase in blood pressure resulting from increasing levels of adiposity independently of insulin resistance. Sympathetic nervous system activation, associated with obesity (34) and molecules released by hypertrophied fat cells are two factors with the potential to promote the formation of angiotensin II (Ang II) and aldosterone. These have a direct vasopressor and antinatriuretic effect (35). A local RAS is present in human adipose tissue and may act as a distinct system from the plasma RAS (36,37). The involvement of adipose tissue RAS in hypertension needs to be confirmed in human. Secondary to the liver, white adipose tissue is an important production site of angiotensinogen (AGT). This hormone is secreted into the circulation and it is conceivable that it increased cardio-metabolic complications.

In accordance, several studies have demonstrated that weight loss induced concomitant reduction in blood pressure and insulin resistance (38,39). In light of these findings, obesity may appear to be an essential, yet complex, factor in the insulin resistance–hypertension relationship. Even if these results need to be prospectively confirmed, this supports obesity as an etiological factor of hypertension via increased insulin resistance. Also, a gene–environment interaction should be considered when looking at different populations. Concordance rates of 15% for dizygotic and 31% for monozygotic twins have been reported in those with both obesity and hypertension (40).

Whatever be the true extent of the influence of obesity, body fat distribution is a crucial determinant of insulin resistance and hypertension. It has been established that abdominal obesity, or android obesity, is an important constituent of insulin resistance, hypertension, type 2 diabetes, and cardiovascular disease (4). Visceral adipose tissue (VAT) secretes numerous biologically active substances (adipokines) that act on insulin resistance and vasculature (41). All components of the RAS system (AGT, AT_1 receptor, and ACE, but neither renin, nor AT_2 receptor) are found in both visceral and subcutaneous adipose tissue (42). Therefore, one could speculate that the contribution of adipose tissue to plasma AGT levels is significant in the overweight or obese subjects. Because plasma AGT levels correlate with blood pressure and are associated with BMI (43), it is tempting to speculate that hypertension is associated with overweight and/or obesity, which may be mediated by AGT produced by the enlarged adipose tissue mass (44). This model implies adipose tissue RAS in the pathogenic alterations of metabolism and hypertension.

There is an increasing evidence from small and large human epidemiological studies that abdominal fat may have a great implication in the link between insulin resistance and hypertension. It was reported that 1 kg increment in visceral fat predicts a 10 mmHg increase

Table 2 Potential Pathophysiological Pathways of Obesity/Insulin Resistance Leading to Systemic Hypertension

Stimulation of the sympathetic nervous system
Stimulation or renal sodium retention
Decreased heart rate variability
Hemodynamic effects
Hypertrophy of smooth muscle by vascular or endothelial resistance

in blood pressure (45). VAT was also associated with blood pressure and hyperinsulinemia in children (46). In postmenopausal women, a negative correlation was observed between blood pressure or insulin and fat leg mass compared to adipose tissue stored in the visceral region, suggesting some degree a protection of peripheral adiposity (47).

Waist circumference (above and beyond BMI) showed a great ability to predict hypertension in a large population (48). Indeed, waist circumference has been reported as the strongest independent predictor (including age, gender, BMI, and insulin resistance) for both systolic and diastolic blood pressure in 413 normoglycemic Chinese individuals (49). A similar association, in a cohort of 563 Japanese Americans, has been recently reported between the prevalence of hypertension and intra-abdominal fat accumulation, but not with waist circumference (50). Recently, a comparative study on different abdominal fat measurement showed that waist circumference correlated better than BMI or percent fat measured by DEXA with insulin, blood pressure as well as glucose concentration, triglycerides, and HDL levels in healthy whites and African-American men and women (51).

Waist circumference may be "central" in the association between insulin resistance and hypertension, but further research is needed to confirm this concept (52). It is plausible that crosstalks exist between VAT, Ang II, and insulin in the overweight/obesity state in humans, in an independent and facilitative manner, depending on a permissive genetic background. This process may contribute to conditions such as the development of cardiovascular diseases and metabolic complications. Central obesity, assessed by waist circumference, has a predominant role, compared to insulin levels, in explaining individual differences in blood pressure, at least in Caucasian (48), Chinese (49), and Japanese (50).

Potential pathophysiological mechanisms linking insulin to hypertension are numerous (Table 2). The presence of abdominal obesity may influence the pathophysiological events linking insulin resistance to hypertension as shown by the association between blood pressure and waist. Nevertheless, the link between insulin resistance and blood pressure suffers from a lack of consistency, and ethnicity may be an important potential confounder.

ADIPOSITY INDICES AND HYPERTENSION

Although excess fatness may contribute to high blood pressure in obese patients, the best indices of adiposity which relate to blood pressure are still unclear. Investigators have reported the relationship between indices of adiposity (BMI, waist circumference, waist/hip and waist/height ratios, percentage of body fat derived from skin-fold thicknesses) and blood pressure in normotensive and untreated hypertensive African-Americans (53). In a stepwise regression analysis, waist/hip ratio was the best adiposity parameter explaining the variation in blood pressure in the whole population, while waist circumference was the best correlate of blood pressure in normotensive individuals.

WEIGHT LOSS

Regardless of the mechanisms involved, weight loss in obese individuals is associated with a decrease in blood pressure. In 50% or more of individuals, the average decrease in diastolic blood pressure is 1–4 mmHg systolic and 1–2 mmHg diastolic per kilogram of weight reduction as normalization of blood pressure (54–56). It is noticed that after the weight loss has ceased, the persistent effect of weight loss on blood pressure may not always be encountered (57,58).

CONCLUSION

Obesity alone does not appear to be responsible for an increase in blood pressure. Even when the obesity is distributed to the upper body and the individuals are morbidly obese, not all individuals are hypertensive. Factors such as genotype, diabetes mellitus, atherosclerosis, etc., and environmental factors are probably responsible, just as they are for lean individuals with systemic hypertension. Regardless of mechanism, weight loss in obese individuals is associated with a decrease in blood pressure. In the search for a "healthy weight," it is very important to inform patients about the results to be expected to avoid unrealistic weight loss expectations. Bodyweight normalization should not be the primary target but rather some weight loss could lead to substantial improvements in blood pressure. There is extensive research directed at the development of new anti-obesity compounds. The effect of these molecules on cardiovascular risk factors has been studied and reported but information regarding their impact on the cardiovascular system is sparse (59).

REFERENCES

1. Stamler R, Stamler J, Riedlinger Wf, et al. Weight and blood pressure. Findings in hypertension screening of 1 million Americans. JAMA 1978; 240:1607–1610.
2. Clinical Guidelines on the Identification, Evaluation, and Treatment of Overweight and Obesity in Adults—The Evidence Report. National Institutes of Health. Obes Res 1998; Suppl. 2:51s–209s.
3. Devereux Rb, Alderman Mh. Role of preclinical cardiovascular disease in the evolution from risk factor exposure to development of morbid events. Circulation 1993; 88:1444–1455.
4. Poirier P, Giles Td, Bray Ga, et al. Obesity and cardiovascular disease: Pathophysiology, evaluation, and effect of weight loss: An update of the 1997 American Heart Association Scientific Statement on Obesity and Heart Disease from the Obesity Committee of the Council on Nutrition, Physical Activity, and Metabolism. Circulation 2006; 113:898–918.
5. Welborn Ta, Breckenridge A, Rubinstein Ah, et al. Serum-insulin in essential hypertension and in peripheral vascular disease. Lancet 1966; 1:1336–1337.
6. Reaven Gm, Lithell H, Landsberg L. Hypertension and associated metabolic abnormalities—The role of insulin resistance and the sympathoadrenal system. N Engl J Med 1996; 334:374–381.
7. Saad Mf, Rewers M, Selby J, et al. Insulin resistance and hypertension: The insulin resistance atherosclerosis study. Hypertension 2004; 43:1324–1331.
8. Lin Mw, Hwu Cm, Huang Yh, et al. Directly measured insulin resistance and the assessment of clustered cardiovascular risks in hypertension. Am J Hypertens 2006; 19:1118–1124.
9. Denker Ps, Pollock Ve. Fasting serum insulin levels in essential hypertension. A meta-analysis. Arch Intern Med 1992; 152:1649–1651.
10. Haffner Sm, Miettinen H, Gaskill Sp, et al. Metabolic precursors of hypertension. The San Antonio Heart Study. Arch Intern Med 1996; 156:1994–2001.
11. Liese Ad, Mayer-Davis Ej, Chambless Le, et al. Elevated fasting insulin predicts incident hypertension: The aric study. Atherosclerosis risk in communities study investigators. J Hypertens 1999; 17:1169–1177.
12. Dyer Ar, Liu K, Walsh M, et al. Ten-year incidence of elevated blood pressure and its predictors: The cardia study. Coronary artery risk development in (young) adults. J Hum Hypertens 1999; 13:13–21.
13. Salonen Jt, Lakka Ta, Lakka Hm, et al. Hyperinsulinemia is associated with the incidence of hypertension and dyslipidemia in middle-aged men. Diabetes 1998; 47:270–275.
14. Goff Dc Jr, Zaccaro Dj, Haffner Sm, et al. Insulin sensitivity and the risk of incident hypertension: Insights from the insulin resistance atherosclerosis study. Diabetes Care 2003; 26:805–809.
15. Ferrannini E, Natali A, Bell P, et al. Insulin resistance and hypersecretion in obesity. European Group for the Study of Insulin Resistance (Egir). J Clin Invest 1997; 100:1166–1173.
16. Falkner B, Sherif K, Sumner Ae, et al. Blood pressure increase with impaired glucose tolerance in young adult American blacks. Hypertension 1999; 34:1086–1090.
17. Tseng Ch. Exogenous insulin use and hypertension in adult patients with type 2 diabetes mellitus. Arch Intern Med 2006; 166:1184–1189.
18. Shimamoto K, Ura N. Mechanisms of insulin resistance in hypertensive rats. Clin Exp Hypertens 2006; 28:543–552.
19. Despres Jp, Lemieux I, Bergeron J, et al. Abdominal obesity and the metabolic syndrome: Contribution to global cardiometabolic risk. Arterioscler Thromb Vasc Biol 2008; 28:1039–1049.
20. Rheaume C, Waib Ph, Kouame N, et al. Effects of intense and prolonged exercise on insulin sensitivity and glycogen metabolism in hypertensive subjects. Circulation 2003; 108:2653–2659.

21. Bianchi S, Bigazzi R, Quinones Ga, et al. Insulin resistance in microalbuminuric hypertension sites and mechanisms. Hypertension 1995; 26:789–795.
22. Natali A, Taddei S, Quinones Ga, et al. Insulin sensitivity, vascular reactivity, and clamp-induced vasodilatation in essential hypertension. Circulation 1997; 96:849–855.
23. Baron Ad, Brechtel-Hook G, Johnson A, et al. Skeletal muscle blood flow. A possible link between insulin resistance and blood pressure. Hypertension 1993; 21:129–135.
24. Hulthen Ul, Endre T, Mattiasson I, et al. Insulin and forearm vasodilation in hypertension-prone men. Hypertension 1995; 25:214–218.
25. Bloomgarden Zt. Second World Congress on the insulin resistance syndrome: Hypertension, cardiovascular disease, and treatment approaches. Diabetes Care 2005; 28:2073–2080.
26. Sharma Am, Chetty Vt. Obesity, hypertension and insulin resistance. Acta Diabetol 2005;42 (Suppl. 1):S3–S8.
27. Zeng G, Quon Mj. Insulin-stimulated production of nitric oxide is inhibited by Wortmannin. Direct measurement in vascular endothelial cells. J Clin Invest 1996; 98:894–898.
28. Lin Mw, Hwu Cm, Huang Yh, et al. Directly measured insulin resistance and the assessment of clustered cardiovascular risks in hypertension. Am J Hypertens 2006; 19:1118–1124.
29. Muller Dc, Elahi D, Pratley Re, et al. An epidemiological test of the hyperinsulinemia–hypertension hypothesis. J Clin Endocrinol Metab 1993; 76:544–548.
30. Rocchini Ap. Insulin resistance, obesity and hypertension. J Nutr 1995; 125:1718s–1724s.
31. Blair D, Habicht Jp, Sims Ea, et al. Evidence for an increased risk for hypertension with centrally located body fat and the effect of race and sex on this risk. Am J Epidemiol 1984; 119:526–540.
32. Modan M, Halkin H, Fuchs Z, et al. Hyperinsulinemia–A link between glucose intolerance, obesity, hypertension, dyslipoproteinemia, elevated serum uric acid and internal cation imbalance. Diabete Metab 1987; 13:375–380.
33. Château-Degat Ml, Poirier, P. Insulin resistance, obesity and hypertension: Is the link waist circumference? Therapy 2007; 4:575–583.
34. Poirier P, Hernandez Tl, Weil Km, et al. Impact of diet-induced weight loss on the cardiac autonomic nervous system in severe obesity. Obes Res 2003; 11:1040–1047.
35. Poirier P, Eckel Rh. Obesity and cardiovascular disease. Curr Atheroscler Rep 2002; 4:448–453.
36. Paul M, Wagner J, Dzau Vj. Gene expression of the renin–angiotensin system in human tissues. Quantitative analysis by the polymerase chain reaction. J Clin Invest 1993; 91:2058–2064.
37. Karlsson C, Lindell K, Ottosson M, et al. Human adipose tissue expresses angiotensinogen and enzymes required for its conversion to angiotensin II. J Clin Endocrinol Metab 1998; 83:3925–3929.
38. Mukasa K. Antihypertensive drugs and insulin resistance in obesity. Intern Med 2005; 44:395–396.
39. Ikeda T, Gomi T, Hirawa N, et al. Improvement of insulin sensitivity contributes to blood pressure reduction after weight loss in hypertensive subjects with obesity. Hypertension 1996; 27:1180–1186.
40. Carmelli D, Cardon Lr, Fabsitz R. Clustering of hypertension, diabetes, and obesity in adult male twins: Same genes or same environments? Am J Hum Genet 1994; 55:566–573.
41. Mathieu P, Pibarot P, Larose E, et al. Visceral obesity and the heart. Int J Biochem Cell Biol 2008; 40:821–836.
42. Giacchetti G, Faloia E, Mariniello B, et al. Overexpression of the renin–angiotensin system in human visceral adipose tissue in normal and overweight subjects. Am J Hypertens 2002; 15:381–388.
43. Umemura S, Nyui N, Tamura K, et al. Plasma angiotensinogen concentrations in obese patients. Am J Hypertens 1997; 10:629–633.
44. Van HV, Elizalde M, Ariapart P, et al. The association of human adipose angiotensinogen gene expression with abdominal fat distribution in obesity. Int J Obes Relat Metab Disord 2000; 24:673–678.
45. Sironi Am, Gastaldelli A, Mari A, et al. Visceral fat in hypertension: Influence on insulin resistance and beta-cell function. Hypertension 2004; 44:127–133.
46. Nishina M, Kikuchi T, Yamazaki H, et al. Relationship among systolic blood pressure, serum insulin and leptin, and visceral fat accumulation in obese children. Hypertens Res 2003; 26:281–288.
47. Van Pelt Re, Evans Em, Schechtman Kb, et al. Contributions of total and regional fat mass to risk for cardiovascular disease in older women. Am J Physiol Endocrinol Metab 2002; 282:E1023–E1028.
48. Poirier P, Lemieux I, Mauriege P, et al. Impact of waist circumference on the relationship between blood pressure and insulin: The Quebec Health Survey. Hypertension 2005; 45:363–367.
49. Thomas Gn, Critchley Ja, Tomlinson B, et al. Obesity, independent of insulin resistance, is a major determinant of blood pressure in normoglycemic Hong Kong Chinese. Metabolism 2000; 49:1523–1528.
50. Hayashi T, Boyko Ej, Leonetti Dl, et al. Visceral adiposity and the prevalence of hypertension in Japanese Americans. Circulation 2003; 108:1718–1723.
51. Shen W, Punyanitya M, Chen J, et al. Waist circumference correlates with metabolic syndrome indicators better than percentage fat. Obesity (Silver Spring) 2006; 14:727–736.
52. Ferrannini E. Insulin and blood pressure: Connected on a circumference? Hypertension 2005; 45:347–348.

53. Kotchen Ta, Grim Ce, Kotchen Jm, et al. Altered relationship of blood pressure to adiposity in hypertension. Am J Hypertens 2008; 21:284–289.
54. Schotte De, Stunkard Aj. The effects of weight reduction on blood pressure in 301 obese patients. Arch Intern Med 1990; 150:1701–1704.
55. Novi Rf, Porta M, Lamberto M, et al. Reductions of body weight and blood pressure in obese hypertensive patients treated by diet. A retrospective study. Panminerva Med 1989; 31:13–15.
56. Staessen J, Fagard R, Amery A. The relationship between body weight and blood pressure. J Hum Hypertens 1988; 2:207–217.
57. Pontiroli Ae, Pizzocri P, Saibene A, et al. Left ventricular hypertrophy and Qt interval in obesity and in hypertension: Effects of weight loss and of normalisation of blood pressure. Int J Obes Relat Metab Disord 2004; 28:1118–1123.
58. Sjostrom Cd, Peltonen M, Wedel H, et al. Differentiated long-term effects of intentional weight loss on diabetes and hypertension. Hypertension 2000; 36:20–25.
59. Drolet B, Simard C, Poirier P. Impact of weight-loss medications on the cardiovascular system: Focus on current and future anti-obesity drugs. Am J Cardiovasc Drugs 2007; 7:273–288.

4 Visceral Adiposity, Liver Fat, and Atherogenic Dyslipidemia

Marja-Riitta Taskinen
Department of Medicine, Helsinki University Central Hospital, Helsinki, Finland

Martin Adiels and Jan Borén
Wallenberg Laboratory, Sahlgrenska University Hospital, Göteborg, Sweden

The dramatic increase of obesity worldwide is the driving force behind the pandemic of the metabolic syndrome, type 2 diabetes, and consequently for the new rise of cardiovascular disease (CVD) morbidity and mortality. Obesity is in most, but not all, subjects associated with excessive visceral fat that clusters with vascular risk factors. A close interaction between visceral obesity, non–alcoholic fatty liver disease (NAFLD), and dyslipidemia have been well documented (1–3). The unique anatomical relation of visceral fat to the hepatic portal circulation and consequently to hepatic lipoprotein metabolism has led to intensive endeavor to unravel the pathophysiology and the initiating factors for dyslipidemia.

SPECIFIC FEATURES OF ATHEROGENIC DYSLIPIDEMIA

Dyslipidemia is characterized by elevation of both fasting and postprandial plasma levels of triglyceride-rich lipoproteins (TRL) together with lowering of high-density lipoprotein (HDL) cholesterol and elevation of small dense low-density lipoprotein (LDL) particles (Fig. 1). It is of note that these components are not isolated, but metabolically closely interrelated. The lipid and lipoprotein abnormalities together comprise the atherogenic lipid profile that predisposes to atherosclerosis and is an ultimate goal for the management. It is important to realize that TRLs are not a homogenous pool of lipoprotein particles. The hypertriglyceridemia, which accompanies abdominal obesity and insulin resistance, is characterized by pronounced increase of large very-low-density lipoprotein (VLDL)1 particles that are the major determinant of plasma triglyceride levels (4). Emerging data indicate that this increase of large VLDL particles is due to excess hepatic production of VLDL particles (5). In contrast, the changes in smaller VLDL2 particles are less marked than those of VLDL1 particles. Similarly, direct hepatic secretion of VLDL2 particles is comparable in insulin-resistant and insulin-sensitive subjects. As apolipoprotein B 100 (apo B100) is the major structural protein of VLDL particles, the atherogenic lipid profile also comprises elevation of apo B100 (6).

In circulation, VLDL, intermediate-density lipoprotein (IDL), and LDL are linked in a delipidation cascade in which triglyceride-rich VLDL particles are converted to cholesterol-rich LDL in a process catalyzed by lipoprotein lipase (LPL) and hepatic lipase (HL) (7). Large VLDL1 particles are an excellent substrate for cholesteryl ester transfer protein (CETP) that mediates the exchange of triglycerides and cholesterol esters (CEs) between VLDL1 and both HDL and LDL particles. Expanded pool of plasma TG and long residence time of TRLs accelerates the exchange process resulting in TG-enriched LDL and HDL particles. In this process, both LDL and HDL become depleted in CEs. Triglyceride-rich LDL and HDL particles are good substrates for HL, which is commonly increased in visceral obesity and insulin resistance (8,9). Lipolysis of large triglyceride-rich LDL results in the formation of small dense LDL. Since each LDL particle contains one molecule of apo B100, the number of LDL particles is increased if particles are small and dense at the same level of LDL cholesterol (6). Consequently, the absolute concentration of LDL cholesterol can be misleading in the evaluation of CVD risk in abdominally obese subjects. This seems to be particularly true in people with the metabolic syndrome, where LDL particle number and concentrations of small LDL particles increase with the number of MetS components despite only trivial changes in LDL cholesterol concentration (10).

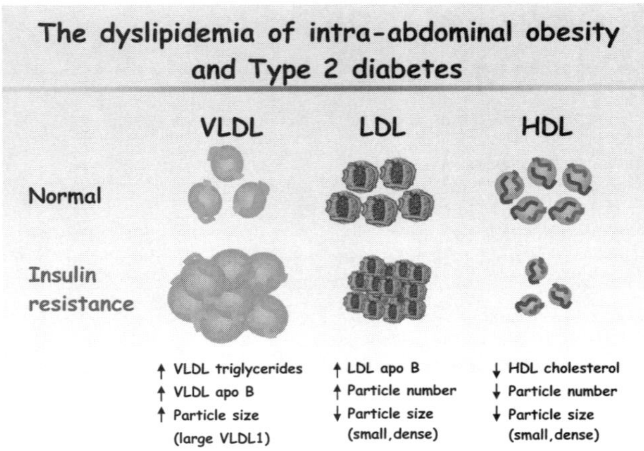

Figure 1 The dyslipidemia of intra-abdominal obesity and type 2 diabetes.

Triglyceride-rich large HDL particles are also a preferred substrate for HL (9). This interaction alters the composition of HDL particles and renders them less stable. Substantial evidence demonstrate that indeed the catabolic rate of HDL is enhanced in subjects with visceral obesity (11). In fact, the amount of intra-abdominal fat measured by MRI shows a close correlation with the clearance rate of HDL apo A-I (12). In this process, free apo A-I molecules are shed from particles and cleared by the kidney. Thus, HDL particles become CEs depleted and contain less apo A-I molecules per particle. Phospholipid transfer protein (PLTP) is another factor remodeling HDL particles in circulation. Similar to CETP activity, PLTP activity has been reported to be increased in obesity and also to correlate with waist-to-hip circumference ratio (13,14). Recent data suggest that PLTP activity may be linked with liver fat (14). The end result of the concerted action of increased HL, CETP, and PLTP activities is decrease in HDL mean particle size, and the HDL profile is characterized by dense HDL3a, 3b, and 3c species. It is important to note that small dense HDL particles in people with metabolic syndrome seem to be dysfunctional, showing impaired antioxidative and defective antiapoptotic activity (15,16). Importantly, the functional abnormalities are associated with compositional changes of neutral core lipid content. In parallel with small dense LDL, HDL mean particle size closely correlates with waist and is considered to be a novel component of the atherogenic dyslipidemia (17,18). Thus, there seems to be a symmetry of mechanism leading to the generation of small dense LDL and HDL particles. These changes are reflected in higher apo B/apo A-I ratio in obese subjects with visceral obesity (6). A high apo B/apo A-I ratio has come up as a superior predictor of CVD risk over the traditional lipid parameters and may thus provide a new tool to identify abdominally obese subjects at high CVD risk (6,19).

INTERACTION OF FATTY LIVER AND VISCERAL OBESITY WITH DYSLIPIDEMIA

The different components of dyslipidemia correlate with measures of visceral fat like waist/hip ratio, waist circumference, and the quantitated intra-abdominal fat volume by using MRI or CT. Similarly, individual lipid abnormalities correlate with different measures of insulin resistance, such as glucose disposal rate, fasting insulin concentration, or the homeostasis model assessment (HOMA) index. Substantial number of studies have reported that the components of dyslipidemia correlate with the liver fat (1,3,20). There is a positive correlation between plasma triglycerides and liver fat, but a negative correlation between HDL cholesterol and liver fat. Recent data confirmed that fatty liver correlates more strongly with HDL2 cholesterol than total HDL cholesterol consistently with the changes of HDL profile observed in subjects with metabolic syndrome (21). In a study, in 2006, we observed a strong relationship between increased liver fat volume and overproduction of large VLDL particles (5). We reported that VLDL1 production rate correlated inversely with LDL size and HDL cholesterol. Thus, overproduction of large VLDL1 particles initiates a sequence of events leading to the generation of small dense LDL particles and increased catabolism of HDL particles. Therefore, it is of key importance to elucidate the mechanisms behind the relationship between fatty liver, visceral obesity, insulin resistance, and how these factors associate with the overproduction of VLDL1 particles.

IMBALANCE OF LIPOREGULATION: THE CULPRIT OF HEPATIC STEATOSIS AND DYSLIPIDEMIA

Non–alcoholic fatty liver disease (NAFLD) is highly prevalent in people with the metabolic syndrome and type 2 diabetes (3,22). Emerging data indicate that fatty accumulation in the liver tightly associates with insulin resistance and visceral fat volume (23). Thus, fatty liver seems to be the hallmark of hepatic insulin resistance. Collectively, the components contribute to the dyslipidemia seen in these people. The fact that VLDL1 overproduction is the central component of dyslipidemia raises the question "What regulates VLDL1 overproduction?" The dynamics of FA metabolism and FA sources [FA flux from adipose tissue, diet, and de novo lipogenesis (DNL)] seem to play the critical role in the pathogenesis of both liver fat and hepatic insulin resistance. The fat of lipids entering the liver may be directed to VLDL triglycerides, β-oxidation, or storage. Recent data indicated that the contribution of FA sources was similar in the VLDL triglycerides and in the liver fat (24). Overall imbalance between FA flux to the liver, DNL, β-oxidation, and VLDL secretion results in the accumulation of TG in hepatocytes. Of note is the fact that about 80% of fatty acids in the plasma FFA pool is derived from adipose tissue in fasting state and even in the fed state 60% originates from adipose tissue highlighting the importance of contribution of plasma FFA (25,26). Importantly, the contribution of visceral adipose tissue lipolysis to FFA pool increases as a function of visceral fat volume. In insulin resistant states, insulin fails to suppress the release of FFAs from adipose tissue resulting in increased flux of FFA to the plasma pool and ultimately to the liver. We recently demonstrated that insulin fails to suppress plasma FFA in subjects with high liver fat and also that the suppression of VLDL1 secretion associates with liver fat content and to the actual suppression of plasma FFA by insulin (27). We also observed that FFA suppression was inversely correlated to intra-abdominal fat volume but not to subcutaneous fat proving evidence for the role of visceral fat as the source of FFA for the liver. This is further supported by the observation that insulin-resistant men have a higher flux of FAs from visceral lipolysis to hepatic VLDL-TG production than insulin-sensitive men in postprandial state (28). Altogether the data clearly pinpoint the role of visceral fat as a source of FA flux to the liver as well as to VLDL secretion.

Excessive flux of FA together with impaired hepatic β-oxidation initiates a deleterious sequence of events directing FAs to harmful nonoxidative pathways (29). Metabolites of fatty acids and intermediate lipids may interfere with insulin signaling, resulting in hepatic insulin resistance. It is important to note that hepatic insulin resistance per se seems to be sufficient to produce derangement of cholesterol metabolism in livers of insulin receptor knock-out (LIRKO) (30) mice. In humans, the coexistence of insulin resistance and hyperinsulinemia encumber to dissect a causal relationship between hepatic insulin resistance and liver fat, leaving this question to be answered by future studies.

PREDICTORS OF VLDL1 OVERPRODUCTION

The fact that VLDL1 overproduction is the central component of dyslipidemia raises the question "What regulates VLDL1 production?" The mechanisms whereby visceral obesity, fatty liver, and insulin resistance can modify VLDL assembly and secretion are multiple and complex and not very well established (20). We have recently shown that features of insulin resistance including insulin, HOMA-IR, adiponectin, intra-abdominal fat, and liver fat were determinants of VLDL apo B and VLDL TG production rates. However, in a multiple regression analysis, only liver fat and fasting glucose remained significant. We also explored the relationship between liver fat and the suppression of VLDL1 production by insulin in subjects with a wide range of liver fat volume. This study showed that insulin downregulates VLDL1 secretion in subjects with low liver fat, but fails to suppress VLDL secretion in subjects with high liver fat resulting in overproduction of VLDL1 (5). Importantly, insulin resistance and visceral obesity lower plasma adiponectin concentrations that modifies both VLDL-TG and HDL concentrations by several mechanisms (31,32). Adiponectin may also impair liver fatty acid β-oxidation via AMPK and PPARα and shift the metabolism of FAs towards TG storage. Finally, recent data has linked liver endocannabinoid (EC) system to lipogenesis and to the regulation of plasma lipids (33,34). CB1 receptor-blockade could have salutary effects directly on hepatic fat metabolism manifested as a weight-independent component of plasma lipids seen in RIO program (35). The potential role of both adiponectin and CB1 receptor in the regulation of hepatic lipid metabolism as well as novel target for therapy remain to be established in humans.

CONCLUSIONS

Recent advances in our knowledge of dyslipidemia in visceral obesity and insulin resistance open new options for management and hopefully will be translated into clinical benefits to reduce cardiometabolic risk.

REFERENCES

1. Nieves DJ, Cnop M, Retzlaff B, et al. The atherogenic lipoprotein profile associated with obesity and insulin resistance is largely attributable to intra-abdominal fat. Diabetes 2003; 52(1):172–179.
2. Van Gaal LF, Mertens IL, De Block CE. Mechanisms linking obesity with cardiovascular disease. Nature 2006; 444(12):875–880.
3. Kotronen A, Yki-Järvinen H. Fatty liver: A novel component of the metabolic syndrome. Arterioscler Thromb Vasc Biol 2007; 27:2276–2283.
4. Hiukka A, Fruchart-Najib J, Leinonen E, et al. Alterations of lipids and apolipoprotein CIII in very low density lipoprotein subspecies in type 2 diabetes. Diabetologia 2005; 48:1207–1215.
5. Adiels M, Taskinen M-R, Packard C, et al. Overproduction of large VLDL particles is driven by increased liver fat content in man. Diabetologia 2006; 49:755–765.
6. Sniderman AD, Faraj M. Apolipoprotein B, apolipoprotein A-I, insulin resistance and the metabolic syndrome. Curr Opin Lipidol 2007; 18:633–637.
7. Taskinen M-R. Type 2 diabetes as a lipid disorder. Curr Mol Med 2005; 5:297–308.
8. Deeb SS, Zambon A, Carr MC, et al. Hepatic lipase and dyslipidemia: interactions among genetic variants, obesity, gender, and diet. J Lipid Res 2003; 44:1279–1286.
9. Després JP, Ferland M, Moorjani S, et al. Role of hepatic-triglyceride lipase activity in the association between intra-abdominal fat and plasma HDL-cholesterol in obese women. Arteriosclerosis 1989; 9:485–492.
10. Kathiresan S, Otvos JD, Sullivan LM, et al. Increase small low-density lipoprotein particle number: a prominent feature of the Metabolic Syndrome in the Framingham Heart Study. Circulation 2006; 113:20–29.
11. Lewis GF, Rader DJ. New insights into the regulation of HDL metabolism and reverse cholesterol transport. Circ Res 2005; 96:1221–1232.
12. Brinton EA, Terry JG. Increased intra-abdominal fat may lower HDL levels by increasing the fractional catabolic rate of Lp A-I in postmenopausal women. Circulation 1996; 94(suppl):I-266.
13. Dallinga-Thie GM, Dullaart RPF, van Tol A. Concerted actions of cholesteryl ester transfer protein and phospholipid transfer protein in type 2 diabetes: Effects of apolipoproteins. Curr Opin Lipidol 2007; 18:251–257.
14. Dullaart RPF, de Vries R, Dallinga-Thie GM, et al. Phospholipid transfer protein activity is determined by type 2 diabetes mellitus and metabolic syndrome, and is positively associated with serum transaminases. Clin Endocrinol 2008; 68:375–381.
15. Hansel B, Giral P, Nobecourt E, et al. Metabolic syndrome is associated with elevated oxidative stress and dysfunctional dense high-density lipoprotein particles displaying impaired antioxidative activity. J Clin Endocrinol Metab 2004; 89(10):4963–4971.
16. De Souza JA, Vindis C, Hansel B, et al. Metabolic syndrome features small, apolipoprotein A-I-poor, triglyceride-rich HDL3-particles with defective anti-apoptotic activity. Atherosclerosis 2008; 197:84–94.
17. Pascot A, Lemieux I, Prud'homme D, et al. Reduced HDL particle size as an additional feature of the atherogenic dyslipidemia of abdominal obesity. J Lipid Res 2001; 42:2007–2014.
18. Watanabe H, Söderlund S, Soro-Paavonen A, et al. Decreased high-density lipoprotein (HDL) particle size, preβ-, and large HDL subspecies concentration in Finnish low-HDL families: Relationship with intima-media thickness. Arterioscler Thromb Vasc Biol 2006; 26:897–902.

19. INTERHEART Study Investigators. Effect of potentially modifiable risk factors associated with myocardial infarction in 52 countries (the INTERHEART study): A case-control study. Lancet 2004; 364:937–952.
20. Adiels M, Taskinen M-R, Borén J. Fatty liver, insulin resistance, and dyslipidemia. Curr Diab Rep 2008; 8:60–64.
21. Kantartzis K, Rittig K, Cegan A, et al. Fatty liver is independently associated with alterations in circulating HDL2 and HDL3 subfractions. Diabetes Care 2008; 31(2):366–368.
22. Musso G, Gambino R, Bo S, et al. Should nonalcoholic fatty liver disease be included in the definition of metabolic syndrome? Diabetes Care 2008; 31(3):562–568.
23. Eguchi Y, Eguchi T, Mizuta T, et al. Visceral fat accumulation and insulin resistance are important factors in nonalcoholic fatty liver disease. J Gastroenterol 2006; 41:462–469.
24. Donnelly KL, Smith CI, Schwarzenberg SJ, et al. Sources of fatty acids stored in liver and secreted via lipoproteins in patients with nonalcoholic fatty liver disease. J Clin Invest 2005; 115(5):1343–1351.
25. Barrows BR, Parks EJ. Contributions of different fatty acid sources to very low-density lipoprotein-triglycerol in the fasted and fed states. J Clin Endocrinol Metab 2006; 91:1446–1452.
26. Tamura S, Shimomura I. Contribution of adipose tissue and de novo lipogenesis to nonalcoholic fatty liver disease. J Clin Invest 2005; 115(5):1139–1142.
27. Adiels M, Westerbacka J, Soro-Paavonen A, et al. Acute suppression of VLDL1 secretion rate by insulin is associated with hepatic fat content and insulin resistance. Diabetologia 2007; 50:2356–2365.
28. Hodson L, Bickerton AST, McQuaid SE, et al. The contribution of splanchnic fat to VLDL triglyceride is greater in insulin-resistant than insulin-sensitive men and women. Diabetes 2007; 56:2433–2441.
29. Holland WL, Knotts TA, Chavez JA, et al. Lipid mediators of insulin resistance. Nutrition Rev 2007; 65(6):S39–S46.
30. Biddinger SB, Hernandez-Ono A, Rask-Madsen C, et al. Hepatic insulin resistance is sufficient to produce dyslipidemia and susceptibility to atherosclerosis. Cell Metab 2008; 7:125–134.
31. Kadowaki T, Yamauchi T. Adiponectin and adiponectin receptors. Endocrine Rev 2005; 26:439–451.
32. Lara-Castro C, Fu Y, Chung BH, et al. Adiponectin and the metabolic syndrome: Mechanisms mediating risk for metabolic and cardiovascular disease. Curr Opin Lipidol 2007; 18:263–270.
33. Osei-Hyiaman D, DePetrillo M, Pacher P, et al. Endocannabinoid activation at hepatic CB1 receptors stimulates fatty acid synthesis and contributes to diet-induced obesity. J Clin Invest 2005; 115(5):1298–1305.
34. Côté M, Matias I, Lemieux I, et al. Circulating endocannabinoid levels, abdominal adiposity and related cardiometabolic risk factors in obese men. Int J Obesity 2007; 31:692–699.
35. Després J-P, Golay A, Sjöström L, et al. Effects of rimonabant on metabolic risk factors in overweight patients with dyslipidemia. N Engl J Med 2005; 353(20):2121–2134.

5 Visceral Adiposity and Inflammation

Ulf Smith

The Lundberg Laboratory for Diabetes Research, Center of Excellence for Cardiovascular and Metabolic Research, Department of Molecular and Clinical Medicine, The Sahlgrenska Academy, University of Gothenburg, Gothenburg, Sweden

VISCERAL FAT—AN ECTOPIC FAT DEPOT

The negative consequences of an excessive accumulation of body fat have long been recognized. However, our acceptance to the concepts that not all obese individuals carry the same risk for type 2 diabetes, dyslipidemia, and cardiovascular diseases are more recent.

Around 20% of obese individuals are characterized as obese but at the same time they are metabolically healthy—in contrast, around 20% of nonobese individuals display several metabolic abnormalities associated with the metabolic syndrome (for review see Ref. 1). A key factor driving the obesity-associated propensity for the various risk factors included in the metabolic syndrome is the dysregulated adipose tissue (reviewed in Ref. 2).

Several studies with genetically engineered animal models have shown that the ability to expand the subcutaneous tissue, to store and appropriately package the lipid droplets, can occur without any obvious metabolic consequences. For instance, overexpression of adiponectin in the subcutaneous adipose tissue allows the mice to become morbidly obese but at the same time metabolically perfectly normal (3). In this case, like in human, the adipose tissue is then characterized by many small adipose cells, that is, a hyperplastic adipose tissue.

In contrast, inability of the subcutaneous adipose tissue to recruit new preadipocytes leads to adipose cell enlargement and inflammation in the adipose tissue, which prevents the normal differentiation of the preadipocytes in the subcutaneous site and also favors the accumulation of lipids in ectopic sites (2). These sites include the liver, skeletal muscle, and other ectopic fat depots like the visceral fat, epicardial fat, and perivascular fat. Several recent studies have also shown that an expanded visceral fat depot is associated with expanded epicardial fat and, conversely, that the amount of epicardial fat is also associated with the various components of the metabolic syndrome as have been reported for amount of visceral fat (4,5).

This line of reasoning is obviously focused on mechanisms and the pathogenesis of the obesity-associated metabolic consequences. It should not, however, be taken as downplaying the clinical importance of defining amount of visceral fat or its surrogate measurement—waist circumference (WC) (6). The important work by Despres and Lemieux (6) has convincingly demonstrated that WC is a highly useful marker of cardiometabolic risk and, indeed, it is now also a key criterion for defining the metabolic syndrome (7).

VISCERAL FAT AND INFLAMMATION

We know that an enlarged WC is frequently associated with an expanded visceral fat depot (and liver fat, epicardial fat, etc.) and that cardiometabolic risk is associated with the WC. The key question is obviously, why! the amount of visceral fat is usually quite small; and the extensive work by Jensen and Koutsari (8) (also reviewed in Ref. 1), clearly indicates that the contribution of this depot to free fatty acid (FFA) release and turnover is quite small. Additionally, there is no convincing evidence in human that the portal FFA levels are higher than the systemic levels. Thus, if it is not through an augmentic lipolytic activity, how can an expanded visceral fat contribute the metabolic syndrome. Obviously, the view that visceral fat is only one, albeit clinically easily accessible, marker of ectopic fat deposition provides a credible answer since it is then also associated with ectopic fat deposition in other depots as well. In addition, however, we know that visceral fat is characterized by a marked proinflammatory profile. Many cell-based studies have shown that visceral adipose tissue has a higher gene expression, and secretion,

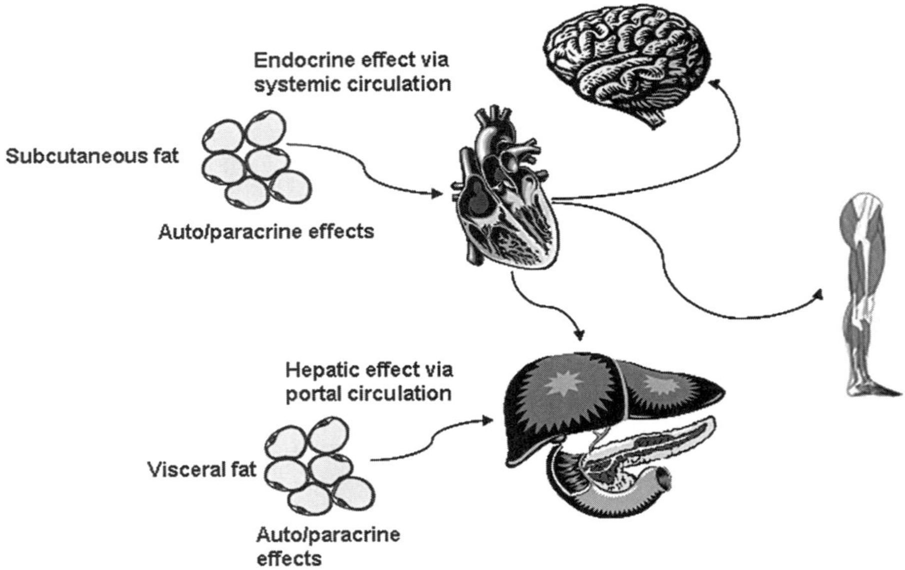

Figure 1 Endocrine effects of cytokines released from visceral or subcutaneous adipose tissue: The cytokines released from visceral depot would primarily alter carbohydrate and lipid metabolism and stimulate production of acute-phase response proteins in the liver, whereas the cytokines produced by subcutaneous depot would mainly affect adipose cell development and function locally as well as exert systemic effects on, for example, the skeletal muscle. *Source*: From Ref. 1.

of IL-6, IL-8, and plasminogen activator inhibitor (9–11) as well as increased infiltration of inflammatory cells, including plasma cells (12).

An increased release of proinflammatory molecules by visceral fat may be particularly relevant for the liver since this depot, in contrast to subcutaneous fat, is drained by the portal vein (Fig. 1). Considering the discussion above, that is, that the visceral fat depot is quite small compared to subcutaneous fat, one may again question what evidence do we have to support a strong systemic proinflammatory potential of the visceral fat. Importantly, however, recent studies have convincingly demonstrated that visceral fat is an important proinflammatory depot (13,14). Fontana et al. (13) measured IL-6, TNFα, MCP-1, resistin, leptin, and adiponectin levels in the portal vein in morbidly obese subjects undergoing bariatric surgery. The key finding was that the IL-6 levels were ~50% higher in portal blood than in the radial artery. All other levels of cytokines and adiponectin were unchanged while, surprisingly, leptin levels were ~20% lower in portal blood. Importantly, arterial C-reactive protein (CRP) levels were positively correlated with the portal vein concentration of IL-6 (13), supporting that the liver was a target, increasing the secretion of acute phase reactants like CRP.

These findings were further corroborated by the recent publication of Cartier et al. (14). These authors measured the circulating levels of IL-6 and TNF-α in a large group of individuals with varying body mass index (BMI). They also compared individuals with a similar BMI but with varying amounts of intra-abdominal adipose tissue. They found that the levels of both IL-6 and TNF-α were increased in obesity. However, individuals with the same BMI but with a larger intra-abdominal fat depot had clearly increased circulating IL-6 levels. Interestingly, a positive correlation was found between circulating IL-6 levels and insulin, similar to a previous study (15). In this latter study, where insulin sensitivity was also measured with the euglycemic clamp technique, it was concluded that the correlation between circulating insulin and IL-6 levels remained even after adjusting for degree of insulin sensitivity (15).

An emerging picture is, thus, that visceral fat is an important producer of IL-6 (and possibly IL-8 although this has not been documented in vivo) which, in turn, can induce peripheral insulin resistance when chronically elevated. Thus, IL-6 impairs insulin signaling and action in the adipose cells as well as in the liver (16,17). The effect in skeletal muscle has been more unclear and short-term positive effects on glucose uptake have been reported (18). However, we have recently overexpressed IL-6 in the skeletal muscle in mice, leading to markedly increased circulating levels (19). When examined after 7 to 14 days of elevated circulating IL-6 levels, we found increased serum amyloid A levels, reduced adiponectin, and a reduced glucose uptake by the skeletal muscle in vivo combined with a reduced GLUT-4 expression. Thus, this study strongly supports the concept that chronically elevated IL-6 levels lead to insulin resistance in vivo combined with a marked proinflammatory response in the liver (19).

In conclusion, expanded visceral fat is also associated with an increased lipid accumulation in other ectopic sites. It is unlikely that the association with the metabolic syndrome and cardiometabolic risk is due to an important contribution of this depot to the portal or circulating FFA levels. Instead, recent studies have consistently shown that visceral fat is an important contributor of circulating, and portal, IL-6 levels and that circulating IL-6 levels are particularly increased in visceral obesity. Chronically elevated IL-6 levels induce insulin resistance in all key target tissues for insulin as well as a marked proinflammatory response in the liver.

REFERENCES

1. Yang X, Smith U. Adipose tissue distribution and risk of metabolic disease: Does thiazolidinedione-induced adipose tissue redistribution provide a clue to the answer? Diabetologia 2007; 50(6):1127–1139.
2. Gustafson B, Hammarstedt A, Andersson CX, et al. Inflamed adipose tissue: A culprit underlying the metabolic syndrome and atherosclerosis. Arterioscler Thromb Vasc Biol 2007; 27(11):2276–2283.
3. Kim JY, van de Wall E, Laplante M, et al. Obesity-associated improvements in metabolic profile through expansion of adipose tissue. J Clin Invest 2007; 117(9):2621–2637.
4. Cikim AS, Topal E, Harputluoglu M, et al. Epicardial adipose tissue, hepatic steatosis and obesity. J Endocrinol Invest 2007; 30(6):459–464.
5. Iacobellis G, Leonetti F. Epicardial adipose tissue and insulin resistance in obese subjects. J Clin Endocrinol Metab 2005; 90(11):6300–6302.
6. Despres JP, Lemieux I. Abdominal obesity and metabolic syndrome. Nature 2006; 444(7121):881–887.
7. Alberti KG, Zimmet P, Shaw J. Metabolic syndrome—A new world-wide definition. A consensus statement from the International Diabetes Federation. Diabet Med 2006; 23(5):469–480.
8. Koutsari C, Jensen MD. Thematic review series: Patient-oriented research. Free fatty acid metabolism in human obesity. J Lipid Res 2006; 47(8):1643–1650.
9. Fain JN, Madan AK, Hiler ML, et al. Comparison of the release of adipokines by adipose tissue, adipose tissue matrix, and adipocytes from visceral and subcutaneous abdominal adipose tissues of obese humans. Endocrinology 2004; 145(5):2273–2282.
10. Bruun JM, Lihn AS, Madan AK, et al. Higher production of IL-8 in visceral vs. subcutaneous adipose tissue. Implication of nonadipose cells in adipose tissue. Am J Physiol Endocrinol Metab 2004; 286(1): E8–E13.
11. Janand-Delenne B, Chagnaud C, Raccah D, et al. Visceral fat as a main determinant of plasminogen activator inhibitor 1 level in women. Int J Obes Relat Metab Disord 1998; 22(4):312–317.
12. Palming J, Gabrielsson BG, Jennische E, et al. Plasma cells and Fc receptors in human adipose tissue—Lipogenic and anti-inflammatory effects of immunoglobulins on adipocytes. Biochem Biophys Res Commun 2006; 343(1):43–48.
13. Fontana L, Eagon JC, Trujillo ME, et al. Visceral fat adipokine secretion is associated with systemic inflammation in obese humans. Diabetes 2007; 56(4):1010–1013.
14. Cartier A, Lemieux I, Almeras N, et al. Visceral obesity and plasma glucose-insulin homeostasis: Contributions of IL-6 and TNF-{alpha} in men. J Clin Endocrinol Metab 2008; 93:1931–1938.
15. Andreozzi F, Laratta E, Cardellini M, et al. Plasma interleukin-6 levels are independently associated with insulin secretion in a cohort of Italian-Caucasian nondiabetic subjects. Diabetes 2006; 55(7):2021–2024.
16. Rotter V, Nagaev I, Smith U. Interleukin-6 (IL-6) induces insulin resistance in 3T3-L1 adipocytes and is, like IL-8 and tumor necrosis factor-alpha, overexpressed in human fat cells from insulin-resistant subjects. J Biol Chem 2003; 278(46):45777–45784.
17. Senn JJ, Klover PJ, Nowak IA, et al. Suppressor of Cytokine Signaling-3 (SOCS-3), a potential mediator of Interleukin-6-dependent insulin resistance in hepatocytes. J Biol Chem 2003; 278(16); 13740–13746.
18. Carey AL, Steinberg GR, Macaulay SL, et al. Interleukin-6 increases insulin-stimulated glucose disposal in humans and glucose uptake and fatty acid oxidation in vitro via AMP-activated protein kinase. Diabetes 2006; 55(10):2688–2697.
19. Franckhauser S, Elias I, Rotter Sopasakis V, et al. Overexpression of Il6 leads to hyperinsulinaemia, liver inflammation and reduced body weight in mice. Diabetologia 2008; 51:1306–1316.

6 Abdominal Obesity and Alterations in Haemostasis—Thrombosis

Irène Juhan-Vague and Marie-Christine Alessi

Laboratoire d'Hématologie, Faculté de Médecine, Université de la Méditerranée, Inserm, Marseille, France

INTRODUCTION

Different prospective epidemiological studies have shown that overweight and obese men and women, especially those with abdominal obesity, experience increased risk of coronary heart disease and type 2 diabetes (1–4). Abdominal obesity belongs to the metabolic syndrome that includes insulin resistance, changes in lipoprotein metabolism (hypertriglyceridemia and hypo HDL cholesterolemia), abnormalities of vascular homeostasis with hypertension, endothelial dysfunction, and a prothrombotic state.

In this review, we describe how visceral adiposity and the features of the metabolic syndrome result in alteration in haemostasis leading to atherothrombosis. We also give some arguments on a reciprocal relationship between haemostasis, endothelial dysfunctions, and the metabolic syndrome (Figs. 1–4).

ABDOMINAL OBESITY AND PLATELET HYPERACTIVITY

Increased platelet response is seen in individuals with abdominal obesity and this increase in platelet may play a role in the cardiovascular risk associated with this type of obesity (5–7).

This platelet hyperactivity may be supported by insulin resistance, inflammation, and adipokines. Insulin resistance, which is well recognized in the muscle, hepatic, and adipose cells during obesity, also develops at the platelet level (8–11). Platelets from obese subjects are resistant to the hypoaggregating effect of insulin (12). Urinary thromboxane metabolite excretion, which reflects platelet activation, is increased in obese women and is mainly determined by insulin resistance (13).

Platelet activation is modulated by inflammatory factors and can lead to the release of proteins with known proinflammatory functions, thus combining haemostasis and the chronic low inflammatory state (14) observed in obesity (Fig. 1).

Lipid abnormalities described in the metabolic syndrome also have an effect on platelet activity. Hypertriglyceridemia and increased concentration of free fatty acids (FFA) induce a proaggregating effect in vitro (15). Hypo HDLemia could also influence platelet aggregation, because HDL opposes the activation properties of LDL on platelets, whereas the effects of chylomicrons, VLDL or IDL on platelet function are debatable (16).

Recently, products of adipose tissue have been shown to modulate platelet function. Leptin is primarily produced by adipocytes, and its circulating levels reflect the amount of energy stored in adipose tissue. In addition to its role as a hormonal regulator of body weight and energy expenditure, leptin is now considered to play a regulatory role in various physiological states. Platelets have leptin receptors and are activated in vitro by leptin (17–19). Leptin promotes human platelet aggregation by potentiating the normal response to adenosine diphosphate and thrombin. This has been suggested as a mechanism for acute thrombotic events in obesity (17–19). In obese humans, however, homozygous or heterozygous leptin deficiency is associated with increased platelet aggregation relative to controls, and in vitro incubation with leptin did not increase platelet aggregation (20). Four-day leptin infusion only slightly increases platelet aggregation in healthy volunteers (21). It is well known that human obesity is characterized by a leptin-resistant state. Thus, one may argue that obesity is associated with impaired platelet sensitivity to leptin, resembling the reduced sensitivity of platelets to insulin in insulin resistance (22,23). This needs to be confirmed in vivo.

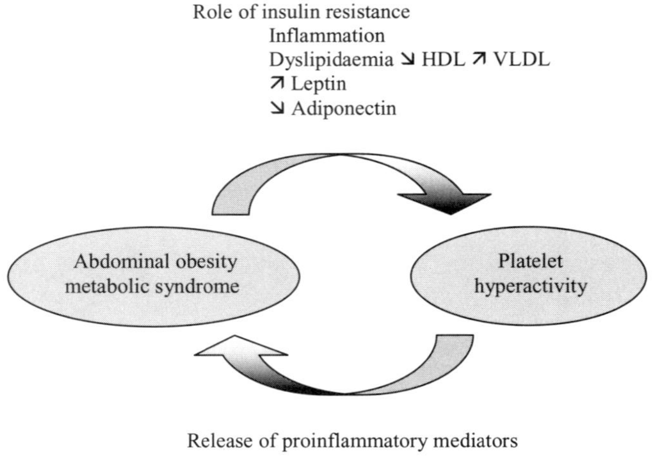

Figure 1 Connections between abdominal obesity and platelet hyperactivity.

Adiponectin is an adipocytokine abundantly present in plasma. Its plasma concentration decreases in obesity, type 2 diabetes, and patients with coronary artery disease. Adiponectin levels are negatively correlated with the percentage of visceral fat and insulin resistance. Results obtained in adiponectin knockout mice clearly indicate that adiponectin acts as an endogenous antithrombotic factor (24). These mice showed an accelerated thrombus formation on carotid arterial injury, which was corrected by adenovirus-mediated supplementation of adiponectin. In vitro platelet aggregation induced by low concentration of agonists was enhanced in adiponectin knockout mice and recombinant adiponectin inhibited the enhanced platelet aggregation. These data suggest that the defect of adiponectin plays a key role in the thrombotic risk observed in obese insulin-resistant patients. This effect, however, has yet to be demonstrated in humans. Preliminary data indicate that addition of human recombinant adiponectin induces no significant antiaggregation effect on platelets from individuals without hypoadiponectinemia (25).

Platelets play a major role in the development of atherothrombosis, and their pharmacological inhibition is at the center of the active cardiovascular disease treatment and in the secondary prevention of cardiovascular events. There is growing view that all patients with type 2 diabetes should receive aspirin (26). There is no consensus regarding antiplatelet therapy in insulin-resistant patients with prognostically important coronary arterial disease. The identification of optimized approaches for the prevention and treatment of heart disease in insulin-resistant, nondiabetic patients remains a major global challenge. A few data are available about the primary protective effect of antiplatelet therapy in both obese and type 2 diabetic patients. In fact, recent trial suggests that antiplatelet therapy is beneficial for patients with symptomatic atherothrombosis but at the same time harmful for patients with multiple risk factors without symptoms (27). It is admitted that the platelet response to antiagregating agent is variable, some patients being resistant to the drug effect (28). It cannot be excluded that platelet hyperactivity, which is present in patients with abdominal obesity, can cause the heterogeneity of response to treatment. Indeed, obesity is associated with a lower sensitivity to aspirin (29) and clopidogrel (30), and the presence of a type 2 diabetes decreases the biological efficiency of the aspirin–clopidogrel (30) association.

ABDOMINAL OBESITY AND HYPERCOAGULABILITY

Abdominal obesity is accompanied by coagulation abnormalities that may favor thrombus propagation.

Tissue factor (TF), the key initiator of coagulation, is widely expressed in atherosclerotic plaques and found in macrophages, smooth muscle cells, extracellular matrix, and acellular lipid-rich core. The blood-borne TF encrypted on the circulating microparticles derived from vascular cells is a marker of vascular injury and a source of procoagulant activity. Evidence indicates that elevated levels of blood-borne or circulating TF have been associated with metabolic

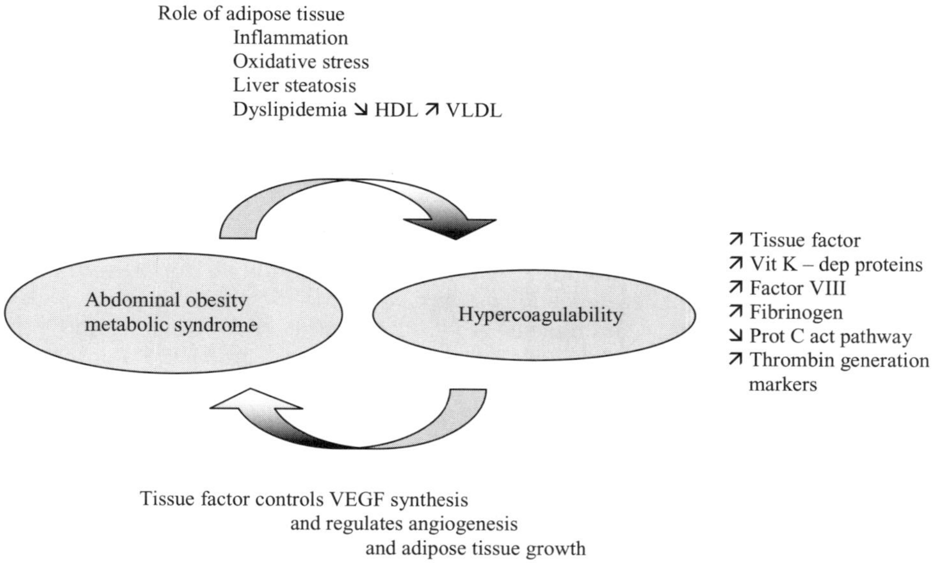

Figure 2 Connections between abdominal obesity and hypercoagulability.

syndrome, type 2 diabetes, and cardiovascular risk factors and are a candidate biomarker for future cardiovascular events (31). Treatment of insulin resistance such as weight loss (32) or thiazolidinediones decreased circulating TF levels. Adipose tissue participating in the TF pool may increase during the metabolic syndrome. Indeed, homogenates of human adipose express TF on macrophages and smooth muscle cells. This elevated TF expression may result from various stimulants, such as C-reactive protein, oxidized LDL, TGF-β, angiotensin II, hyperglycemia, and adipocytokines, which accompany abdominal obesity. Among them, hyperinsulinemia may be of particular relevance. Adipose TF expression is potentiated by insulin administration in obese mice (33,34). In human volunteers, a 24-hour hyperinsulinemic or hyperglycemic clamp produces a strong increase in TF procoagulant expression in circulating monocytes with a parallel increase in plasma thrombin–antithrombin complexes and other markers of thrombin generation. Effects of selective hyperinsulinemia or hyperglycemia were less striking but were additive (35).

More than a consequence of abdominal obesity, TF could indirectly affect the development of adipose tissue. It is involved in the maintenance of vascular integrity and angiogenesis (36). An accelerated angiogenesis could favor a pathological development of adipose tissue. Recent studies have shown that vascular endothelial growth factor (VEGF) synthesis is controlled by TF, and the blocking of VEGF can inhibit adipose tissue growth [(37); Fig. 2].

Plasma concentrations of vitamin K–dependent proteins are increased during obesity and decreased after weight loss (38,39). In obese nondiabetic patients, increased levels of vitamin K–dependent coagulation proteins are clustered with dyslipidemia and inflammation, whereas they are not related to anthropometric parameters or arterial pressure or glucidic metabolism (40). These results may be in favour of a potentiation of hepatic synthesis of vitamin K–dependent proteins during obesity. Accumulation of fat in the liver could play an important role in this process, as a strong relationship has been reported between circulating levels of vitamin K–dependent proteins and the hepatic enzyme gamma glutamyl transferase (41). Moreover, it has been reported that VLDL produced in excess during abdominal obesity supports activation of factor VII by the Xa/Va complex—this could slow down the clearance of factor VII (42).

High factor VIII levels correlate with measures of obesity (43). This elevation must be brought closer to that of von Willebrand factor, produced by endothelial cells (vide infra), since factor VIII circulates as an inactive procofactor in complex with von Willebrand factor, which slows down factor VIII elimination.

High fibrinogen level is associated with an increased prevalence and incidence of primary and recurrent coronary heart disease (44). Fibrinogen promotes thrombus formation and platelet aggregation. The plasma concentration of fibrinogen is increased in obesity, especially in women. Its plasma concentration depends on the fat mass and not on fat repartition (45,46). It is proposed that the increase in IL-6 level produced by macrophages of adipose tissue, and adipocytes themselves, is responsible for the slight increase in hepatic synthesis of fibrinogen in obese persons (47,48).

Interestingly, it was shown that HDL attenuates the expression of TF and downregulates thrombin generation via the enhancement of the anticoagulant protein C pathway (49). Therefore, the hypo HDLaemia, which accompanies abdominal obesity, could again be involved in the thrombotic risk by increasing thrombin generation.

In summary, the increase in local and systemic TF concentration, factor VIII, vitamin K–dependent proteins, and fibrinogen levels in patients with the metabolic syndrome may support an exacerbated tendency to thrombosis. Abdominal obesity may be independently involved directly or indirectly through its capacity to produce haemostatic factors or inflammatory mediators and its association with several other well-known cardiovascular risk factors such as insulin resistance and dyslipidemia.

ABDOMINAL OBESITY AND HYPOFIBRINOLYSIS

Hypofibrinolysis, due to an increased level of plasminogen activator inhibitor 1 (PAI-1), is the most important and visible change of the haemostatic system in the metabolic syndrome. PAI-1 is the predominant inhibitor of the fibrinolytic system. Increased concentration of PAI-1 in the circulation leads to impairment of the removal of thrombi from the vascular system (50) and may influence the development of atherosclerotic lesions as well (51). In large epidemiological studies, elevated plasma levels of PAI-1 proved to be predictors of myocardial infarction (for review see Ref. 52). Remarkably, the predictive ability of PAI-1 disappears after adjustment for markers of the metabolic syndrome (53). These results suggest that the presence of abdominal obesity and insulin resistance are a prerequisite for the increased PAI-1 levels in patients at risk of atherothrombosis and have led to the proposal that increased PAI-1 level can be considered as a true component of the metabolic syndrome (52,54).

The increase in plasma PAI-1 levels associated with abdominal obesity may be attributed to PAI-1 production by ectopic adipose tissues (55–57) (Fig. 3). PAI-1 is localized mainly in the stromal compartment of human adipose tissue (58,59). Macrophages infiltrating adipose tissue (60) express PAI-1 (56) as well as adipocytes in response to PAI-1 inducers (61). Thus, adipose

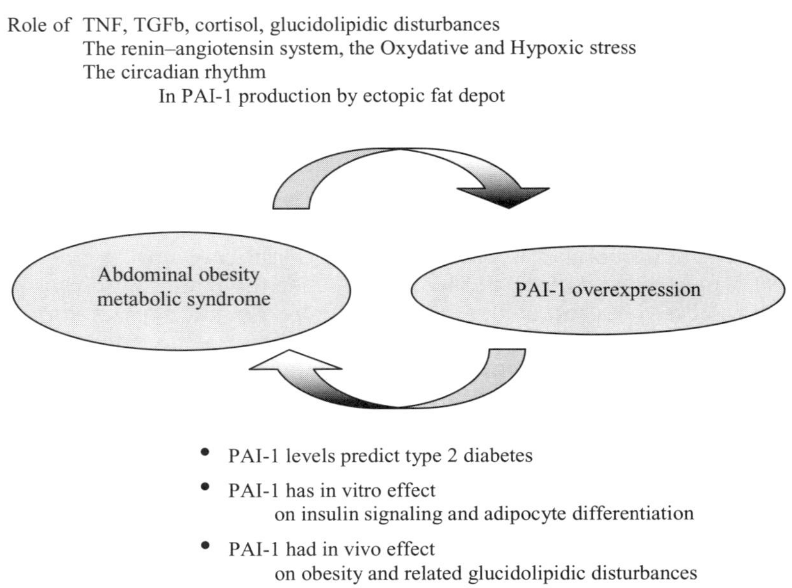

Figure 3 Connections between abdominal obesity and hypofibrinolysis.

tissue has evolved into a PAI-1 producing organ, with PAI-1 being produced by macrophages and adipocytes when they gain the capacity to respond to inducers of PAI-1 synthesis. This may be particularly relevant in the visceral fat, which is strongly infiltrated by macrophages (62). Ectopic fat accumulation in liver is also associated with strong PAI-1 expression close to the fat cells (63). Overall these findings suggest that circulating PAI-1 levels reflect fat redistribution and may be considered a biomarker of ectopic fat storage disease.

Tissue expression of PAI-1 is not constitutive but mainly inducible. Many inducers of PAI-1 synthesis during obesity have been identified that may exert their effect locally or more remotely. The TNF and TGF-β pathways (64,65), reactive oxygen species (ROS) (66,67), and local cortisol production within adipose tissue (68,69) may all be involved in PAI-1 overproduction during abdominal obesity. Alteration of the self-regulated circadian clock may also dysregulate PAI-1 synthesis in obese patients. Several groups as well as ours have observed in vitro that high insulin, high glucose, or high triglyceride concentration and elevated levels of FFA contribute to PAI-1 synthesis (for review see Ref. 52). However, in vivo, acute changes in insulin or triglyceride levels (postprandial period, in vivo administration) are not accompanied by changes in PAI-1 levels.

The involvement of the renin–angiotensin system, which is fully expressed in adipose tissue, may be important because inhibition of angiotensin-converting enzyme significantly reduces plasma PAI-1 levels in obese individuals (70).

Therefore, the causes of PAI-1 overexpression in metabolic syndrome are complex, with much interference between biological systems. Establishment of inflammation or oxidative stress at the macrophage level as fundamental precursors is tempting and may reveal interesting approaches to elucidate the link between atherosclerosis and metabolic syndrome.

Contribution of PAI-1 to the Development of Adipose Tissue and Insulin Resistance

Circulating PAI-1 levels predict development of type 2 diabetes, suggesting that PAI-1 may causally be related to development of obesity (71–74). Carriers of the -675 4G PAI-1 allele were more prone to obesity and metabolic syndrome in some studies but not in all (75–77). We recently showed that patients with the highest pro-insulin levels were at risk for developing a myocardial infarction only if they were homozygous for the 4G allele, suggesting that PAI-1 genotype may influence the vascular risk associated with hyperinsulinaemia (78). All together these findings indicate that PAI-1 gene variability plays a role in modulating obesity-associated phenotypes.

In vivo in mice and in vitro studies support the role of PAI-1 in obesity development. Three groups found that fat accumulation was prevented in mice lacking PAI-1 in both a nutritionally induced (79,80) and a genetic (81) murine model of obesity. Results obtained by our group (82–84) followed this direction, showing an effect of pharmacological inhibition of PAI-1 on weight gain and on insulin sensitivity.

In addition, PAI-1 deficiency may exert beneficial effects through improved insulin sensitivity within adipose tissue. Adipocytes from PAI-$1^{-/-}$ mice exhibited enhanced basal as well as insulin-stimulated glucose uptake. In agreement, 3T3 adipocytes treated with PAI-1 neutralizing antibodies exhibited greater differentiation than wild-type or untreated 3T3 adipocytes (85). This effect may be mediated through the ability of PAI-1 to interfere with insulin signaling by preventing binding of vitronectin to integrin $\alpha_V\beta3$ and thus cooperation between integrin and insulin signaling (86,87). PAI-1 deficiency may also block the deleterious effect of TNF on insulin sensitivity of adipocytes. Indeed, PAI-1 deficiency blunted the deleterious effect of TNF on glucose uptake and on adipocyte differentiation marker expression (85). Finally, it was recently hypothesized that PAI-1 could exert its deleterious effect through inhibition of the proprotein convertase furin, which is involved in TGF-β activation and insulin receptor processing (88).

Mice overexpressing murine PAI-1 in adipocytes and macrophages exhibited adipocyte hypotrophy, a higher mRNA level of a preadipocyte marker in adipose tissue, and reduced feeding efficiency compared with wild-type mice (89). These findings suggest that targeted PAI-1 overexpression in macrophages and adipocytes impairs adipose tissue growth, which agrees with the recently described inhibitory effect of PAI-1 on murine adipocyte differentiation (85). This finding may, at first glance, appear to be at odds with that obtained in PAI-1 deficient mice, but it must be interpreted in connection with the multiple facets of PAI-1, which render it a serpin that acts locally at various sites and perhaps systemically through endocrine effects. Interestingly, when one looks at metabolic parameters, it appears that old transgenic mice overexpressing PAI-1 that are maintained on standard fat diet exhibit significantly higher insulinaemia and a tendency toward higher triglyceride levels, despite lower body fat (84). These data are not inconsistent with those obtained in PAI-1 deficient mice and indicate that PAI-1 overexpression might worsen the metabolic profile. This requires confirmation, because this deleterious effect was not found in younger transgenic mice fed a diet high in fat (89). Note that two studies from the same group were unable to demonstrate any effect of PAI-1 deficiency on adipocyte differentiation (90) or weight gain (91).

In vitro and in vivo studies have indicated that PAI-1 might be involved in the development of obesity. Overall, these data support the concept that PAI inhibition has the potential to reduce obesity and improve insulin sensitivity, and may represent a new therapeutic target. This requires confirmation in different experimental models, and the mechanisms involved should be precisely defined.

ABDOMINAL OBESITY AND ENDOTHELIAL DYSFUNCTION

Endothelial dysfunction contributes to cardiovascular diseases, including hypertension and coronary artery disease (92) (Fig. 4).

It has become clear that the metabolic syndrome is associated with endothelial dysfunction (93), with inadequate vasodilatation and/or paradoxical vasoconstriction in coronary and peripheral arteries in response to stimuli that release nitric oxide (NO). Endothelial dysfunction during obesity may also result from impaired NO bioavailability due to increased endogenous endothelin levels (94) in addition to the direct vasoconstrictor effects of endothelin (95). The metabolic syndrome leads not only to endothelial dysfunction through the frequent association with traditional cardiovascular risk factors (49) but also to insulin resistance. In healthy conditions, insulin promotes glucose disposal and stimulates the production of NO, which in turn, through NO-dependent increases in blood flow to skeletal muscle and may account for 25% to 40% of the increase in glucose uptake in response to insulin stimulation (96). A physiologic increment in plasma insulin concentration particularly increased microvascular blood volume, consistent with a mechanism of capillary recruitment (97).

Metabolic insulin resistance is characterized by pathway-specific impairment in phosphatidylinositol 3-kinase–dependent signaling, which in endothelium may cause imbalance between production of NO and secretion of endothelin-1, leading to decreased blood flow, which worsens insulin resistance (98–100). Experimental inhibition of phosphatidylinositol 3-kinase with wortmannin not only blocked the ability of insulin to stimulate increased expression of endothelial NO synthase but also increased expression of vascular cellular adhesion molecules-1 (VCAM1) and E-selectin, and increased rolling interactions of monocytes with endothelial

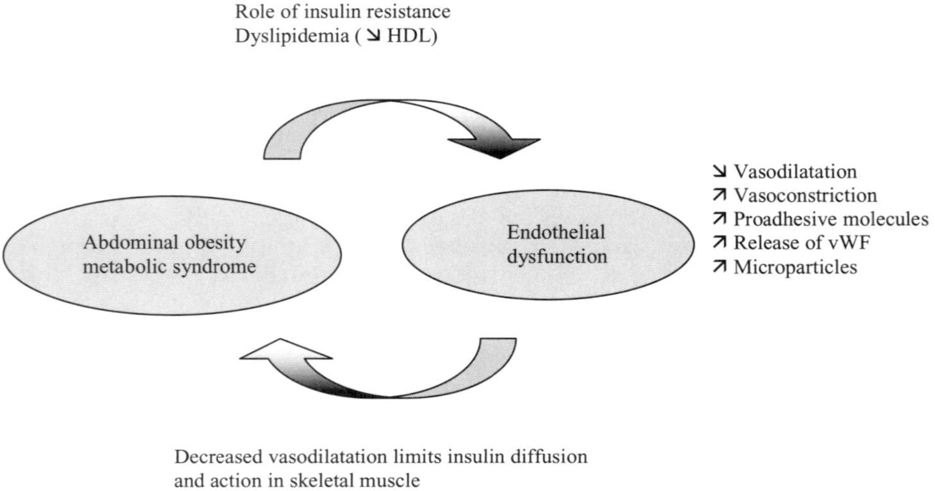

Figure 4 Connections between abdominal obesity and endothelial dysfunction.

cells, showing that inhibition of the metabolic branch of insulin signaling leads to an enhanced atherogenic action of insulin in endothelial cells (101).

In parallel with inadequate vasodilatation, in obesity, endothelial cells take a proinflammatory phenotype with increased expression of VCAM1, ICAM1, E-selectin, a release of microparticles (102) and shedding products, and an increased synthesis and release of von Willebrand factor (VWF); the latter plays a major role in the adhesion of platelets to the vascular wall. VWF levels are correlated with parameters of the insulin resistance syndrome (45,103) and inflammatory parameters (40,45,104,105). These endothelial disorders may arise at a very early age in obese children who display significantly elevated values for sICAM-1, VWF in parallel with inflammatory, and insulin resistance markers (106).

Interestingly, some recent clinical studies demonstrated that nonpharmacological and pharmacological strategies targeting obesity and/or insulin resistance ameliorate endothelial function and low-grade inflammation whereas improving endothelial function ameliorates insulin resistance (98,100), underscoring the reciprocal connection between endothelial dysfunction and insulin resistance.

CONCLUSION

Abdominal obesity is accompanied by important changes in the haemostatic system that favor not only the development of arterial but also venous thrombosis (107). Hyperactivity of platelets and hypercoagulability favor platelet and fibrin deposits, and hypofibrinolysis due to the PAI-1 excess prevents their elimination. The increased PAI-1 expression that accompanies abdominal obesity is the main abnormality in haemostasis, with an original regulation. As PAI-1 could also be directly involved in the physiopathology of obesity, it represents an original target for preventing both the vascular and metabolic risks.

REFERENCES

1. Lakka HM, Laaksonen DE, Lakka TA, et al. The metabolic syndrome and total cardiovascular disease mortality in middle-aged men. JAMA 2002; 288:2709–2716.
2. Hu G, Qiao Q, Tuomilehto J, Balkau B, et al. DECODE Study Group. Prevalence of the metabolic syndrome and its relation to all-cause and cardiovascular mortality in nondiabetic European men and women. Arch Intern Med 2004; 164:1066–1076.
3. Meigs JB, Wilson PW, Nathan DM, et al. Prevalence and characteristics of the metabolic syndrome in the San Antonio. Heart and Framingham Offspring Studies. Diabetes 2003; 52:2160–2167.
4. Ford ES. Risks for all-cause mortality, cardiovascular disease, and diabetes associated with the metabolic syndrome, a summary of the evidence. Diabetes Care 2005; 28:1769–1778.
5. Trovati M, Mularoni EM, Burzacca S, et al. Impaired insulin-induced platelet antiaggregating effect in obesity and in obese NIDDM patients. Diabetes 1995; 44:1318–1322.
6. Anfossi G, Trovati M. Pathophysiology of platelet resistance to anti-aggregating agents in insulin resistance and type 2 diabetes: Implications for anti-aggregating therapy. Cardiovasc Hematol Agents Med Chem 2006; 4:111–128.
7. Davi G, Guagnano MT, Ciabattoni G, et al. Platelet activation in obese women: Role of inflammation and oxidant stress. JAMA 2002; 288:2008–2014.
8. Trovati M, Anfossi G. Influence of insulin and of insulin resistance on platelet and vascular smooth muscle cell function. J Diabetes Complications 2002; 16:35–40.
9. Falcon C, Pfliegler G, Deckmyn H, et al. The platelet insulin receptor: Detection, partial characterization, and search for a function. Biochem Biophys Res Commun 1988; 157:1190–1196.
10. Ferreira IA, Mocking AI, Feijge MA, et al. Platelet inhibition by insulin is absent in type 2 diabetes mellitus. Arterioscler Thromb Vasc Biol 2006; 26:417–422.
11. Westerbacka J, Yki-Jarvinen H, Turpeinen A, et al. Inhibition of platelet–collagen interaction: An in vivo action of insulin abolished by insulin resistance in obesity. Arterioscler Thromb Vasc Biol 2002; 22:167–172.
12. Russo I, Del Mese P, Doronzo G, et al. Platelet resistance to the antiaggregatory cyclic nucleotides in central obesity involves reduced phosphorylation of vasodilator-stimulated phosphoprotein. Clin Chem 2007; 53:1053–1060.
13. Basili S, Pacini G, Guagnano MT, et al. Insulin resistance as a determinant of platelet activation in obese women. J Am Coll Cardiol 2006; 48:2531–2538.

14. Von Hundelshausen P, Weber C. Platelets as immune cells: Bridging inflammation and cardiovascular disease. Circ Res 2007; 100:27–40, review.
15. Englyst NA, Taube JM, Aitman TJ, et al. A novel role for CD36 in VLDL-enhanced platelet activation. Diabetes 2003; 52:1248–1255.
16. Korporaal SJ, Akkerman JW. Platelet activation by low density lipoprotein and high density lipoprotein. Pathophysiol Haemost Thromb 2006; 35:270–280.
17. Konstantinides S, Schafer K, Loskutoff DJ. The prothrombotic effects of leptin possible implications for the risk of cardiovascular disease in obesity. Ann N Y Acad Sci 2001; 947:134–141.
18. Konstantinides S, Schafer K, Koschnick S, et al. Leptin-dependent platelet aggregation and arterial thrombosis suggests a mechanism for atherothrombotic disease in obesity. J Clin Invest 2001; 108:1533–1540.
19. Nakata M, Yada T, Soejima N, et al. Leptin promotes aggregation of human platelets via the long form of its receptor. Diabetes 1999; 48:426–429.
20. Ozata M, Avcu F, Durmus O, et al. Leptin does not play a major role in platelet aggregation in obesity and leptin deficiency. Obes Res 2001; 9:627–630.
21. Canavan B, Salem RO, Schurgin S, et al. Effects of physiological leptin administration on markers of inflammation, platelet activation, and platelet aggregation during caloric deprivation. J Clin Endocrinol Metab 2005; 90:5779–5785.
22. Giandomenico G, Dellas C, Czekay RP, et al. The leptin receptor system of human platelets. J Thromb Haemost 2005; 3:1042–1049.
23. Corsonello A, Perticone F, Malara A, et al. Leptin-dependent platelet aggregation in healthy, overweight and obese subjects. Int J Obes Relat Metab Disord 2003; 27:566–573.
24. Kato H, Kashiwagi H, Shiraga M, et al. Adiponectin acts as an endogenous antithrombotic factor. Arterioscler Thromb Vasc Biol 2006; 26:224–230.
25. Stejskal D, Proskova J, Solichova P. Adiponectin added into the plasma of healthy probands does not affect platelet aggregability. Biomed Pap Med Fac Univ Palacky Olomouc Czech Repub 2006; 150:89–90.
26. American Diabetes Association: Standards of Medical Care in Diabetes. Diabetes Care 2005; 28(Suppl. 1):S4–S36.
27. Bhatt DL, Fox KA, Hacke W, et al. CHARISMA Investigators. Clopidogrel and aspirin versus aspirin alone for the prevention of atherothrombotic events. N Engl J Med 2006; 354:1706–1717.
28. Anfossi G, Trovati M. Pathophysiology of platelet resistance to anti-aggregating agents in insulin resistance and type 2 diabetes: Implications for anti-aggregating therapy. Cardiovasc Hematol Agents Med Chem 2006; 4:111–128.
29. Tamminen M, Lassila R, Westerbacka J, et al. Obesity is associated with impaired platelet-inhibitory effect of acetylsalicylic acid in nondiabetic subjects. Int J Obes Relat Metab Disord 2003; 27:907–911.
30. Angiolillo DJ, Bernardo E, Ramirez C, et al. Insulin therapy is associated with platelet dysfunction in patients with type 2 diabetes mellitus on dual oral antiplatelet treatment. J Am Coll Cardiol 2006; 48:298–304.
31. Meerarani P, Moreno PR, Cimmino G, et al. Atherothrombosis: Role of tissue factor; link between diabetes, obesity and inflammation. Indian J Exp Biol 2007; 45:103–110.
32. Kopp CW, Kopp HP, Steiner S, et al. Weight loss reduces tissue factor in morbidly obese patients. Obes Res 2003; 11:950–956.
33. Samad F, Pandey M, Loskutoff DJ. Tissue factor gene expression in the adipose tissues of obese mice. Proc Natl Acad Sci USA 1998; 95:7591–7596.
34. Samad F, Pandey M, Loskutoff DJ. Regulation of tissue factor gene expression in obesity. Blood 2001; 98:3353–3358.
35. Vaidyula VR, Rao AK, Mozzoli M, et al. Effects of hyperglycemia and hyperinsulinemia on circulating tissue factor procoagulant activity and platelet CD40 ligand. Diabetes 2006; 55:202–208.
36. Belting M, Dorrell MI, Sandgren S, et al. Regulation of angiogenesis by tissue factor cytoplasmic domain signaling. Nat Med 2004; 10:502–509.
37. Fukumura D, Ushiyama A, Duda DG, et al. Paracrine regulation of angiogenesis and adipocyte differentiation during in vivo adipogenesis. Circ Res 2003; 93:e88–e97.
38. Folsom AR, Qamhieh HT, Wing RR, et al. Impact of weight loss on plasminogen activator inhibitor (PAI-1), factor VII, and other hemostatic factors in moderately overweight adults. Arterioscler Thromb 1993; 13:162–169.
39. Primrose JN, Davies JA, Prentice CR, et al. Reduction in factor VII, fibrinogen and plasminogen activator inhibitor-1 activity after surgical treatment of morbid obesity. Thromb Haemost 1992; 68:396–399.
40. Sakkinen PA, Wahl P, Cushman M, et al. Clustering of procoagulation, inflammation, and fibrinolysis variables with metabolic factors in insulin resistance syndrome. Am J Epidemiol 2000; 152:897–907.
41. Godsland IF, Crook D, Proudler AJ, et al. Hemostatic risk factors and insulin sensitivity, regional body fat distribution, and the metabolic syndrome. J Clin Endocrinol Metab 2005; 90:190–197.

42. Carvalho de Sousa J, Bruckert E, Giral P, et al. Coagulation factor VII and plasma triglycerides. Decreased catabolism as a possible mechanism of factor VII hyperactivity. Haemostasis 1989; 19:125–130.
43. Folsom AR, Conlan MG, Davis CE, et al. Relations between hemostasis variables and cardiovascular risk factors in middle-aged adults. Atherosclerosis Risk in Communities (ARIC) Study. Ann Epidemiol 1992; 2:481–494.
44. Fibrinogen Studies Collaboration. Plasma fibrinogen level and the risk of major cardiovascular diseases and nonvascular mortality: An individual participant meta-analysis. JAMA 2005; 294:1799–1809.
45. Juhan-Vague I, Thompson SG, Jespersen J. Involvement of the hemostatic system in the insulin resistance syndrome. A study of 1500 patients with angina pectoris. The ECAT Angina Pectoris Study Group. Arterioscler Thromb 1993; 13:1865–1873.
46. Juhan-Vague I, Morange P, Renucci JF, et al. Fibrinogen, obesity and insulin resistance. Blood Coagul Fibrinolysis 1999; 10 (Suppl. 1):S25–S28.
47. Fain JN, Madan AK, Hiler ML, et al. Comparison of the release of adipokines by adipose tissue, adipose tissue matrix, and adipocytes from visceral and subcutaneous abdominal adipose tissues of obese humans. Endocrinology 2004; 145:2273–2282.
48. Yudkin JS, Kumari M, Humphries SE, et al. Inflammation, obesity, stress and coronary heart disease: Is interleukin-6 the link? Atherosclerosis 2000; 148:209–214.
49. Mineo C, Deguchi H, Griffin JH, et al. Endothelial and antithrombotic actions of HDL. Circ Res 2006; 98:1352–1364.
50. Eren M, Painter CA, Atkinson JB, et al. Age-dependent spontaneous coronary arterial thrombosis in transgenic mice that express a stable form of human plasminogen activator inhibitor-1. Circulation 2002; 106:491–496.
51. Sobel BE. Increased plasminogen activator inhibitor-1 and vasculopathy. A reconcilable paradox. Circulation 1999; 99:2496–2498.
52. Alessi MC, Juhan-Vague I. PAI-1 and the metabolic syndrome: Links, causes, and consequences. Arterioscler Thromb Vasc Biol 2006; 26:2200–2207.
53. Juhan-Vague I, Pyke SDM, Alessi MC, et al. Fibrinolytic factors and the risk of myocardial infarction or sudden death in patients with angina pectoris. Circulation 1996; 94:2057–2063.
54. Mertens I, Verrijken A, Michiels JJ, et al. Among inflammation and coagulation markers, PAI-1 is a true component of the metabolic syndrome. Int J Obes 2006; 30:1308–1314.
55. Morange PE, Alessi MC, Verdier M, et al. PAI-1 produced ex vivo by human adipose tissue is relevant to PAI-1 blood level. Arterioscler Thromb Vasc Biol 1999; 19:1361–1365.
56. Alessi MC, Peiretti F, Morange P, et al. Production of plasminogen activator inhibitor 1 by human adipose tissue: Possible link between visceral fat accumulation and vascular disease. Diabetes 1997; 46:860–867.
57. Shimomura I, Funahashi T, Takahashi M, et al. Enhanced expression of PAI-1 in visceral fat: Possible contributor to vascular disease in obesity. Nat Med 1996; 2:800–803.
58. Bastelica D, Morange P, Berthet B, et al. Stromal cells are the main plasminogen activator inhibitor-1 producing cells in human fat: Evidence of differences between visceral and subcutaneous deposits. Arterioscler Thromb Vasc Biol 2002; 22:173–178.
59. Fain JN, Madan AK, Hiler ML, et al. Comparison of the release of adipokines by adipose tissue, adipose tissue matrix, and adipocytes from visceral and subcutaneous abdominal adipose tissues of obese humans. Endocrinology 2004; 145:2273–2282.
60. Cancello R, Henegar C, Viguerie N, et al. Reduction of macrophage infiltration and chemoattractant gene expression changes in white adipose tissue of morbidly obese subjects after surgery-induced weight loss. Diabetes 2005; 54:2277–2286.
61. Venugopal J, Hanashiro K, Nagamine Y. Regulation of PAI-1 gene expression during adipogenesis. J Cell Biochem 2007; 101:369–380.
62. Curat CA, Wegner V, Sengenes C, et al. Macrophages in human visceral adipose tissue: Increased accumulation in obesity and a source of resistin and visfatin. Diabetologia 2006; 49:744–747.
63. Alessi MC, Bastelica D, Mavri A, et al. Plasma PAI-1 levels are more strongly related to liver steatosis than to adipose tissue accumulation. Arterioscler Thromb Vasc Biol 2003; 23:1262–1268.
64. Samad F, Yamamoto K, Loskutoff DJ. Distribution and regulation of plasminogen activator inhibitor-1 in murine adipose tissue in vivo. Induction by tumor necrosis factor-alpha and lipopolysaccharide. J Clin Invest 1996; 97:37–46.
65. Alessi MC, Bastelica D, Morange P, et al. Plasminogen activator inhibitor 1, transforming growth factor-beta1, and BMIare closely associated in human adipose tissue during morbid obesity. Diabetes 2000; 49:1374–1380.
66. Ferroni P, Guagnano MT, Manigrasso MR, et al. Increased plasminogen activator inhibitor-1 levels in android obesity: Correlation with oxidative stress. J Thromb Haemost 2005; 3:1086–1087.

67. Furukawa S, Fujita T, Shimabukuro M, et al. Increased oxidative stress in obesity and its impact on metabolic syndrome. J Clin Invest 2004; 114:1752–1761.
68. Ayachi SE, Paulmyer-Lacroix O, Verdier M, et al. 11 beta-Hydroxysteroid dehydrogenase type 1-driven cortisone reactivation regulates plasminogen activator inhibitor type 1 in adipose tissue of obese women. J Thromb Haemost 2006; 4:621–627.
69. Hermanowski-Vosatka A, Balkovec JM, Cheng K, et al. 11 beta-HSD1 inhibition ameliorates metabolic syndrome and prevents progression of atherosclerosis in mice. J Exp Med 2005; 202:517–527.
70. Vaughan DE, Lazos SA, Tong K. Angiotensin II regulates the expression of plasminogen activator inhibitor-1 in cultured endothelial cells. A potential link between the renin–angiotensin system and thrombosis. J Clin Invest 1995; 95:995–1001.
71. Festa A, D'Agostino R Jr, Tracy RP, et al. Insulin Resistance Atherosclerosis Study. Elevated levels of acute-phase proteins and plasminogen activator inhibitor-1 predict the development of type II diabetes: The insulin resistance atherosclerosis study. Diabetes 2002; 51:1131–1137.
72. Festa A, Williams K, Tracy RP, et al. Progression of plasminogen activator inhibitor-1 and fibrinogen levels in relation to incident type II diabetes. Circulation 2006; 113:1753–1759.
73. Kanaya AM, Wassel Fyr C, Vittinghoff E, et al. Adipocytokines and incident diabetes mellitus in older adults: The independent effect of plasminogen activator inhibitor 1. Arch Intern Med 2006; 166:350–356.
74. Meigs JB, O'donnell CJ, Tofler GH, et al. Hemostatic markers of endothelial dysfunction and risk of incident type 2 diabetes: The Framingham Offspring Study. Diabetes 2006; 55:530–537.
75. Hoffstedt J, Andersson IL, Persson L, et al. The common -675 4G/5G polymorphism in the plasminogen activator inhibitor -1 gene is strongly associated with obesity. Diabetologia 2002; 45:584–587.
76. Lopes C, Dina C, Durand E, et al. PAI-1 polymorphisms modulate phenotypes associated with the metabolic syndrome in obese and diabetic Caucasian population. Diabetologia 2003; 46:1284–1290.
77. Freeman MS, Mansfield MW. Comment on: The common -675 4G/5G polymorphism in the plasminogen activator inhibitor-1 gene is strongly associated with obesity. Diabetologia 2002; 45:1602–1603.
78. Juhan-Vague I, Morange PE, Frere C, et al. HIFMECH Study Group. The plasminogen activator inhibitor-1 -675 4G/5G genotype influences the risk of myocardial infarction associated with elevated plasma proinsulin and insulin concentrations in men from Europe: The HIFMECH study. J Thromb Haemost 2003; 1:2322–2329.
79. Ma LJ, Mao SL, Taylor KL, et al. Prevention of obesity and insulin resistance in mice lacking plasminogen activator inhibitor 1. Diabetes 2004; 53:336–346.
80. De Taeye BM, Novitskaya T, Gleaves L, et al. Bone marrow plasminogen activator inhibitor-1 influences the development of obesity. J Biol Chem 2006; 281:32796–32805.
81. Schafer K, Fujisawa K, Konstantinides S, et al. Disruption of the plasminogen activator inhibitor 1 gene reduces the adiposity and improves the metabolic profile of genetically obese and diabetic ob/ob mice. FASEB J 2001; 15:1840–1842.
82. Crandall DL, Quinet EM, El Ayachi S, et al. Modulation of adipose tissue development by pharmacologic inhibition of PAI-1. Arterioscler Thromb Vasc Biol 2006; 26:2209–2215.
83. Lijnen HR, Alessi MC, Frederix L, et al. Tiplaxtinin impairs nutritionally induced obesity in mice. Thromb Haemost 2006; 96:731–737.
84. Lijnen HR, Alessi MC, Van Hoef B, et al. On the role of plasminogen activator inhibitor-1 in adipose tissue development and insulin resistance in mice. J Thromb Haemost 2005; 3:1174–1179.
85. Liang X, Kanjanabuch T, Mao SL, et al. Plasminogen activator inhibitor-1 modulates adipocyte differentiation. Am J Physiol Endocrinol Metab 2006; 290:E103–E113.
86. Lebrun P, Baron V, Hauck CR, et al. Cell adhesion and focal adhesion kinase regulate insulin receptor substrate-1 expression. J Biol Chem 2000; 275:38371–38377.
87. Lopez-Alemany R, Redondo JM, Nagamine Y, et al. Plasminogen activator inhibitor type-1 inhibits insulin signaling by competing with alphavbeta3 integrin for vitronectin binding. Eur J Biochem 2003; 270:814–821.
88. Griffiths SL, Grainger DJ. Proposal of a novel diabetogenic mechanism involving the serpin PAI-1. Bioessays 2006; 28:629–641.
89. Lijnen HR, Maquoi E, Morange P, et al. Nutritionally induced obesity is attenuated in transgenic mice overexpressing plasminogen activator inhibitor-1. Arterioscler Thromb Vasc Biol 2003; 23:78–84.
90. Scroyen I, Christiaens V, Lijnen HR. No functional role of plasminogen activator inhibitor-1 in murine adipogenesis or adipocyte differentiation. J Thromb Haemost 2007; 5:139–145.
91. Morange PE, Lijnen HR, Alessi MC, et al. Influence of PAI-1 on adipose tissue growth and metabolic parameters in a murine model of diet-induced obesity. Arterioscler Thromb Vasc Biol 2000; 20:1150–1154.
92. Schachinger V, Britten MB, Zeiher AM. Prognostic impact of coronary vasodilator dysfunction on adverse long-term outcome of coronary heart disease. Circulation 2000; 101:1899–1906.
93. Steinberg HO, Chaker H, Leaming R, et al. Obesity/insulin resistance is associated with endothelial dysfunction. Implications for the syndrome of insulin resistance. J Clin Invest 1996; 97:2601–2610.

94. Mather KJ, Lteif A, Steinberg HO, et al. Interactions between endothelin and nitric oxide in the regulation of vascular tone in obesity and diabetes. Diabetes 2004; 53:2060–2066.
95. Mather KJ, Mirzamohammadi B, Lteif A, et al. Endothelin contributes to basal vascular tone and endothelial dysfunction in human obesity and type 2 diabetes. Diabetes 2002; 51:3517–3523.
96. Baron AD, Steinberg H, Brechtel G, et al. Skeletal muscle blood flow independently modulates insulin-mediated glucose uptake. Am J Physiol 1994; 266:E248–E253.
97. Coggins M, Lindner J, Rattigan S, et al. Physiologic hyperinsulinemia enhances human skeletal muscle perfusion by capillary recruitment. Diabetes 2001; 50:2682–2690.
98. Baron AD, Tarshoby M, Hook G, et al. Interaction between insulin sensitivity and muscle perfusion on glucose uptake in human skeletal muscle, evidence for capillary recruitment. Diabetes 2000; 49:768–774.
99. Lteif A, Vaishnava P, Baron AD, et al. Endothelin limits insulin action in obese/insulin-resistant humans. Diabetes 2007; 56:728–734.
100. Kim JA, Montagnani M, Koh KK, et al. Reciprocal relationships between insulin resistance and endothelial dysfunction: Molecular and pathophysiological mechanisms. Circulation 2006; 113:1888–1904.
101. Montagnani M, Golovchenko I, Kim I, et al. Inhibition of phosphatidylinositol 3-kinase enhances mitogenic actions of insulin in endothelial cells. J Biol Chem 2002; 277:1794–1799.
102. Arteaga RB, Chirinos JA, Soriano AO, et al. Endothelial microparticles and platelet and leukocyte activation in patients with the metabolic syndrome. Am J Cardiol 2006; 98:70–74.
103. Meigs JB, Mittleman MA, Nathan DM, et al. Hyperinsulinemia, hyperglycemia, and impaired hemostasis: The Framingham Offspring Study. JAMA 2000; 283:221–228.
104. Ziccardi P, Nappo F, Giugliano G, et al. Reduction of inflammatory cytokine concentrations and improvement of endothelial functions in obese women after weight loss over one year. Circulation 2002; 105:804–849.
105. Picchi A, Gao X, Belmadani S, et al. Tumor necrosis factor-alpha induces endothelial dysfunction in the prediabetic metabolic syndrome. Circ Res 2006; 99:69–77.
106. Valle Jimenez M, Estepa RM, Camacho RM, et al. Endothelial dysfunction is related to insulin resistance and inflammatory biomarker levels in obese prepubertal children. Eur J Endocrinol 2007; 156:497–502.
107. Ageno W, Prandoni P, Romualdi E, et al. The metabolic syndrome and the risk of venous thrombosis: A case-control study. J Thromb Haemost 2006; 4:1914–1918.

7 Physiological and Metabolic Characteristics of Visceral Adipocytes

Alain Veilleux and André Tchernof

Molecular Endocrinology and Oncology Research Center & Department of Nutrition, Laval University Medical Research Center and Laval University, Québec, Canada

INTRODUCTION

Abdominal obesity is recognized as a strong predictor of the metabolic disorders associated with obesity (1,2). Excess visceral fat accumulation, also known as intra-abdominal or visceral obesity, is strongly and independently associated with metabolic alteration such as insulin resistance, hypertension, and dyslipidemia, which are important risk factors for cardiovascular disease (1,3). Specific features of the visceral adipose tissue depots, which include omental, mesenteric, and retroperitoneal fat, have been shown to be related or lead to metabolic alterations. In this chapter, we provide an overview of the biological nature of the visceral adipocyte and its potential links with the metabolic disturbances associated with visceral fat accumulation.

ADIPOCYTE SIZE

According to the size of their triglyceride droplets, the mature adipocyte population of a given depot will show important differences in cell size. These differences vary as a function of the nutritional status of the individual (4). The mean adipocyte size also varies according to sex, adiposity level, and anatomical location of the adipose tissue depot (5–8). In both sexes, omental and subcutaneous adipocytes become larger with obesity, but adipocyte size reaches a plateau in massively obese subject (5,8,9). In normal weight to moderately obese women (5,8,9), omental adipocytes are 20% to 30% smaller than those of subcutaneous adipocytes. Omental and subcutaneous adipocytes actually reach a similar size at very elevated BMI values ($>60kg/m^2$) (5,8,9). As women reach menopause, the omental–subcutaneous depot difference seems to be attenuated because omental, but not subcutaneous, adipocyte size is increased (10). In men, omental and subcutaneous adipocytes have a similar cell size through most of the adiposity range. In addition, maximal adipocyte size is lower in men (~120 μm) than in women (~140 μm) (9). Since fat cell size is a critical determinant of adipocyte function (4), these sex-, depot-, and adiposity-related differences might play an important role in the variation of adipose cell function in various fat compartments.

ADIPOCYTE METABOLISM

The response of adipose tissue to lipolytic agonists is known to be different in the visceral and subcutaneous compartments (5,8,11–13). Again, one of the main determinants of these regional differences is adipocyte size (4,5,8). Studies assessing differences in adipocyte metabolism between small and large adipocytes from the same adipose tissue depot of a given individual showed that lipolysis, lipid synthesis, and glucose uptake (4,14,15), as well as gene expression (16), are strongly influenced by adipocyte size. Consequently, adipocyte hypertrophy in a given adipose tissue depot lead to high rates of lipid synthesis, increased lipolysis, and therefore increased fatty acid flux across the cell membrane (17). Consistent with the fact that adipocytes from the omental fat compartment are smaller than that of the subcutaneous fat compartment in women, basal lipolysis in this depot is lower in the former than in the latter (8,11–13). Thus, in women and possibly in very lean men, visceral adipose tissue is not believed, at least in the basal condition, to be a major contributor to circulating free fatty acids (FFA) (18). However, compared to the subcutaneous adipose tissue depot, lipolysis in omental fat is more responsive to β-adrenergic agonist stimulation (8,11–13) and less to insulin suppression (19,20). Since abdominal obesity is characterized by excess of positive lipolytic stimuli and insulin resistance, the contribution of this highly responsive tissue to the circulating pool of FFA is likely to be increased in such condition (18). In consequence, the increased FFA flux may preferentially alter liver metabolism as this depot is drained by the portal vein system (21). In men, lipolytic activity is higher than that observed in women, but no regional difference is observed (5,8). Thus, in absolute values, more FFA are released into the portal vein circulation by visceral adipose tissues in men (18). Compared to women, this may increase the impact of omental adipose tissue on the metabolism and lead to a greater cardiovascular disease risk (5). In women, at menopause, visceral fat lipolysis rates tend to increase in parallel to visceral fat cell size (10), which could partially offset the apparent protection of women against cardiovascular disease.

Accumulation of triglycerides in adipose tissue relies mainly on the hydrolysis of triglyceride-rich lipoproteins by lipoprotein lipase (LPL) and on triglyceride synthesis inside the adipocyte. The regional differences in the rate of these processes are also tightly associated with adipocyte size. Many studies including both sexes failed to find differences in omental versus subcutaneous LPL activity (22,23). However, higher LPL activity in subcutaneous adipose tissue is observed in studies including mostly women (8,20,24), and the opposite is observed in studies including mostly men (5,24,25). Thus, we propose that regional differences in LPL activity are sex-specific and likely reflect the propensity of each compartment to accumulate lipids in each sex. Concordant with these observations, triglyceride synthesis in women is reduced in omental adipose tissue (11,26), and is similar in both abdominal subcutaneous and omental adipose tissue depots in men (11).

In summary, adipocyte metabolism seems to favor greater accumulation of lipid in the visceral fat compartment and higher release of FFA in the portal vein of men compared to women. Adipocyte size appears to be a major correlate of these differences.

ADIPOKINES

In addition to the lipid-storage function, adipose tissue is known to produce a number of cytokines, termed adipokines, as well as many other factors involved in the regulation of several biological processes (27). Adipokines are mainly secreted not only by adipocytes or preadipocytes, but also, especially in obesity, by macrophages invading the tissue (27). Recent studies have observed that visceral and subcutaneous adipose tissue did not contribute equally to the secretion of these factors (28–31). The literature also suggests that adipocyte size has an important influence on the secretion pattern of these factors (32). Similar to adipocyte metabolism, sex- and depot-specific differences in adipocyte size may modulate the secretion pattern of some adipokines.

Circulating levels of adiponectin, an adipokine with insulin-sensitizing and anti-inflammatory properties, are inversely associated to adiposity (33). The decrease in adiponectin concentration with obesity is believed to have negative consequences on whole-body glucose homeostasis (33). Studies suggested that visceral adipose tissue accumulation assessed by computed tomography is an independent predictor of circulating adiponectin levels (34,35). Omental adipose tissue also seems to be a critical determinant of serum adiponectin levels. Indeed, omental adipocyte adiponectin secretion is primarily reduced in obesity, while subcutaneous adipocyte adiponectin secretion is maintained in abdominally obese women (36).

Interleukin-6 (IL-6), a proinflammatory cytokine, is positively associated with obesity and especially with visceral fat accumulation (37,38). IL-6 is also tightly linked to C-reactive protein (CRP) production and other markers of cardiovascular disease (39). As it accounts for one-third of IL-6 production, it is suggested that adipose tissue–derived IL-6 may have systemic effects on metabolism (39). In addition, local production and accumulation of this cytokine can alter lipid metabolism of the adipose tissue itself (32,39,40). Indeed, elevated plasma IL-6 is associated with increased omental fat cell β-adrenergic lipolytic responsiveness (41), and β-adrenergic–dependent lipolysis is increased by high levels of IL-6 (42). Moreover, LPL activity is reduced by half in subcutaneous and omental adipose tissue depots by chronic IL-6 treatment (42,43). Although metabolism of both adipose tissue depots is affected by IL-6, this effect is more pronounced in visceral fat since this tissue releases 2 to 3 times more IL-6 than subcutaneous adipose tissue (40). In menopausal women, higher visceral fat accumulation also seems to be related to higher circulating levels of IL-6 (41). In consequence, increased secretion of IL-6 in obesity could alter lipid metabolism of visceral adipose tissue and possibly increase the release of FFA into the portal vein (39).

Tumor necrosis factor alpha (TNF-α) is a proinflammatory cytokine mainly secreted by immune cell such as macrophages (39). Obesity is associated with increased circulating and adipose tissue TNF-α (44). This increase is mainly imputable to infiltration of macrophages in adipose tissue and to increased secretion by adipocytes (32,45). In addition to its role in immunity, chronically high levels of TNF-α tend to reduce fat mass accumulation through the induction of lipolysis and the impairment of insulin-induced lipogenesis and glucose uptake (30,46). Moreover, TNF-α may be associated with insulin resistance in muscle through the induction of nitric oxide production (47). Since TNF-α correlates positively with visceral fat accumulation, TNF-α could alter fat partitioning between the visceral and subcutaneous compartment through the regulation of adipocyte metabolism (48,49). However, this remains controversial (30,38). In this regard, studies measuring regional expression differences in TNF-α and its receptor failed to find consistent results (29,30), and the alteration of fat disposal by this cytokine seems to be greater in subcutaneous adipose tissue (30). Taken together with the fact that tissues with hypertrophic adipocytes may contain higher levels of TNF-α (32), it may be suggested that TNF-α could limit fat accumulation in subcutaneous adipose tissue and drive the lipid overflow to the visceral and ectopic fat compartments.

Impairment of fibrinolysis by an enhanced plasma activity of the plasminogen activator inhibitor-1 (PAI-1) may be involved in the development of cardiovascular disease (50). PAI-1 is expressed by hepatocytes and endothelial cells, although preadipocytes and mature adipocytes also secrete significant amounts of PAI-1 (50). The release of this cytokine in omental adipose tissue is higher compared to subcutaneous adipose tissue and this regional difference is even more pronounced in the presence of obesity (31,51,52). Indeed, strong positive correlations have been observed between plasma PAI-1 levels and measures of visceral obesity (53). Specific accumulation of visceral adipose tissue may contribute to increased plasma levels of PAI-1 and consequently to the impaired fibrinolysis associated to abdominal obesity (50). Therefore, PAI-1 secretion by the visceral adipocyte could contribute to visceral obesity-associated metabolic disturbances.

As described above, adipose tissue can secrete numerous adipokines which can alter metabolic pathways and lead to an increased risk of developing metabolic diseases. Several studies support the hypothesis that visceral adipocyte hypertrophy is accompanied with deleterious changes in the expression and/or secretion pattern of some key adipokines such as adiponectin, IL-6, TNF-α, and PAI-1. These studies tend to confirm that visceral obesity is characterized by a proinflammatory and proatherogenic state, at least partly created by abnormal adipokine secretion.

GENOMICS AND GENE EXPRESSION

Few studies have compared gene expression profiles of visceral and subcutaneous adipose tissue to highlight the intrinsic properties of abdominal adipocytes and other cell types found within these fat depots (54–57). It appears that the interindividual variability of gene expression within each depot is relatively low even if physiological, metabolic, and environmental factors are not controlled (54).

Moreover, less than 10% of the genes are differentially expressed in omental versus subcutaneous adipose tissue (55). This highly similar expression pattern suggests that the primary characteristics of adipose tissue are generally conserved regardless of anatomical localization and habitus of the individual in whom the sample is taken (54,55). However, specific biological functions, including cell differentiation, lipolysis, and cytokine secretion, show clear differential regulation in visceral versus subcutaneous adipose tissue (55,56). Furthermore, the identification of genes specifically prone to high interindividual variation lead to pathways of the inflammatory response, cell death regulation, and lipid metabolism (57). None of these genomic studies have assessed the consequences of obesity on gene expression patterns in visceral and subcutaneous adipose tissue. Nevertheless, Jernas et al. have identified gene expression differences in large adipocytes compared to small adipocytes (16). In that study, immune and structure-related genes showed higher expression levels in larger adipocyte. Thus, based on the increase in mean adipocyte size with obesity, we may suggest that adipocyte gene expression patterns would also change with obesity. Macrophage infiltration in adipose tissue of obese individuals could also significantly affect gene expression patterns (45). Future studies will be necessary to better evaluate the contribution of nonadipocyte cells and the impact of obesity on adipose tissue gene expression profiles.

LINK BETWEEN PHYSIOLOGICAL AND METABOLIC CHARACTERISTICS OF THE VISCERAL ADIPOCYTE AND METABOLIC ALTERATIONS

The development of metabolic alterations in obesity is closely linked to visceral fat accumulation. The greater negative impact of this depot on metabolic pathways appears to be attributable, at least partly, to the physiological and metabolic nature of visceral adipocytes. Visceral adipocyte lipolysis is more sensitive to β-adrenergic agonists and less to its suppression by insulin. Even if this visceral fat is not a major contributor to whole-body FFA production, its altered lipolytic responsiveness, amplified by the release of FFA directly in the portal vein of abdominally obese individuals may play a significant role. As previously described, the visceral adipocyte or visceral fat reveals a distinct secretion pattern of proinflammatory and anti-inflammatory adipokines compared to adipocytes located in subcutaneous adipose tissue. The greater proinflammatory potential of visceral adipose tissue may alter local and systemic metabolism. Indeed, visceral adipocytes and surrounding cells secrete more proinflammatory adipokines such as TNF-α, IL-6, and PAI-1 which can alter lipolysis, insulin sensitivity, and fibrinolysis. Moreover, in abdominally obese individuals, this depot secretes less adiponectin, which acts as an anti-inflammatory and insulin-sensitizing molecule. Taken together, the proinflammatory adipokine profile and altered lipolysis in visceral adipose tissue may contribute to metabolic alterations observed in abdominally obese individuals, and subsequently to the increased risk of developing type 2 diabetes and cardiovascular disease.

REFERENCES

1. Third Report of the National Cholesterol Education Program (NCEP) Expert Panel on Detection, Evaluation, and Treatment of High Blood Cholesterol in Adults (Adult Treatment Panel III)—final report. Circulation 2002; 106:3143–3421.
2. Despres JP, Lemieux I. Abdominal obesity and metabolic syndrome. Nature 2006; 444:881–887.
3. Despres JP. Is visceral obesity the cause of the metabolic syndrome? Ann Med 2006; 38:52–63.
4. Farnier C, Krief S, Blache M, et al. Adipocyte functions are modulated by cell size change: Potential involvement of an integrin/ERK signalling pathway. Int J Obes Relat Metab Disord 2003; 27:1178–1186.
5. Boivin A, Brochu G, Marceau S, et al. Regional differences in adipose tissue metabolism in obese men. Metabolism 2007; 56:533–540.
6. Fried SK, Kral JG. Sex differences in regional distribution of fat cell size and lipoprotein lipase activity in morbidly obese patients. Int J Obes 1987; 11:129–140.
7. Salans LB, Cushman SW, Weismann RE. Studies of human adipose tissue. Adipose cell size and number in nonobese and obese patients. J Clin Invest 1973; 52:929–941.
8. Tchernof A, Belanger C, Morisset AS, et al. Regional differences in adipose tissue metabolism in women: Minor effect of obesity and body fat distribution. Diabetes 2006; 55:1353–1360.
9. Caron-Jobin M, Nadeau M, Mailloux J, et al. Omental and subcutaneous adipocyte size in men and women. Obesity 2008; In press.
10. Tchernof A, Desmeules A, Richard C, et al. Ovarian hormone status and abdominal visceral adipose tissue metabolism. J Clin Endocrinol Metab 2004; 89:3425–3430.
11. Edens NK, Fried SK, Kral JG, et al. In vitro lipid synthesis in human adipose tissue from three abdominal sites. Am J Physiol 1993; 265:E374–E379.
12. Reynisdottir S, Dauzats M, Thorne A, et al. Comparison of hormone-sensitive lipase activity in visceral and subcutaneous human adipose tissue. J Clin Endocrinol Metab 1997; 82:4162–4166.
13. Richelsen B, Pedersen SB, Moller-Pedersen T, et al. Regional differences in triglyceride breakdown in human adipose tissue: Effects of catecholamines, insulin, and prostaglandin E2. Metabolism 1991; 40:990–996.
14. Zinder O, Shapiro B. Effect of cell size on epinephrine- and ACTH-induced fatty acid release from isolated fat cells. J Lipid Res 1971; 12:91–95.

15. Franck N, Stenkula KG, Ost A, et al. Insulin-induced GLUT4 translocation to the plasma membrane is blunted in large compared with small primary fat cells isolated from the same individual. Diabetologia 2007; 50:1716–1722.
16. Jernas M, Palming J, Sjoholm K, et al. Separation of human adipocytes by size: Hypertrophic fat cells display distinct gene expression. FASEB J 2006; 20:1540–1542.
17. Smith J, Al Amri M, Dorairaj P, et al. The adipocyte life cycle hypothesis. Clin Sci (Lond) 2006; 110:1–9.
18. Nielsen S, Guo Z, Johnson CM, et al. Splanchnic lipolysis in human obesity. J Clin Invest 2004; 113:1582–1588.
19. Zierath JR, Livingston JN, Thorne A, et al. Regional difference in insulin inhibition of non-esterified fatty acid release from human adipocytes: Relation to insulin receptor phosphorylation and intracellular signalling through the insulin receptor substrate-1 pathway. Diabetologia 1998; 41:1343–1354.
20. Mauriege P, Marette A, Atgie C, et al. Regional variation in adipose tissue metabolism of severely obese premenopausal women. J Lipid Res 1995; 36:672–684.
21. Tchernof A. Visceral adipocytes and the metabolic syndrome. Nutr Rev 2007; 65:S24-S29.
22. Fried SK, Russell CD, Grauso NL, et al. Lipoprotein lipase regulation by insulin and glucocorticoid in subcutaneous and omental adipose tissues of obese women and men. J Clin Invest 1993; 92:2191–2198.
23. Panarotto D, Poisson J, Devroede G, et al. Lipoprotein lipase steady-state mRNA levels are lower in human omental versus subcutaneous abdominal adipose tissue. Metabolism 2000; 49:1224–1227.
24. Rebuffe-Scrive M, Andersson B, Olbe L, et al. Metabolism of adipose tissue in intraabdominal depots of nonobese men and women. Metabolism 1989; 38:453–458.
25. Marin P, Andersson B, Ottosson M, et al. The morphology and metabolism of intraabdominal adipose tissue in men. Metabolism 1992; 41:1242–1248.
26. Maslowska MH, Sniderman AD, MacLean LD, et al. Regional differences in triacylglycerol synthesis in adipose tissue and in cultured preadipocytes. J Lipid Res 1993; 34:219–228.
27. Trayhurn P, Wood IS. Signalling role of adipose tissue: Adipokines and inflammation in obesity. Biochem Soc Trans 2005; 33:1078–1081.
28. Drolet R, Bélanger C, Fortier M, et al. Fat depot-specific impact of visceral obesity on adipocyte adiponectin release in women. Obesity 2008; In press.
29. Hube F, Birgel M, Lee YM, et al. Expression pattern of tumour necrosis factor receptors in subcutaneous and omental human adipose tissue: Role of obesity and non-insulin-dependent diabetes mellitus. Eur J Clin Invest 1999; 29:672–678.
30. Good M, Newell FM, Haupt LM, et al. TNF and TNF receptor expression and insulin sensitivity in human omental and subcutaneous adipose tissue—Influence of BMI and adipose distribution. Diab Vasc Dis Res 2006; 3:26–33.
31. He G, Pedersen SB, Bruun JM, et al. Differences in plasminogen activator inhibitor 1 in subcutaneous versus omental adipose tissue in non-obese and obese subjects. Horm Metab Res 2003; 35:178–182.
32. Skurk T, Alberti-Huber C, Herder C, et al. Relationship between adipocyte size and adipokine expression and secretion. J Clin Endocrinol Metab 2007; 92:1023–1033.
33. Whitehead JP, Richards AA, Hickman IJ, et al. Adiponectin—A key adipokine in the metabolic syndrome. Diabetes Obes Metab 2006; 8:264–280.
34. Cnop M, Havel PJ, Utzschneider KM, et al. Relationship of adiponectin to body fat distribution, insulin sensitivity and plasma lipoproteins: Evidence for independent roles of age and sex. Diabetologia 2003; 46:459–469.
35. Park KG, Park KS, Kim MJ, et al. Relationship between serum adiponectin and leptin concentrations and body fat distribution. Diabetes Res Clin Pract 2004; 63:135–142.
36. Motoshima H, Wu X, Sinha MK, et al. Differential regulation of adiponectin secretion from cultured human omental and subcutaneous adipocytes: Effects of insulin and rosiglitazone. J Clin Endocrinol Metab 2002; 87:5662–5667.
37. Bastard JP, Jardel C, Bruckert E, et al. Elevated levels of interleukin 6 are reduced in serum and subcutaneous adipose tissue of obese women after weight loss. J Clin Endocrinol Metab 2000; 85:3338–3342.
38. Fenkci S, Rota S, Sabir N, et al. Relationship of serum interleukin-6 and tumor necrosis factor alpha levels with abdominal fat distribution evaluated by ultrasonography in overweight or obese postmenopausal women. J Investig Med 2006; 54:455–460.
39. Wisse BE. The inflammatory syndrome: The role of adipose tissue cytokines in metabolic disorders linked to obesity. J Am Soc Nephrol 2004; 15:2792–2800.
40. Fried SK, Bunkin DA, Greenberg AS. Omental and subcutaneous adipose tissues of obese subjects release interleukin-6: Depot difference and regulation by glucocorticoid. J Clin Endocrinol Metab 1998; 83:847–850.
41. Morisset A-S, Huot C, Légaré D, et al. Circulating IL-6 levels and abdominal fat cell metabolism in women. Obesity 2008; 16:1487–1492.
42. Trujillo ME, Sullivan S, Harten I, et al. Interleukin-6 regulates human adipose tissue lipid metabolism and leptin production in vitro. J Clin Endocrinol Metab 2004; 89:5577–5582.

43. Greenberg AS, Nordan RP, McIntosh J, et al. Interleukin 6 reduces lipoprotein lipase activity in adipose tissue of mice in vivo and in 3T3-L1 adipocytes: A possible role for interleukin 6 in cancer cachexia. Cancer Res 1992; 52:4113–4116.
44. Hotamisligil GS, Arner P, Caro JF, et al. Increased adipose tissue expression of tumor necrosis factor-alpha in human obesity and insulin resistance. J Clin Invest 1995; 95:2409–2415.
45. Weisberg SP, McCann D, Desai M, et al. Obesity is associated with macrophage accumulation in adipose tissue. J Clin Invest 2003; 112:1796–1808.
46. Grunfeld C, Feingold KR. The metabolic effects of tumor necrosis factor and other cytokines. Biotherapy 1991; 3:143–158.
47. Perreault M, Marette A. Targeted disruption of inducible nitric oxide synthase protects against obesity-linked insulin resistance in muscle. Nat Med 2001; 7:1138–1143.
48. Park HS, Park JY, Yu R. Relationship of obesity and visceral adiposity with serum concentrations of CRP, TNF-alpha and IL-6. Diabetes Res Clin Pract 2005; 69:29–35.
49. Tsigos C, Kyrou I, Chala E, et al. Circulating tumor necrosis factor alpha concentrations are higher in abdominal versus peripheral obesity. Metabolism 1999; 48:1332–1335.
50. Alessi MC, Juhan-Vague I. PAI-1 and the metabolic syndrome: links, causes, and consequences. Arterioscler Thromb Vasc Biol 2006; 26:2200–2207.
51. Gottschling-Zeller H, Birgel M, Rohrig K, et al. Effect of tumor necrosis factor alpha and transforming growth factor beta 1 on plasminogen activator inhibitor-1 secretion from subcutaneous and omental human fat cells in suspension culture. Metabolism 2000; 49:666–671.
52. Alessi MC, Peiretti F, Morange P, et al. Production of plasminogen activator inhibitor 1 by human adipose tissue: Possible link between visceral fat accumulation and vascular disease. Diabetes 1997; 46:860–867.
53. Kockx M, Leenen R, Seidell J, et al. Relationship between visceral fat and PAI-1 in overweight men and women before and after weight loss. Thromb Haemost 1999; 82:1490–1496.
54. van Beek EA, Bakker AH, Kruyt PM, et al. Intra- and interindividual variation in gene expression in human adipose tissue. Pflugers Arch 2007; 453:851–861.
55. Vohl MC, Sladek R, Robitaille J, et al. A survey of genes differentially expressed in subcutaneous and visceral adipose tissue in men. Obes Res 2004; 12:1217–1222.
56. Montague CT, Prins JB, Sanders L, et al. Depot-related gene expression in human subcutaneous and omental adipocytes. Diabetes 1998; 47: 1384–1391.
57. Zhang Y, Bossé Y, Marceau P, et al. Gene expression variability in subcutaneous and omental adipose tissue of obese men. Gene Expr 2007; 14:35–46.

8 The Endocrine Function of Adipose Tissue: Implications of Visceral Obesity for Patients With Cardiometabolic Risk

Max Lafontan

Unité Inserm 858, Institut de Médecine Moléculaire de Rangueil, Hôpital Rangueil and Université Paul Sabatier, Toulouse Cedex, France

The topography of fat distribution plays an important role in the development of health risks. Patients with abdominal obesity exhibiting fat accumulation in subcutaneous and particularly in intraabdominal deposits (i.e., those with expanded visceral depots) are the one who are most prone to metabolic and cardiovascular problems (1–3). In humans, omentectomy (i.e., removal of the omentum), when performed together with adjustable gastric banding, has significant positive and long-term effects on the metabolic profiles of glucose and insulin in obese subjects (4). Regional differences in fat depots are intriguing and far-reaching, and the mechanisms leading to the deleterious effects of visceral fat remain controversial (working hypothesis in Fig. 1).

Originally, adipose tissue was considered to be the biological system that stored triglycerides (TG) and released nonesterified fatty acids (NEFA) and glycerol. Understanding the site-related differences in the regulation of lipolysis and lipid mobilization have been clarified for insulin and catecholamines and validated in vivo (5). In addition to these functions, adipose tissue is now recognized as expressing and secreting a large variety of biological compounds—details of which can be found in a number of recently published reviews (5–9). The other important point that has expanded our views is that most of the scientists studying adipose tissue have now clearly integrated the fact that adipose tissue not only consists of fat cells but also contains the cells present in the stroma-vascular fraction (SVF). SVF is the fraction usually removed after collagenase digestion of adipose tissue for the preparation of isolated fat cells. The SVF includes a number of cell types, such as fat cell progenitors (i.e., the preadipocytes), microvascular endothelial cells, pericytes, lymphocytes, monocytes, and macrophages. It is also a site where human adipose–derived stem cells, capable of differentiating along the adipocyte, chondrocyte, and osteoblast pathways (10,11) are found. The crosstalk between the various cell types in adipose tissue and the nature of paracrine messages between them is an intense area of research. Blood monocyte–derived macrophages infiltrate the adipose tissue of obese patients and their number correlate directly with obesity (12,13). Finally, each fat deposit is also characterized by its vascular bed and its innervations that could also interfere with the control of the fat-storage function (14). Why is it more risky for health to accumulate fat in the visceral area than in other regions? Although the answer is not yet entirely clear, biochemical and physiological explanations will be proposed here with particular attention paid to the production of visceral adipose tissue. Do visceral adipocytes possess unusual or special properties that could be at the origin of metabolic disturbances? Do other visceral adipose tissue elements such as the SVF play any role? Is visceral fat (i.e., omental and mesenteric fat) a major culprit or simply an innocent bystander as posed by Frayn (15)? This review will focus on the endocrine components of visceral fat compared with other fat deposits. A brief overview of the cell populations of visceral fat will introduce the review.

THE CELLULAR CONTEXT OF VISCERAL ADIPOSE TISSUE

Visceral fat deposits represent the minor component of total body fat; they occupy the body cavity and surround most of the visceral organs and abdominal vessels. Mesenteric and omental depots represent 5–8% and 20% of the total body fat in women and men, respectively; and the total body fat increases during obesity in both the sexes. Visceral adipocytes are smaller

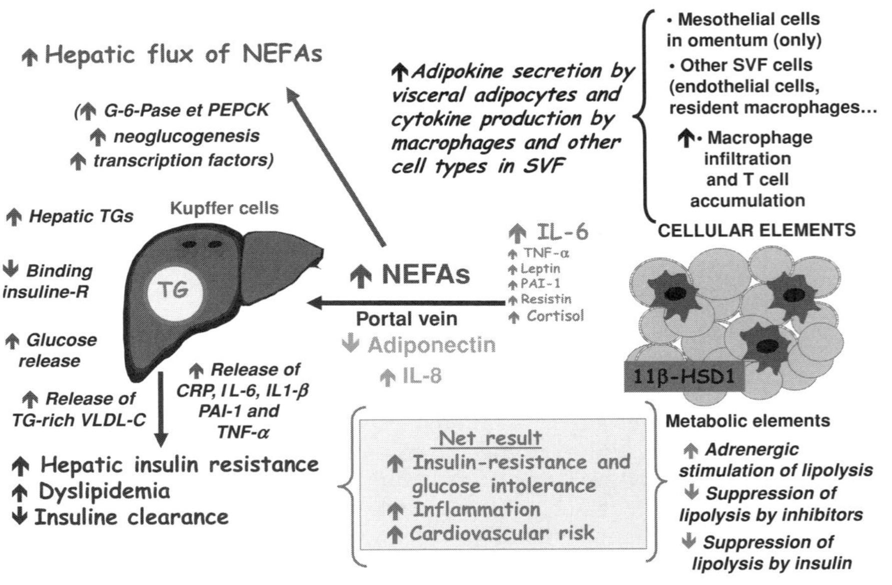

Figure 1 Working hypothesis for the mechanism(s) involved in the privileged visceral adipose tissue–liver interactions leading to the appearance of obesity-related diseases. Major factors involved in the control adipocyte metabolism and adipose tissue secretions are depicted. Putative incidence of adipose tissue productions on liver dysfunctions is pinpointed. Visceral fat deposits represent only 5% to 20% of body fat mass. Visceral adipose tissue contains visceral adipocytes, mesothelial cells (specific of the omentum), and a number of different fat cell types in the stroma-vascular fraction (SVF) [i.e., macrophages, lymphocytes (T cells), microvascular endothelial cells, and adipose-derived stem cells]. Most of these cell types possess secreting activities which largely remain to be identified but mainly quantified. The interleukin IL-6 is the unique factor which is increased in the portal vein of obese patients. Adipokines, growth factors, chemokines, and interleukins secreted by visceral fat deposits are still poorly characterized in human obesity. It is essential to delineate those which appear in portal vein from those devoted to paracrine/autocrine effects. Non-esterified fatty acids (NEFAs) are directly delivered by visceral adipocytes to liver and impact on a number of metabolic parameters in liver. Note that the upper subcutaneous fat depot is also a site of NEFA release. *Abbreviation*: 11β-HSD1: Type 1, 11β-hydroxysteroid dehydrogenase (in humans, converts the inactive 11-keto metabolite, cortisone into the active glucocortocoid cortisol).
(↑) Increased (activity or secretion)
(↓) Decreased (activity or secretion).

than subcutaneous adipocytes in lean men and women. Regional differences in fat cell size disappear in obese men while being preserved in obese women. Omental adipose tissue is characterized by the presence of mesothelial cells that surround fat lobules and do not exist in subcutaneous deposits (16). In the SVF fraction, there are more macrophages in visceral adipose tissue than in abdominal subcutaneous fat of some obese populations (17–19). With adipose tissue expansion, adipocyte hypertrophy cannot account for the entire gain of fat in obesity or in the variations in regional fat gain. Regional adipocyte hyperplasia occurs in humans and is related to the pattern of proliferation and differentiation of fat cell precursors. According to some in vitro results, subcutaneous preadipocytes, replicate and differentiate more rapidly than the visceral ones (omental and mesenteric) (20,21). The replication decreases with aging in subcutaneous fat while it is maintained in visceral fat. A higher population of progenitors and/or maintenance of their replication in visceral fat, as well as increased sensitivity to insulin growth factor-1 (IGF-1), could contribute to the late development of visceral fat that is observed with aging. A study has revealed that ability to differentiate remain stable in both types of fat deposits (22). Nevertheless, other studies have shown that omental preadipocytes have a reduced responsiveness to pro-differentiating agents, such as peroxisome proliferator-activated receptor-γ (PPAR-γ) and retinoid X receptor-α (RXRα) agonists. Reduction of responsiveness is probably related to lower expression and activity of PPAR-$\gamma_{1/2}$ and RXRα receptors (23–25). Other contradictory results, which will not be discussed here in detail, exist, but these results are probably related to discrepancies in the techniques used to collect fat cell precursors and in the culture techniques used to promote differentiation. The fate of the other cell types present in the SVF together with fat cell precursors will also depend on the composition of the culture media. SVF cells secretion will also be able to impact differently on the differentiation processes (26–28). A useful method in the future for isolating enriched fat cell progenitor (i.e., preadipocytes) populations from the SVF fraction could be using cell surface markers, such as CD34- and CD31-coupled magnetic microbeads. The $CD34^+/CD31^-$ cell population in the SVF of human adipose tissue displays progenitor cell properties that are different from adult mesenchymal cells and hematopoietic stem cells (29). They can exhibit adipocyte and endothelial-like phenotypes under appropriate differentiating stimuli, and their migration and differentiation are modulated by factors originating from capillary endothelial cells in adipose tissue (30). The results are too preliminary to come to any final conclusions on the cell dynamics in visceral fat deposits. It will be interesting to determine in the near future, using optimized methods, how the composition of the SVF is affected in fat depots. Biological studies of the SVF cell population are required to accurately establish the regional differences in the recruitment, accumulation, and proliferation of progenitor cells and their development into adipocytes or other cell types (i.e., vascular endothelial cells) in normal weight and obese patients.

AN OVERVIEW OF THE ENDOCRINE FACTORS AND CYTOKINES SECRETED BY ADIPOSE TISSUE

The induction of insulin resistance and the appearance of vascular disorders through the altered production and release of numerous bioactive molecules from adipose tissue remains an open question. The factors expressed and/or secreted by adipose tissue, as well as their major biological impact are listed in Table 1. Some factors are strictly limited to adipocyte activity, that is, the adipokines. A number of other products that are secreted originate mainly from the various cell types of the SVF, although sometimes they may be weakly secreted by adipocytes (31). Leptin, adiponectin (Acrp30), retinol binding protein 4 (RBP-4), tumor necrosis factor-α (TNF-α), interleukin-6, -8, and -10 (IL-6, IL-8, and IL-10), plasminogen activator inhibitor-1 (PAI-1), resistin, monocyte chemoattractant protein-1 (MCP-1; also known as CCL2), angiotensinogen and angiotensin II, macrophage inflammatory protein-1β (MIP-1β IL-1 receptor antagonist (IL-1Ra), visfatin, angiopoietin-like peptide 4 (ANGPTL4), vaspin, serum amyloid A (SAA), apelin, omentin and some others still poorly studied are new candidates among the growing number of factors found to be secreted by adipose tissue (see reviews in Refs. 5 and 7). Leptin and adiponectin are primary adipokines mainly secreted by adipocytes. RBP-4 (32–34) and apelin (35) are not only secreted by the adipocytes but they are also secreted by other tissues. TNF-α, IL-6, IL-7, IL-8, IL-10, MCP-1, visfatin, and PAI-1 are expressed in adipocytes and in activated macrophages and immune cells. Resistin is produced by peripheral mononuclear cells in humans while it is secreted by the adipocytes in rodents. A general tendency to overestimate the importance of the adipocyte secretions is linked to a number of original studies that were carried out on adipose tissue explants instead of isolated adipocytes. Moreover, the definition of some factors was often limited to RT-PCR identification of mRNAs without identification of proteins. As this field is expanding rapidly, a recent study has reported changes in six newly identified secretory products of omental adipose tissue, which were deregulated with obesity. These six changes are as follows: three chemokines (growth-related oncogene factor, regulated on activation, normal T cell expressed and secreted protein (RANTES) and MIF-1β), one interleukin (IL-7), one tissue inhibitor of metalloproteinases (TIMP-1), and one growth factor (thrombopoietin) (36). The relative and quantitative contribution of adipocytes and other cells of the SVF fraction (i.e., macrophages, lymphocytes, microvascular endothelial cells, and adipose-derived stem cells) as well as mesothelial cells in the omentum (16) to the total secretion of the adipose tissue still remains unclear. Further studies are needed to clarify this important point. In terms of adipocyte secretions, cell size seems to be an important determinant. Enlarged adipocytes are associated with insulin resistance and are independent predictors of type 2 diabetes. A differential expression of pro- and anti-inflammatory factors was observed with increasing adipocyte size with a shift toward the dominance of proinflammatory adipokines appearing as a dysregulation of the hypertrophic fat cell (37,38).

LEPTIN AND ADIPONECTIN: THE GOLD STANDARD OF ADIPOKINES

Leptin is the well-known satiety factor playing a role in energy regulation. Syndromes produced as a result of deficient leptin signaling (i.e., leptin deficiency, mutated leptin receptors, and

Table 1 Adipose Tissue Productions

- Lipid and lipoprotein metabolism
  - Lipoprotrein lipase (LPL)
  - Acylation stimulating protein (ASP/C3desARG))
  - Prostaglandin E2 (PGE2), prostaglandins F2α (PGF2α), prostacyclin (PGI2)
  - Autotaxin (lysophospholipase D) and production of lysophosphatidic acid (LPA)
  - Retinol binding protein-4 (RBP4)
  - Cholesterol ester transport protein (CETP)
- Food intake and activation of sympathetic nervous system
  - Leptin
- Metabolism and energy homeostasy
  - Leptin
  - Adiponectin
  - Resistin
  - Interleukin-6 and Interleukin-8 (IL-6 and IL-8)
- Vessels and angiogenesis
  - Vascular endothelial growth factor (VEGF), thrombopoietin
  - Monobutyrin
  - Leptin, apelin
  - Fasting-induced adipose factor (FIAF) or peroxisome proliferator-activated receptor γ angiopoietin-related gene (PGAR)
  - Angiopoietin-2, angiotensinogen/angiotensin-2, adrenomedullin
- Metabolism of extracellular matrix
  - Type 6 collagen
  - Plasminogen activator inhibitor-1 (PAI-1)
  - Metalloproteases (gelatinases MMP-2 and MMP-9)
  - Tissue inhibitors of metalloproteases (TIMP-1 toTIMP-3)
- Immune system, acute phase reactants and inflammation
  - Tumor necrosis factor α (TNFα)
  - Interleukins 1β, -6, -8, -10 (IL-1β,IL-6,IL-8, IL-10)
  - Interleukin-1 receptor antagonist (IL-1Ra), macrophage inflammatory protein-1β (MIP-1β)
  - Regulated on activation, normal T cell expressed and secreted (RANTES)
  - Adipsin, factors C3, B, and D of alternate complement system
  - Monocyte chemoattractant protein-1 (MCP-1)
  - α1-Acid glycoprotein
  - Serum amyloïd A3 (SAA-3)
  - Haptoglobin, pentraxin-3, lipocalin 24p3
  - Metallothionein
  - Cathepsin S and L
- Insulin sensitivity of muscle, hepatocyte and adipocyte
  - Leptin
  - Adiponectin
  - Resistin
  - Visfatin
  - Omentin
  - Vaspin
  - Interleukine-6 (IL-6)
  - Adipsin/ASP
  - Apelin
- Growth factors influencing adipose tissue development
  - Insulin growth factor-1 (IGF-1),
  - Nerve growth factor (NGF)
  - VEGF
  - Thrombopoietin

This list of productions/secretions originating from adipocyte and/or various cells of the stroma-vascular fraction is nonexhaustive. The factors are grouped according to their contribution in the control of major functions.

altered function of signaling pathways) have been reported in human beings. The current situation regarding the actions of leptin in the brain, with particular emphasis on transport across the blood–brain barrier, signal transduction, neuropeptide targets, and role during fasting and obesity has recently been reviewed (39). Leptin is a highly pleiotropic molecule that regulates a number of other endocrine and immune functions in peripheral organs and vessels (9). Levels of leptin mRNA (40,41) and leptin secretion rates are higher in subcutaneous than in visceral adipocytes, and in these two fat depots, there is a strong correlation between fat cell size and the leptin secretion rate (42). Regional differences in adipocyte leptin secretion are marked and presented during different stages of preadipocyte differentiation and seem to be determined by intrinsic (i.e., primary) factors (43). The subcutaneous fat depot is the major source of leptin due to the combination of a mass effect (subcutaneous fat being the major depot in men and women) and a higher secretion rate. Most of the circulating leptin originate from peripheral fat deposits, with the contribution from visceral fat being very limited. The leptin concentration was 20% lower in the portal vein than in the radial artery in obese subjects (44).

Adiponectin is a plasma protein, abundantly secreted from adipocytes, that assembles into a number of different complexes of higher orders. It exhibits a number of actions on skeletal muscle, liver, and vessels. Adiponectin exerts insulin-sensitizing effects, and thus its administration results in improved insulin sensitivity and glucose tolerance and it can correct the hyperglycemia associated with obesity (45). A number of studies in rodents have shown that adiponectin exerts anti-inflammatory and anti-atherogenic effects on vessels, and thus prevents cardiovascular diseases (46). Although it operates on various peripheral organs, its effects on the central nervous system (CNS) cannot be ruled out since adiponectin receptors have been identified in the paraventricular nucleus, area postrema, amygdala, with more in the periventricular areas. A CNS action for peripheral adiponectin was recently described. Adiponectin stimulates food intake and decreases energy expenditure during fasting through its effects in the CNS (47). Plasma adiponectin decreases in parallel with the progression of obesity and type 2 diabetes. Low plasma adiponectin concentrations in different ethnic groups indicate that the level of hypoadiponectinemia is more closely related to the degree of insulin resistance and hyperinsulinemia than on adiposity and glucose intolerance (45). The administration of adiponectin to rodents decreases body fat mass by stimulation of fatty acid oxidation in muscle (48). The action on muscle fatty acid oxidation involves stimulation of adiponectin receptors (i.e., AdipoR1), activation of AMP-activated protein kinase, and inactivation of acyl-CoA carboxylase via intracellular signal transduction proteins (see review in Ref. 49). A 3-fold increase in circulating adiponectin levels in response to a targeted mutation of the adiponectin gene enhanced insulin sensitivity and decreased hepatic glucose output (50). Moreover, long-term adenovirus-mediated overexpression of adiponectin ameliorates glycemic and lipid parameters, and reduces obesity in rats.

The mechanisms controlling adiponectin maturation and its secretion are still unclear (51). The secretion of adiponectin by omental fat cells is generally higher than by subcutaneous fat cells; and a strong negative correlation exists with body mass index (BMI). Adiponectin concentrations were similar in the portal vein and radial artery in obese subjects (44). Adiponectin gene expression is repressed by TNF-α in human preadipocytes. Adiponectin secretion from omental fat cells was increased by insulin, thiazolidinedione, and rosiglitazone, while secretion from subcutaneous fat cells was unaffected. The reduced secretion of adiponectin from omental adipose tissue, associated with the lower production by subcutaneous adipocytes, may account for the decline in plasma adiponectin often observed in obesity (52). An increase in adiponectin production from adipose tissue could be highly beneficial for glucose and lipid homeostasis although visceral fat does not appear to be the unique determinant of systemic adiponectin levels.

MEDIATORS OF INSULIN RESISTANCE IDENTIFIED IN ADIPOSE TISSUE AND VISCERAL FAT

A number of studies in rodents have provided details of the molecular links between obesity, inflammation, and insulin resistance, and are described and discussed in recently published reviews (53,54). The NF-κB pathway [activated by an inhibitor of NF-κB (IκB) kinase β (IKKβ)] and the c-jun NH2-terminal kinase (JNK) pathway have been identified as the link between

Table 2 Differences in Expression/Secretion of Various Factors Between Visceral and Subcutaneous Human Adipocytes

Effects and factors	Regional differences
Miscellaneous secreted factors and hormone receptors	
Leptin mRNA and protein secretion	scAT > vAT
Plasminogen activator inhibitor 1 (PAI-1)	vAT > scAT
11β-Hydroxysteroid dehydrogenase Type1 activity (cortisone → cortisol)	vAT > scAT
Adiponectin (ACRP30)	vAT > scAT
Growth-related oncogen factor-α (GRO-α)	vAT > scAT
Regulated upon activation normal T cell expressed and secreted (RANTES)	vAT > scAT
Inhibitor of apoptosis cIAP2 mRNA	vAT > scAT
Macrophage inflammatory protein-1β (MIP-1β)	vAT > scAT
Interleukin-7 (IL-7)	vAT > scAT
Tissue inhibitor of metalloproteinases-1 (TIMP-1)	vAT > scAT
Thrombopoietin	vAT > scAT
Peroxisome proliferator-activated receptor-γ (PPAR-γ) mRNA	vAT > scAT
Tumor necrosis factor-α (TNF-α) secretion	vAT = scAT
Interleukin-6 (IL-6) secretion	vAT > scAT
Omentin	vAT > scAT
Insulin-like growth factor-1 and IGF-binding protein-3	vAT > scAT
Angiotensinogen	vAT > scAT

Some of the differences mentioned in this table can be increased or reduced according to the extent of the fat mass and adipocyte hypertrophy. Moreover, some sex-related differences have not been detailed. All the references are included in the text.
Abbreviations: vAT, visceral adipocytes; scAT, subcutaneous adipocytes.

the proinflammatory effect of obesity and insulin resistance. They are activated by a number of cytokines and chemokines secreted by adipose tissue. Epidemiologic studies have clearly demonstrated that obesity represents a "low-grade" inflammatory condition, a state proposed to represent a common denominator in the genesis of obesity-associated pathologies. Some of these molecules are secreted in a depot-specific manner (Table 2). Regional secretion in human adipose tissue will be summarized below. TNF-α and IL-6 are the most widely studied cytokines produced by adipose tissue.

Tumor Necrosis Factor-α (TNF-α)

In the case of insulin resistance, overproduction of TNF-α from adipose tissue has been proposed to explain its origin, at least in rodents (55–57). Adipose TNF-α may be an important specific and local factor in adipose tissue, influencing the ability of insulin to stimulate glucose transport into human fat cells, at least in obese women (58). In human adipose tissue, although TNF-α mRNA was identified in adipocytes and SVF cells, it is not found in the veins draining the subcutaneous adipose tissue (59). There is no difference in TNF-α expression between visceral and subcutaneous adipose tissues—TNF-α is essentially produced by the cells of the SVF in human adipose tissue (18,60,61). Macrophages that infiltrate the adipose tissue of obese subjects are able to release TNF-α and IL-6 and IL-8, when activated. They are putative candidate cells of the SVF that could account for the insulin resistance of large fat cells of obese patients. Although increased levels of circulating TNF-α has been observed in insulin-resistant subjects by some groups, a systemic effect of the adipose tissue–derived TNF-α cannot be sustained, since the cytokine is not released into the veins draining fat deposits. The role of TNF-α originating from visceral adipose tissue remains to be established. Plasma TNF-α levels are similar in the portal vein and the radial artery (44) and moreover, since TNF-α is bound to specific binding proteins, it is not certain that it is an important endocrine signal.

Interleukin-6 (IL-6)

Increased IL-6 levels have been reported in patients with type 2 diabetes, while IL-6 levels decrease with weight loss. Plasma IL-6 levels are correlated to the level of insulin sensitivity in patients. Since excess IL-6 in rodents inhibits the autophosphorylation of insulin receptors and downstream signaling, a similar mechanism is expected in humans. Interleukin-6 is an important systemic signal in inflammatory situations and it is also released by skeletal muscle during exercise. Interleukin-6 found in human adipose tissue is mainly produced by cells of the SVF, with a higher expression in visceral than in subcutaneous fat (62). Visceral fat is clearly a site of IL-6 secretion since increased levels of the cytokine are found in the portal vein of obese patients (44). Based on results obtained in rodents, and on its increased production in the visceral fat of the obese patients, IL-6 from visceral fat could represent a potential mechanistic link between visceral fat and systemic inflammation in patients with abdominal obesity. Interleukin-6 is the major cytokine regulating the production of C-reactive protein (CRP) and acute-phase proteins by the liver (63).

Interleukin-8 (IL-8)

Interleukin-8 is a chemokine that promotes the recruitment of polymorphonuclear leukocytes to sites of inflammation and activation of monocytes. Circulating IL-8 in obese subjects is primarily due to the release of IL-8 from nonfat cells from adipose tissue with a 4-fold higher release from visceral fat than from subcutaneous fat. Interleukin-8 mRNA was 2-fold higher in visceral compared with subcutaneous fat. High levels of IL-8 are released from human adipose tissue and may account for some increase in circulating IL-8, observed in obese patients (64,65).

Monocyte Chemoattractant Protein-1 (MCP-1)

Monocyte chemoattractant protein-1 (also called CCL2) recruits immune cells at sites of inflammation. Two studies have focused attention on its putative role in macrophage recruitment in adipose tissue. Overexpression of MCP-1 in mice adipocytes is sufficient to initiate macrophage recruitment into adipose tissue (66,67). Mice deficient in the receptor for MCP-1 (i.e., CCR2) are protected against diet-induced obesity and have fewer macrophages recruited into adipose tissue (68). In human adipose tissue, MCP-1 expression is increased with adiposity (69) and decreased after bariatric surgery (70). MCP-1 production is higher in SVF cells versus adipocytes and correlates with macrophage markers in both adipose tissue compartments. MCP-1 release is higher in obese subjects and in abdominal obesity, but after adjusting for the macrophages resident within adipose tissue, the difference disappears. MCP-1 is stimulated by IL-1β, TNF-α, IL-8, IL-4, and IL-6, and is decreased by metformin and TZD, suggesting that these agents have anti-inflammatory properties (61).

Serum Retinol–Binding Protein-4 (RBP-4)

Under normal conditions, hepatocytes are regarded as the major source of this recently characterized adipokine, that is, a 21-kDa secreted protein that was thought to deliver vitamin A (retinol) to tissues through its transport activity (71). Adipose tissue had previously been reported to contain relatively high levels of the specific mRNA for retinol-binding protein (RBP) with a level of approximately 20% of that of liver (72). Retinol-binding protein is expressed almost exclusively in the adipocytes and only weakly in the SVF cells. Cultured adipocytes synthesized RBP-4 protein and secreted it into the medium (73). Studies in mice have focused attention on an unsuspected role of the RBP form, RBP-4, in insulin resistance. Injection of RBP-4 in normal mice caused insulin resistance, while genetic deletion of RBP-4 enhanced insulin sensitivity. RBP-4 knockout mice show enhanced insulin sensitivity, and pharmacological treatment, which lowers serum RBP-4, improves insulin sensitivity (34). Serum RBP-4 levels are elevated in insulin-resistant mice and in humans with obesity, impaired glucose tolerance or type 2 diabetes (74). Three other studies have not confirmed the initial observations (75–77). Severe calorie restriction, reduced adipose tissue and plasma levels of RBP-4, but there was no evidence for a role for RBP-4 in the regulation of diet-induced changes in insulin sensitivity (77). The reasons for the discrepancies between the various research groups are not clear and require further investigations. Treatment with the insulin sensitizing agent rosiglitazone lowered serum RBP-4 (78) and a recent report has shown that in man, RBP-4 is preferentially expressed in visceral versus subcutaneous fat. RBP-4 expression is considerably increased in the visceral fat of obese patients and its circulating levels are also increased. RBP-4 mRNA correlated inversely with GLUT-4 mRNA in visceral fat and positively with adipocyte size in both fat depots. Compared with the other proteins secreted by adipocytes (i.e., IL-6, adiponectin, visfatin, and leptin), RBP-4 was the best predictor of insulin resistance and the best marker of visceral fat mass (79). In rodents, increasing serum RBP-4 levels induce hepatic expression of phosphoenolpyruvate carboxykinase (PEPCK) and impair insulin signaling in muscle. The degree to which RBP-4 contributes to insulin resistance in humans is not known, but RBP-4 seems to be an adipocyte-derived signaling molecule highly expressed by visceral adipocytes that may contribute to the pathogenesis of liver dysfunction and type 2 diabetes. In a recent report, serum RBP-4 was not associated with the amount of fat including the visceral depot, but correlated positively with liver fat. Metabolic measures support the close relationship between circulating RBP-4 with liver fat and, presumably, hepatic insulin resistance (80). In the face of the heterogeneity of the clinical reports concerning the links between RBP-4 and insulin resistance, further studies are still necessary with paying particular attention to the various groups of patients.

RESISTIN, VISFATIN, OMENTIN, VASPIN, AND OTHER MOLECULES SECRETED BY ADIPOSE TISSUE

Resistin is a member of the family of resistin-like molecules (RELM) that is found in inflammatory zones. Initial studies in rodents have given promising results that this hormone, secreted by rodent adipocytes, and increased during obesity, reduced insulin sensitivity. It was claimed to represent a putative link between obesity and diabetes (81). In mouse models, systemic administration or transgenic expression of resistin antagonizes insulin action in the liver. Elevated resistin levels in normal rats fed a regular chow diet produced many features of metabolic syndrome (82). Resistin is expressed in human visceral adipose tissue and probably released by the macrophages of the SVF (18). Inflammation is a state associated with an increase in resistin in human macrophages, being induced by inflammatory endotoxin together with proinflammatory cytokines of the macrophages. In patients with type 2 diabetes, serum resistin levels correlate with levels of soluble TNF-α receptor, an inflammatory marker linked to obesity and insulin resistance. In fact, resistin may contribute to insulin resistance in endotoxemia, other inflammatory states, and obesity (83). The clinical relevance of resistin is still under investigation.

Visfatin [known previously as pre-B-cell colony-enhancing factor (PBEF) and expressed in lymphocytes] has recently been identified as an adipokine that is secreted by the adipocytes in visceral fat (84). It has also been found in the cells of the SVF (18). Visfatin lowered plasma glucose levels in mice and exerted insulin-mimetic effects in cultured cells, and has been shown to bind to and activate the insulin receptor. Targeted mutation in the visfatin gene led to a modest increase in plasma glucose in mice heterozygous for the mutation relative to wild-type littermates. An increase in subcutaneous adipose tissue visfatin mRNA was promoted by exercise, but was not however, accompanied by an increase in plasma visfatin (85). Further studies of the physiological role of visfatin in humans are required to clarify its incidence upon glucose homeostasis and its possible relevance to the development of new therapies for metabolic disorders, such as diabetes.

Vaspin (visceral adipose tissue–derived serine protease inhibitor), a member of the serpin superfamily, was found to improve insulin sensitivity and possess anti-inflammatory properties. Administration of vaspin to obese mice fed with a high-fat/high-sucrose diet improved glucose tolerance and insulin sensitivity. It also led to the reversal of the altered gene expression of factors relevant to insulin resistance, for example, leptin, resistin, TNF-α, glucose transporter-4 (GLUT-4), and adiponectin. DNA chip analyses revealed that vaspin treatment resulted in the reversal of expression of approximately 50% of the genes in white adipose tissue that were induced by a high-fat/high-sucrose diet (86). In a population of (#200) normal patients, the expression of vaspin mRNA was only detectable in 23% of the visceral and in 15% of the subcutaneous adipose tissue samples. Vaspin mRNA expression was not detectable in lean subjects but was frequently detected in the adipose tissue of patients with type 2 diabetes. No significant correlations were found between visceral vaspin gene expression and the area of visceral fat or subcutaneous vaspin expression. Nevertheless, visceral vaspin expression significantly correlates with BMI, percentage body fat, and plasma glucose after a 2-hour oral glucose tolerance test. It should be noted that until now all the studies are limited to determinations of vaspin mRNA (87).

Omentin, also named intelectin, was previously known to be expressed in intestinal Paneth cells and endothelial cells (88). It was then identified as a novel fat depot-specific secreted factor that was highly expressed in omental fat in humans and nonhuman primates. It is not found in subcutaneous adipose tissue but it is a secreted product that is detectable in serum. Omentin is mainly expressed in the SVF fraction of adipose tissue. It is biologically active, enhancing insulin-induced glucose transport, and Akt phosphorylation in human adipocytes; however, it does not stimulate basal glucose transport on its own (89). Two omentin genes, omentin 1 and omentin 2, are localized adjacent to each other in the 1q22–q23 chromosomal region that has previously been linked to type 2 diabetes. The expression of both omentin genes is decreased in obesity and is highly correlated with each other in visceral adipose tissue. Decreased omentin levels are associated with increasing obesity and insulin resistance (90). Further investigation is required to elucidate the roles of these new adipose tissue productions (i.e., visfatin and omentin) in the development of obesity and type 2 diabetes.

Angiopoietin-like peptide 4 (ANGPTL4), also known as fasting-induced adipose factor (FIAF), is a member of the fibrinogen/angiopoietin-like protein family initially identified in liver. It is expressed at high levels in adipocytes and induced by thiazolidinedione treatment and is elevated in genetic models of obesity. Hormone-dependent adipocyte differentiation coincides with a dramatic early induction of the ANGPTL4 transcript (91). In rodents, ANGPTL4 is a powerful regulator of lipid metabolism and adiposity; where its overexpression caused a 50% reduction in adipose tissue weight, partly by stimulating fatty acid oxidation and uncoupling. A possible role for ANGPTL4 in the regulation of systemic lipid metabolism or glucose homeostasis has been postulated (92). Although expressed by adipocytes, the molecular targets, and mechanisms of action of ANGPTL4 and related molecules are still unclear.

Plasminogen activator inhibitor-1 (PAI-1), a member of the serpin family, is the primary inhibitor of fibrinolysis. Although identified in adipose tissue, its expression is not limited as it is expressed in various cell types of SVF (65). PAI-1 expression and secretion is higher in visceral adipose tissue than in subcutaneous. Increased circulating levels of PAI-1 are strongly associated with visceral obesity. A decrease in circulating levels of PAI-1 is correlated with an improvement of insulin resistance in patients treated with thiazolidinediones or after bariatric surgery. PAI-1 has a number of impacts: in addition to its role in fibrinolysis, it inactivates urokinase-type and tissue-type plasminogen activator. It is also involved in angiogenesis and atherogenesis. The regional contribution of adipose tissue to the circulating levels of PAI-1 is not obvious.

Cathepsins are cysteine proteases, which play an important role in extracellular matrix (ECM) remodeling. Expressed and secreted by the preadipocytes and the adipocytes they are upregulated in the obese. Changes in the expression of some members of the cathepsin family have been reported during fat cell differentiation (i.e., cathepsin K and L are increased, while cathepsin S and B are decreased). Cathepsins are released into the extracellular milieu and degrade matrix proteins. Major changes in the expression and function of ECM components take place during adipogenesis and contribute to ECM remodeling in adipose tissue. Cathepsin L and cathepsin S have been shown to be involved in the control of adipogenesis and glucose tolerance (93) and human preadipocyte differentiation (94).

Acute Phase Reactants or Acute Phase Proteins: Acute Phase Reactants or Acute Phase

Proteins are required during the acute phase response following an inflammatory stimulus. Several acute phase reactants are produced by adipose tissue [complement factor C, PAI-1, lipocaline 24p3, α1-acid glycoprotein, pentraxine-3, and serum amyloid-A (SAA)]. Some of these factors are expressed not only in adipocytes but also in cells of the SVF. Hyperglycemia, and the production of the associated reactive oxygen species (ROS), upregulated the production of adipocyte acute phase reactants (95). SAA-3 and pentraxine-3 are produced within adipose tissue. SAA-3 is a proinflammatory and lipolytic adipokine in humans. The increased expression of SAA-3 by adipocytes in obesity suggests that it may play a critical role in local and systemic inflammation and free fatty acid production, and could be a direct link between obesity and its comorbidities, such as insulin resistance and atherosclerosis (96). The production of acute phase reactants could also represent a contribution of the adipose tissue to the immune response; a role of adipose tissue which remains to be clarified.

PRODUCTION OF STEROID HORMONES IN THE ADIPOSE TISSUE REGIONAL DIFFERENCES

Various enzymes controlling steroid synthesis have been described in adipose tissue: cytochrome P450-aromatase, 3β-hydroxysteroid dehydrogenase (HSD), 3α-HSD, 11β-HSD type 1, 17β-HSD, 7α-hydroxylase, 17α-hydroxylase, and 5α-reductase. Therefore, when there is an excess of adipose tissue, significant amounts of steroid hormones could be produced. As a result of the promising results reported in rodents, a link was made between increased 11β-HSD1 activity in adipose tissue and the metabolic syndrome (97); our attention will be focused on cortisol in human adipose tissue. 11β-HSD1 catalyzes the conversion of inactive 11β-ketoglucocorticoid metabolites to active 11β-hydroxylated metabolites; thus, the production of cortisol from cortisone exists in human adipose tissue. 11β-HSD1 is abundantly expressed in rodent visceral adipose depots where it increases the local production of corticosterone without affecting its circulating levels. 11β-HSD1 activity in man shows tissue-specific differences. Increased expression and activity of 11β-HSD1 has been reported in human adipose tissue in some studies. However, discrepancies still exist in the results, and comparison between visceral and subcutaneous deposits has yet to be determined in obese subjects. A recent report has shown that tissues draining into the portal vein, including visceral adipose tissue, contribute substantially to the regeneration of cortisol. Thus, in addition to free fatty acids and adipokines, the portal vein delivers cortisol to the liver (98).

CONCLUSIONS, OUTLOOK, AND FUTURE TRENDS

This overview has focused attention on the diversity of factors secreted by adipose tissue. An important and emerging conceptual point is that a number of the secretions previously attributed to the adipocyte originate, in fact, from various cell types of the SVF (i.e., at least monocytes, macrophages, microvascular endothelial cells, lymphocytes, and adipose-derived stem cells). Although neglected for a long time, the population of the various cells composing the adipose tissue SVF is a matter of renewed interest for investigators in adipose tissue biology. Except for adiponectin and leptin, a large part of the adipokine release by adipose tissue can be attributed to the nonfat cells of the SVF. Most of the adipokines released by this heterogeneous nonfat cell population is due to cells retained in the tissue matrix after collagenase digestion. The definition of the biology of resident macrophages and of the other cell types, which infiltrate the adipose tissue of the obese, will provide valuable information on the putative crosstalk between adipocytes and the other cell types and its effects on adipose tissue function.

Although the number of factors identified in adipose tissue is increasing rapidly, the definition of their physiological/pathological role is slower. It may be a little disappointing for the reader to note that, although differences in the expression of adipokines and cytokines exist between visceral and subcutaneous fat deposits, it is rather difficult to assert that they represent a determining element in the metabolic disorders observed in visceral obesity. There are few data on the concentration of the various secretions in the portal vein that is draining a large part of the visceral fat. A recent study, which certainly requires further confirmation, has provided some clues in obese subjects. Leptin levels were lower in the portal vein of obese subjects, which fits with the lower level of expression of the leptin gene in visceral fat. The fact that plasma TNF-α, resistin, MCP-1, and adiponectin concentrations are similar in the portal vein and radial artery in massively obese patients does not argue for a significant role for these visceral adipose tissue–derived factors. It is only levels of IL-6 that are increased in the portal vein in massive obesity. This observation fits with the results of several studies on IL-6 expression showing increased expression and secretion of IL-6 in the visceral adipose tissue. It is a result suggesting that increased IL-6 secretion in visceral fat of the massively obese patients could be involved in the pathogenesis of metabolic abnormalities associated with abdominal obesity. Proteomics and microarray technologies are providing a large number of new putative adipocyte produced compounds. Demonstration of their physiological/pathological relevance is a time-consuming process and the full characterization of the properties of a new adipokine is a very long exploit. Moreover, due to species-specific differences, results obtained in rodents must be then confirmed by clinical studies.

The "portal paradigm" proposed that visceral adipocytes will release portal NEFAs, which disturb liver metabolism as a result of the increase in lipolysis due to the conjunction of reduced insulin-induced antilipolysis, on the one hand, and the enhancement of the lipolytic potencies of catecholamines, on the other (99). This paradigm has been replaced by a tendency for a number of investigators during the last decade to shift, probably too rapidly, toward an emerging "endocrine paradigm" to explain all the metabolic and cardiovascular problems in abdominal obesity. It is necessary to supplement our knowledge of the physiological/pathological role of the numerous secreted products. Considering the present state of knowledge, the reality is probably in between (Fig. 1). It is clear that chronic excessive fat intake and excess plasma NEFA, quite rapidly leads to glucose intolerance, hyperinsulinemia, hepatic insulin resistance, and dyslipidemia. These various events could occur before any change in the expression of a number of visceral adipokines and cytokines. This view was recently validated in a dog model (100). The contribution of all the newly identified secreted factors (i.e., adipokines, cytokines, and other secreted products) to the origin of the adverse metabolic consequences of the increase in visceral fat in abdominal obesity remains largely an open question.

ACKNOWLEDGMENTS

The author thanks Coralie Sengenes, Jean Galitzky, Virginie Bourlier, and Anne Bouloumié for valuable comments and suggestions. The author apologizes for the omission of many relevant references due to space limitations.

REFERENCES

1. Kissebah A, Krakower GR. Regional adiposity and morbidity. Physiol Rev 1994; 74:761–811.
2. Wajchenberg BL. Subcutaneous and visceral adipose tissue: Their relation to the metabolic syndrome. Endocrine Rev 2000; 21:697–738.
3. Despres JP, Lemieux I. Abdominal obesity and metabolic syndrome. Nature 2006; 444:881–887.
4. Thorne A, Lonnqvist F, Apelman J, et al. A pilot study of long-term effects of a novel obesity treatment: Omentectomy in connection with adjustable gastric banding. Int J Obes Relat Metab Disord 2002; 26:193–199.
5. Lafontan M. Fat cells: Afferent and efferent messages define new approaches to treat obesity. Annu Rev Pharmacol Toxicol 2005; 45:119–146.
6. Kershaw EE, Flier JS. Adipose tissue as an endocrine organ. J Clin Endocrinol Metab 2004; 89:2548–2556.
7. Trujillo ME, Scherer PE. Adipose tissue-derived factors: Impact on health and disease. Endocr Rev 2006; 27:762–778.
8. Tilg H, Moschen AR. Adipocytokines: Mediators linking adipose tissue, inflammation and immunity. Nat Rev Immunol 2006; 6:772–783.
9. Badman MK, Flier JS. The adipocyte as an active participant in energy balance and metabolism. Gastroenterology 2007; 132:2103–2115.
10. Zuk PA, Zhu M, Ashjian P, et al. Human adipose tissue is a source of multipotent stem cells. Mol Biol Cell 2002; 13:4279–4295.
11. Gimble JM, Katz AJ, Bunnell BA. Adipose-derived stem cells for regenerative medicine. Circ Res 2007; 100:1249–1260.
12. Weisberg SP, McCann D, Desai M, et al. Obesity is associated with macrophage accumulation in adipose tissue. J Clin Invest 2003; 112:1796–1608.
13. Curat CA, Miranville A, Sengenes C, et al. From blood monocytes to adipose-tissue-resident macrophages: Induction of diapedesis by human mature adipocytes. Diabetes 2004; 53:1285–1292.
14. Bartness TJ, Song CK. Thematic review series: Adipocyte Biology. Sympathetic and sensory innervation of white adipose tissue. J Lipid Res 2007; 48:1655–1672.
15. Frayn KN, Samra JS, Summers, LKM. Visceral fat in relation to health: Is it a major culprit or simply an innocent bystander. Int J Obesity 1997; 21;1191–1192.
16. Darimont C, Avanti O, Blancher F, et al. Contribution of mesothelial cells in the expression of inflammatory-related factors in omental adipose tissue of obese subjects. Int J Obes (Lond) 2007; 32:112–120.
17. Bornstein SR, Abu-Asab M, Glasgow A, et al. Immunohistochemical and ultrastructural localization of leptin and leptin receptor in human white adipose tissue and differentiating human adipose cells in primary culture. Diabetes 2000; 49:532–538.
18. Curat CA, Wegner V, Sengenes C, et al. Macrophages in the human visceral adipose tissue: Increased accumulation with obesity and source of resistin and visfatin. Diabetologia 2006; 49:744–747.
19. Cancello R, Tordjman J, Poitou C, et al. Increased infiltration of macrophages in omental adipose tissue is associated with marked hepatic lesions in morbid human obesity. Diabetes 2006; 55:1554–1561.
20. Tchkonia T, Tchoukalova YD, Giorgadze N, et al. Abundance of two human preadipocyte subtypes with distinct capacities for replication, adipogenesis, and apoptosis varies among fat depots. Am J Physiol Endocrinol Metab 2004; 288:E267–E277.

21. Grohmann M, Sabin M, Holly J, et al. Characterization of differentiated subcutaneous and visceral adipose tissue from children: The influences of TNF-alpha and IGF-I. J Lipid Res 2005; 46:93–103.
22. Van Harmelen V, Röhring K, Hauner H. Comparison of proliferation and differentiation capacity of human adipocyte precursor cells from the omental and subcutaneous adipose tissue depot of obese subjects. Metabolism 2004; 53:632–637.
23. Adams M, Montague CT, Prins JB, et al. Activators of peroxisome proliferator-activated receptor gamma have depot-specific effects on human preadipocyte differentiation. J Clin Invest 1997; 100:3149–3153.
24. Sewter CP, Blows F, Vidal-Puig A, et al. Regional differences in the response of human pre-adipocytes to PPARgamma and RXRalpha agonists. Diabetes 2002; 51:718–723.
25. Sauma L, Franck N, Paulsson JF, et al. Peroxisome proliferator activated receptor gamma activity is low in mature primary human visceral adipocytes. Diabetologia 2007; 50:195–201.
26. Rehman J, Traktuev D, Li J, et al. Secretion of angiogenic and antiapoptotic factors by human adipose stromal cells. Circulation 2004; 109;1292–1298.
27. Planat-Bénard V, Silvestre J-S, Cousin B, et al. Plasticity of human adipose lineage cells toward endothelial cells. Physiological and therapeutic perspectives. Circulation 2004; 109:656–663.
28. Kilroy GE, Foster SJ, Wu X, et al. 2007. Cytokine profile of human adipose-derived stem cells: Expression of angiogenic, hematopoietic, and pro-inflammatory factors. J Cell Physiol 2004; 212:702–709.
29. Sengenes C, Lolmède K, Zakaroff-Girard A, et al. Preadipocytes in the human subcutaneous adipose tissue display distinct features from the adult mesenchymal and hematopoietic stem cells. J Cell Physiol 2005; 205;114–122.
30. Sengenes C, Miranville A, Maumus M, et al. Chemotaxis and differentiation of human adipose tissue CD34+/CD31- progenitor cells: Role of SDF-1 released by adipose tissue capillary endothelial cells. Stem Cells 2007; 25:2269–2276.
31. Fain JN. Release of interleukins and other inflammatory cytokines by human adipose tissue is enhanced in obesity and primarily due to the nonfat cells. Vitam Horm 2006; 74:443–477.
32. Rajala MW, Scherer PE. Minireview: The adipocyte at the crossroads of energy homeostasis, inflammation and atherosclerosis. J Clin Endocrinol Metab 2003; 144:3765–3773.
33. Trayhurn P, Wood IS. Adipokines: Inflammation and the pleiotropic role of white adipose tissue. Br J Nutr 2004; 92:347–355.
34. Yang Q, Graham TE, Mody N, et al. Serum retinol binding protein 4 contributes to insulin resistance in obesity and type 2 diabetes. Nature 2005; 436:356–362.
35. Boucher J, Masri B, Daviaud D, et al. Apelin, a newly identified adipokine up-regulated by insulin and obesity. Endocrinology 2005; 146:1764–1771.
36. Maury E, Ehala-Aleksejev K, Guiot Y, et al. Adipokines oversecreted by omental adipose tissue in human obesity. Am J Physiol Endocrinol Metab 2007; 293:E656–665.
37. Jernas M, Palming J, Sjoholm K, et al. 2006. Separation of human adipocytes by size: Hypertrophic fat cells display distinct gene expression. FASEB J 2007; 20:1540–1542.
38. Skurk T, Alberti-Huber C, Herder C, et al. Relationship between adipocyte size and adipokine expression and secretion. J Clin Endocrinol Metab 2007; 92:1023–1033.
39. Ahima RS. Central actions of leptin. Trends Endocrinol Metab 2005; 16:307–313.
40. Montague CT, Prins JB, Sanders L, et al. Depot and sex-specific differences in human leptin mRNA expression. Implications for the control of regional fat distribution. Diabetes 1997; 46:342–347.
41. Lefebvre AM, Laville M, Vega N, et al. Depot-specific differences in adipose tissue gene expression in lean and obese subjects. Diabetes 1998; 47:98–103.
42. van Harmelen V, Reynisdottir S, Eriksson P, et al. Leptin secretion from subcutaneous and visceral adipose tissue in women. Diabetes 1998; 47:913–917.
43. van Harmelen V, Dicker A, Rydén M, et al. Increased lipolysis and decreased leptin production by human omental as compared with subcutaneous preadipocytes. Diabetes 2002; 51:2029–2036.
44. Fontana L, Eagon JC, Trujillo ME, et al. Visceral fat adipokine secretion is associated with systemic inflammation in obese humans. Diabetes 2007; 56:1010–1013.
45. Kadowaki T, Yamauchi T, Kubota N, et al. Adiponectin and adiponectin receptors in insulin resistance, diabetes, and the metabolic syndrome. J Clin Invest 2006; 116:1784–1792.
46. Han SH, Quon MJ, Kim JA, et al. Adiponectin and cardiovascular disease: Response to therapeutic interventions. J Am Coll Cardiol 2007; 49:531–538.
47. Kubota N, Yano W, Kubota T, et al. Adiponectin stimulates AMP-activated protein kinase in the hypothalamus and increases food intake. Cell Metab 2007; 6:55–68.
48. Tomas E, Tsao TS, Saha AK, et al. Enhanced muscle fat oxidation and glucose transport by ACRP30 globular domain: Acetyl-CoA carboxylase inhibition and AMP-activated protein kinase activation. Proc Natl Acad Sci U S A 2002; 99:16309–16313.
49. Lafontan M, Viguerie N. Role of adipokines in the control of energy metabolism: Focus on adiponectin. Curr Opin Pharmacol 2006; 6:580–585.

50. Shklyaev S, Aslanidi G, Tennant M, et al. Sustained peripheral expression of transgene adiponectin offsets the development of diet-induced obesity in rats. Proc Natl Acad Sci U S A 2003; 100:14217–14222.
51. Wang ZV, Schraw TD, Kim JY, et al. Secretion of the adipocyte-specific secretory protein adiponectin critically depends on thiol-mediated protein retention. Mol Cell Biol 2007; 27:3716–3731.
52. Motoshima H, Wu X, Sinha MK, et al. Differential regulation of adiponectin secretion from cultured human omental and subcutaneous adipocytes: Effects of insulin and rosiglitazone. J Clin Endocrinol Metab 2002; 87:5662–5667.
53. Hotamisligil GS. Inflammation and metabolic disorders. Nature 2006; 444:860–867.
54. Shoelson SE, Lee J, Goldfine AB. Inflammation and insulin resistance. J Clin Invest 2006; 116:1793–1801.
55. Feinstein R, Kanety H, Papa MZ, et al. Tumor necrosis factor-alpha suppresses insulin-induced tyrosine phosphorylation of insulin receptor and its substrates. J Biol Chem 1993; 268:26055–26058.
56. Hotasmiligil GS, Peraldi P, Budavari A, et al. IRS-1-mediated inhibition of insulin receptor tyrosine kinase activity in TNFα- and obesity-induced insulin resistance. Science 1996; 271:665–668.
57. Uysal KT, Wiesbrock SM, Marino MW, et al. Protection from obesity-induced insulin resistance in mice lacking TNF-α function. Nature 1997; 389:610–614.
58. Löfgren P, Harmelen VV, Reynisdottir S, Näslund E, et al. Secretion of tumor necrosis factor-a shows a strong relationship to insulin-stimulated glucose transport in human adipose tissue. Diabetes 2000; 49:688–692.
59. Mohamed-Ali V, Goodrick S, Rawesh A, et al. Subcutaneous adipose tissue releases interleukin-6 but not tumor necrosis factor-a, in vivo. J Clin Endocrinol Metab 1997; 82:4196–4200.
60. Fain J, Bahouth SW, Madan AK. TNF-a release by the nonfat cells of human adipose tissue. Int J Obes 2004; 28:616–622.
61. Bruun JM, Linh AS, Pedersen SB, et al. Monocyte chemoattractant protein-1 release is higher in visceral than subcutaneous human adipose tissue (AT): Implications of macrophages resident in the adipose tissue. J Clin Endocrinol Metab 2005; 90:2282–2289.
62. Fried SK, Bunkin DA, Greenberg AS. Omental and subcutaneous adipose tissues of obese subjects release interleukin-6: Depot difference and regulation by glucocorticoids. J Clin Endocrinol Metab 1998; 83:847–850.
63. Yudkin JS, Kumari M, Humphries SE, et al. Inflammation, obesity, stress and coronary heart disease: Is interleukin-6 the link? Atherosclerosis 2000; 148:209–214.
64. Bruun JM, Lihn AS, Madan AK, et al. Higher production of IL-8 in visceral vs. subcutaneous adipose tissue. Implication of nonadipose cells in adipose tissue. Am J Physiol Endocrinol Metab 2004; 286:E8–E13.
65. Fain JN, Madan AK, Hiler ML, et al. Comparison of the release of adipokines by adipose tissue, adipose tissue matrix, and adipocytes from visceral and subcutaneous abdominal adipose tissues of obese humans. Endocrinology 2004; 145:2273–2282.
66. Kanda H, Tateya S, Tamori Y, et al. MCP-1 contributes to macrophage infiltration into adipose tissue, insulin resistance, and hepatic steatosis in obesity. J Clin Invest 2006; 116:1494–1505.
67. Kamei N, Tobe K, Suzuki R, et al. Overexpression of monocyte chemoattractant protein-1 in adipose tissues causes macrophage recruitment and insulin resistance. J Biol Chem; 2006 281:26602–26614.
68. Weisberg SP, Hunter D, Huber R, et al. CCR2 modulates inflammatory and metabolic effects of high fat feeding. J Clin Invest 2006; 116:115–124.
69. Di Gregorio GB, Yao-Borengasser A, Rasouli N, et al. Expression of CD68 and macrophage chemoattractant protein-1 genes in human adipose and muscle tissues: Association with cytokine expression, insulin resistance, and reduction by pioglitazone. Diabetes 2005; 54:2305–2313.
70. Schernthaner GH, Kopp HP, Kriwanek S, et al. Effect of massive weight loss induced by bariatric surgery on serum levels of interleukin-18 and monocyte-chemoattractant-protein-1 in morbid obesity. Obes Surg 2006; 16:709–715.
71. Blaner WS. Retinol-binding protein: The serum transport protein for vitamin A. Endocr Rev 1989; 10:308–316.
72. Makover A, Soprano DR, Wyatt ML, et al. Localization of retinol-binding protein messenger RNA in the rat kidney and in perinephric fat tissue. J Lipid Res 1989; 30:171–180.
73. Tsutsumi C, Okuno M, Tannous L, et al. Retinoids and retinoid-binding protein expression in rat adipocytes. J Biol Chem 1992; 267:1805–1810.
74. Graham TE, Yang Q, Bluher M, et al. Retinol-binding protein 4 and insulin resistance in lean, obese, and diabetic subjects. N Engl J Med 2006; 354:2552–2563.
75. Janke J, Engeli S, Boschmann M, et al. Retinol-binding protein 4 in human obesity. Diabetes 2006; 55:2805–2810.
76. Silha JV, Nyomba BL, Leslie WD, et al. Ethnicity, insulin resistance, and inflammatory adipokines in women at high and low risk for vascular disease. Diabetes Care 2007; 30:286–291.

77. Vitkova M, Klimcakova E, Kovacikova M, et al. Plasma levels and adipose tissue messenger ribonucleic acid expression of retinol-binding protein 4 are reduced during calorie restriction in obese subjects but are not related to diet-induced changes in insulin sensitivity. J Clin Endocrinol Metab 2007; 92:2330–2335.
78. Haider DG, Schindler K, Mittermayer F, et al. Effect of rosiglitazone on visfatin and retinol-binding protein-4 plasma concentrations in HIV-positive patients. Clin Pharmacol Ther 2007; 81:580–585.
79. Kloting N, Graham TE, Berndt J, et al. Serum retinol-binding protein is more highly expressed in visceral than in subcutaneous adipose tissue and is a marker of intra-abdominal fat mass. Cell Metab 2007; 6:79–87.
80. Stefan N, Hennige AM, Staiger H, et al. High circulating retinol-binding protein 4 is associated with elevated liver fat but not with total, subcutaneous, visceral, or intramyocellular fat in humans. Diabetes Care 2007; 30:1173–1178.
81. Steppan C, Bailey ST, Bath S, et al. The hormone resistin links obesity to diabetes. Nature 2001; 409:307–312.
82. Satoh H, Nguyen MT, Miles PD, et al. Adenovirus-mediated chronic "hyper-resistinemia" leads to in vivo insulin resistance in normal rats. J Clin Invest 2004; 114:224–231.
83. Lehrke M, Reilly MP, Millington SC, et al. An inflammatory cascade leading to hyperresistinemia in humans. PLoS Med 2004; 1:e45.
84. Fukuhara A, Matsuda M, Nishizawa M, et al. Visfatin: A protein secreted by visceral fat that mimics the effects of insulin. Science 2005; 307:426–430.
85. Frydelund-Larsen L, Akerstrom T, Nielsen S, et al. Visfatin mRNA expression in human subcutaneous adipose tissue is regulated by exercise. Am J Physiol Endocrinol Metab 2007; 292:E24–E31.
86. Hida K, Wada J, Eguchi J, et al. Visceral adipose tissue-derived serine protease inhibitor: A unique insulin-sensitizing adipocytokine in obesity. Proc Natl Acad Sci U S A 2005; 102:10610–10615.
87. Kloting N, Berndt J, Kralisch S, et al. Vaspin gene expression in human adipose tissue: Association with obesity and type 2 diabetes. Biochem Biophys Res Commun 2006; 339:430–436.
88. Komiya T, Tanigawa Y, Hirohashi S. Cloning of the novel gene intelectin, which is expressed in intestinal paneth cells in mice. Biochem Biophys Res Commun 1998 251;759–762.
89. Yang RZ, Lee MJ, Hu H, et al. Identification of omentin as a novel depot-specific adipokine in human adipose tissue: Possible role in modulating insulin action. Am J Physiol Endocrinol Metab 2006; 290:E1253–E1261.
90. de Souza Batista CM, Yang RZ, Lee MJ, et al. Omentin plasma levels and gene expression are decreased in obesity. Diabetes 2007; 56:1655–1661.
91. Yoon JC, Chickering TW, Rosen ED, et al. Peroxisome proliferator-activated receptor gamma target gene encoding a novel angiopoietin-related protein associated with adipose differentiation. Mol Cell Biol 2000; 20:5343–5349.
92. Mandard S, Zandbergen F, van Straten E, et al. The fasting-induced adipose factor/angiopoietin-like protein 4 is physically associated with lipoproteins and governs plasma lipid levels and adiposity. J Biol Chem 2006; 281:934–944.
93. Yang M, Zhang Y, Pan J, et al. Cathepsin L activity controls adipogenesis and glucose tolerance. Nat Cell Biol 2007; 9:970–977.
94. Taleb S, Cancello R, Clement K, et al. Cathepsin s promotes human preadipocyte differentiation: Possible involvement of fibronectin degradation. Endocrinology 2006; 147:4950–4959.
95. Lin Y, Rajala MW, Berger JP, et al. Hyperglycemia-induced production of acute phase reactants in adipose tissue. J Biol Chem 2001; 276:42077–42083.
96. Yang RZ, Lee MJ, Hu H, et al. Acute-phase serum amyloid A: An inflammatory adipokine and potential link between obesity and its metabolic complications. PLoS Med 2006; 3:e287.
97. Masuzaki H, Yamamoto H, Kenyon CJ, et al. Transgenic amplification of glucocorticoid action in adipose tissue causes high blood pressure. J Clin Invest 2003; 112;83–90.
98. Andrew R, Westerbacka J, Wahren J, et al. The contribution of visceral adipose tissue to splanchnic cortisol production in healthy humans. Diabetes 2005; 54:1364–1370.
99. Bergman RN, Ader M. Free fatty acids and pathogenesis of type 2 diabetes mellitus. Trends Endocrinol Metab 2000; 11;351–356.
100. Bergman RN, Kim SP, Catalano KJ, et al. Why visceral fat is bad: Mechanisms of the metabolic syndrome. Obesity (Silver Spring) 2006; 14(Suppl. 1):16S–19S.

9 Free Fatty Acid Metabolism in Visceral Obesity

Asem Ali and Michael D. Jensen
Mayo Clinic, Rochester, Minnesota, U.S.A.

INTRODUCTION

In the postabsorptive state free fatty acids (FFA) are the primary circulating lipid fuel for many organs, including heart, liver, and kidney (Fig. 1). Adipose tissue is the proximate source of ≥95% of FFA, except under postprandial conditions, when spillover of fatty acids released from lipoprotein lipase (LPL)-mediated hydrolysis of chylomicrons (Fig. 1) can account for up to 50% of circulating FFA, although at suppressed levels. The ability of adipose tissue to modulate lipolysis to accommodate for fuel needs in different situations is remarkable. In healthy adults, FFA concentrations may vary across an immense range, from <20 to >3000 μmol/L. In addition, lipolysis/FFA concentrations can change rapidly over relatively short periods of time, as might be expected for a substrate with a half life of <4 minutes. Systemic FFA availability is regulated through a complex system of hormonal, neural, and perhaps substrate interactions that modulate the adipose tissue FFA release. FFA concentrations in turn reflect the balance between release and uptake.

Chronically elevated plasma FFA concentrations are associated with reduced insulin-mediated glucose uptake in muscle, impaired suppression of hepatic glucose production, excess VLDL secretion, impaired β-cell insulin secretion, and endothelial dysfunction. We now know that excess release of FFA by adipose tissue is the cause of elevated postabsorptive FFA concentrations. Individuals with upper body/visceral obesity are more likely to have increased FFA, insulin resistance, dyslipidemia, and greater cardiovascular risk. In contrast, equally obese individuals with a predominantly lower body fat distribution tend to have normal FFA and much less in the way of metabolic abnormalities. The link between fat distribution, fatty acid metabolism, and metabolic risk has become an interesting focus of research in the recent years. Understanding the characteristics of different adipose tissue beds with respect to fatty acid metabolism has helped clarify the role of visceral fat. At least with respect to FFA metabolism, we now have a good idea as to the link between visceral obesity and metabolic abnormalities associated with increased cardiovascular risk and insulin resistance. This chapter will briefly review FFA metabolism and regulation of lipolysis, changes that occur with different obesity phenotypes as well as effects that lead to increased cardiovascular risk, and metabolic as well pathophysiological consequences of these changes.

FFA METABOLISM

The main focus in this chapter is on FFA, particularly long-chain fatty acids. Free fatty acids circulate nonesterified and are highly albumin bound. The major site of esterified fatty acid storage is in adipocytes in the form of triglyceride. Triglyceride stores are present in other cell types, although the current concept is that these pools normally serve as local (intracellular) buffer against the wide variations in plasma FFA concentrations and do not in themselves contribute to plasma FFA availability.

Free Fatty Acid Release from Adipose Tissue

Circulating plasma FFA concentrations are largely related to the rate of release, although at comparable FFA concentrations women have ~40% greater FFA flux than men (1). Other exceptions to the good link between FFA release and FFA concentration are: (1) exercise, where greater uptake of FFA (presumably by muscle) masks increases in lipolysis (2,3) and (2) treatment with thiazolidinediones, which lower concentrations by increasing clearance (4).

The flux of FFA through the systemic circulation in the resting, postabsorptive state is most strongly related to resting energy expenditure (REE) (1). Interindividual variations in plasma

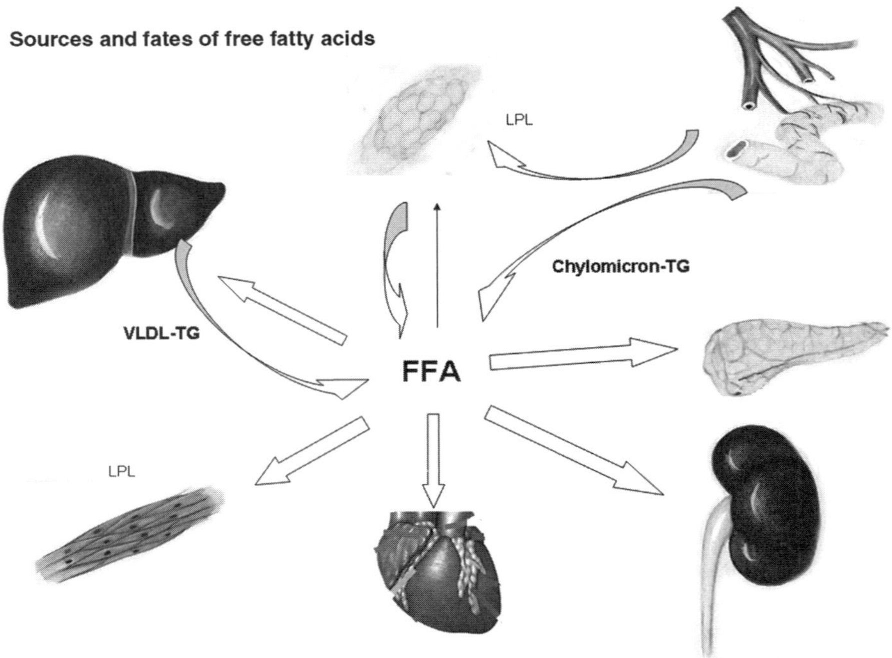

Figure 1 The vast majority of FFA originate from adipose tissue lipolysis, although spillover of fatty acids from chylomicron hydrolysis can also contribute to the FFA pool. Sites of FFA uptake include liver, heart, kidney, muscle, and adipocytes themselves. A small, but biologically important site of FFA uptake are pancreatic β cells. The effects of excess FFA on tissue function is discussed.

epinephrine concentrations account for some of the interindividual differences in plasma FFA flux not attributable to REE and sex (1). Of interest, variability in body fat is not a good predictor of FFA flux, which means that those with less body fat have greater FFA release rates relative to fat mass. Because of this, expressing FFA flux relative to total body fat mass to make comparisons between lean and obese can lead to problematic conclusions. The factors that have been shown to have an important role in regulating FFA release in vivo in humans are listed in Table 1, together with an estimate of their potency (how changes in concentrations are relative to the usual range of plasma concentrations) and rapidity of onset of action. The potency of insulin (5,6), catecholamines (7), growth hormone (8), cortisol (9), and atrial natriuretic peptide (10) have been examined in vivo. Only recently has it been discovered that the nicotinic acid receptor GPR109 A (HM74 A or PUMA-G) also mediates the inhibition of lipolysis by ketone bodies (11) and therefore information on potency and timing of the action of ketone bodies is not published.

Contribution of Fat Depots to Systemic FFA Release

The statistical link between elevated FFA concentrations and visceral obesity logically lead to the idea that visceral fat is a main source of elevated circulating FFA. To address this hypothesis, a series of studies involving femoral artery, femoral vein and hepatic vein catheterization, leg and splanchnic blood flow measures, and systemic and regional FFA kinetics have been conducted.

Table 1 Regulators of lipolysis in humans—circulating factors

	Effect	Potency	Onset of action
Insulin	Inhibition	Very high	Minutes
Catecholamines	Stimulation	Very high	Minutes
Growth hormone	Stimulation	Medium	Hours
Cortisol	Stimulation	Low	Hours
Atrial natriuretic peptide	Stimulation	Low	Minutes
Ketone bodies	Inhibition	Unknown	Unknown

These studies allowed investigators to compare the contribution of different fat depots to the systemic FFA circulating pool. Upper body subcutaneous fat was found to contribute the greatest fraction (~65%) of systemic FFA release (12–16). Leg fat contributes ~20%, and splanchnic fat (which represents visceral fat) contributed about ~15%. The problem with measurement of visceral fat contribution is the difficulty in accessing the portal vein, especially in human subjects. In studying different obesity phenotypes, leg contribution was similar between upper and lower body obese women. However, upper body subcutaneous fat was a greater contributor in upper body obesity (12,14,16). Therefore, the differences in most of the studies relate to upper body subcutaneous fat. A major distinction between nonobese or lower body obese groups and upper body obesity is that postprandial suppression of adipose tissue lipolysis is markedly defective in the later group. Systemic FFA release is almost 3-times greater in upper body obesity, despite higher insulin concentrations (12).

Although the contribution of visceral fat to hepatic FFA delivery does increase in those with greater amounts of visceral fat, this does not translate in substantially greater splanchnic FFA release. This suggests that visceral fat does not directly contribute to peripheral insulin resistance, at least with regards to fatty acid toxicity.

Obesity and Lipolysis

The regulation of lipolysis associated in obesity and different obesity phenotypes has been studied to some extent. The ability of insulin to suppress lipolysis is reduced in adults with greater amounts of body fat (17,18) and reduced in those with upper body obesity compared with lower body obesity (19,20). Somewhat surprisingly, epinephrine (20) and exercise (21) do not increase lipolysis as much in upper body obese women as they do in nonobese or lower body obese women.

The independent effect of insulin on suppression of lipolysis in different fat depots has been studied in nonobese, but not in obese adults. In nonobese adults, splanchnic FFA release is less readily suppressed by insulin as compared to lower body fat (6).

SYSTEMIC EFFECTS OF ELEVATED FFA

Free Fatty Acid Metabolism and the Liver

The delivery of excess FFA to the liver acts to prevent the normal insulin–mediated suppression of glucose output by the liver. There is some controversy as to whether the effects of elevated FFA are on hepatic gluconeogenesis or a combination of gluconeogenesis and glycogenolysis. It is proposed that FFA influence glucose output by creating surpluses of factors, such as acetyl-CoA, NADH, ATP, and citrate, perhaps with intrahepatic triglyceride as the intermediate step. Elevated FFA have also been shown to stimulate VLDL-triglyceride production (22).

Effect of Free Fatty Acids on Vasculature and Blood Pressure Regulation

Hypertension is one of the risk factors for cardiovascular disease and is tightly associated with insulin resistance and visceral obesity. Many mechanisms are thought to fit hypertension into the circle. These mechanisms include impaired (*i*) insulin-mediated vasodilatation in vascular beds (23), (*ii*) α-adrenergic stimulation (24), and (*iii*) nitric oxide and endothelial dysfunction (25,26).

Many of the studies have been conducted at levels of FFA that are high- or supraphysiologic (25,26). Further studies to determine the effect of chronic, more physiologic elevated levels of FFA are required.

Elevated Systemic Free Fatty Acids and β-Cell Dysfunction

It is established that fatty acids can have adverse effects on islet insulin content (27,28). One theory is that type 2 diabetes develops as part of a biphasic β cell response to excess FFA (28,29) (Fig. 1). A number of mechanisms have been proposed to mediate the toxic effects of excess intracellular fatty acids, but species differences in how β cells respond make it difficult to directly translate animal and cell model systems to human type 2 diabetes.

Muscle and Free Fatty Acids

In the 1960s, the discovery that increased fatty acids can preferentially be oxidized by muscle mitochondria and "out-compete" glucose (the Randle cycle), suggested a mechanism for fatty acid–induced insulin resistance (30). More recently, FFA elevation has been shown to interrupt muscle insulin receptor substrate and PI3K insulin–mediated glucose uptake independent of their oxidative role, contributing to peripheral resistance in a novel pathway (31). Intramyocellular triglyceride (imTG) accumulation may provide a link between extracellular FFA and the intramyocellular environment, as imTG correlates well with insulin resistance and FFA are a precursor of imTG (32,33). The precise mechanism(s) are not entirely known at present, but interesting possibilities include actions of diacylglycerols, ceramides, and long-chain acyl-CoA's themselves as intracellular mediators of impaired insulin signaling.

SUMMARY

To summarize, abnormalities of FFA metabolism are highly complex and are closely associated with insulin resistance. This is very commonly associated with visceral obesity. The reason why upper body subcutaneous fat appears dysregulated in visceral obesity is not yet known. The implication of understanding this association, however, is that treatments targeted towards creating healthy subcutaneous fat may alleviate some of the metabolic abnormalities of visceral obesity.

REFERENCES

1. Nielsen S, Guo Z, Albu JB, et al. Energy expenditure, sex, and endogenous fuel availability in humans. J Clin Invest 2003; 111:981–988.
2. Turcotte LP, Richter EA, Kiens B. Increased plasma FFA uptake and oxidation during prolonged exercise in trained vs. untrained humans. Am J Physiol 1992; 262:E791–E799.
3. Burguera B, Proctor DN, Dietz W, et al. Leg FFA kinetics during exercise in men and women. Am J Physiol Endocrinol Metab 2000; 278:E113–E117.
4. Shadid S, Jensen MD. Pioglitazone increases non-esterified fatty acid clearance in upper body obesity. Diabetologia 2006; 49:149–157.
5. Jensen MD, Caruso M, Heiling V, et al. Insulin regulation of lipolysis in nondiabetic and IDDM subjects. Diabetes 1989; 38:1595–1601.
6. Meek S, Nair KS, Jensen MD. Insulin regulation of regional free fatty acid metabolism. Diabetes 1999; 48:10–14.
7. Divertie GD, Jensen MD, Cryer PE, et al. Lipolytic responsiveness to epinephrine in nondiabetic and diabetic humans. Am J Physiol 1997; 272:E1130–E1135.
8. Cersosimo E, Danou F, Persson M, et al. Effects of pulsatile delivery of basal growth hormone on lipolysis in humans. Am J Physiol 1996; 271:E123–E126.
9. Divertie GD, Jensen MD, Miles JM. Stimulation of lipolysis in humans by physiological hypercortisolemia. Diabetes 1991; 40:1228–1232.
10. Birkenfeld AL, Boschmann M, Moro C, et al. Lipid mobilization with physiological atrial natriuretic peptide concentrations in humans. J Clin Endocrinol Metab 2005; 90:3622–3628.
11. Taggart AK, Kero J, Gan X, et al. (D)-Beta-hydroxybutyrate inhibits adipocyte lipolysis via the nicotinic acid receptor PUMA-G. J Biol Chem 2005; 280:26649–26652.
12. Guo ZK, Hensrud DD, Johnson CM, et al. Regional postprandial fatty acid metabolism in different obesity phenotypes. Diabetes 1999; 48:1586–1592.
13. Jensen MD. Gender differences in regional fatty acid metabolism before and after meal ingestion. J Clin Invest 1995; 96:2297–2303.
14. Martin ML, Jensen MD. Effects of body fat distribution on regional lipolysis in obesity. J Clin Invest 1991; 88:609–613.
15. Nielsen S, Guo ZK, Johnson CM, et al. Splanchnic lipolysis in human obesity. J Clin Invest 2004; 113:1582–1588.
16. Basu A, Basu R, Shah P, et al. Systemic and regional free fatty acid metabolism in type 2 diabetes. Am J Physiol Endocrinol Metab 2001; 280:E1000–E1006.
17. Shadid S, Kanaley JA, Sheehan MT, et al. Basal and insulin-regulated free fatty acid and glucose metabolism in humans. Am J Physiol Endocrinol Metab 2007; 292:E1770–E1774.
18. Bonadonna RC, Groop L, Zych K, et al. Dose-dependent effect of insulin on plasma free fatty acid turnover and oxidation in humans. Am J Physiol 1990; 259:E736–E750.
19. Jensen MD. Regulation of forearm lipolysis in different types of obesity. In vivo evidence for adipocyte heterogeneity. J Clin Invest 1991; 87:187–193.
20. Jensen MD, Haymond MW, Rizza RA, et al. Influence of body fat distribution on free fatty acid metabolism in obesity. J Clin Invest 1989; 83:1168–1173.

21. Kanaley JA, Cryer PE, Jensen MD. Fatty acid kinetic responses to exercise. Effects of obesity, body fat distribution, and energy-restricted diet. J Clin Invest 1993; 92:255–261.
22. Lewis GF, Uffelman KD, Szeto LW, et al. Interaction between free fatty acids and insulin in the acute control of very low density lipoprotein production in humans. J Clin Invest 1995; 95:158–166.
23. Laakso M, Edelman SV, Brechtel G, et al. Decreased effect of insulin to stimulate skeletal muscle blood flow in obese man. J Clin Invest 1990; 85:1844–1852.
24. Stepniakowski K, Sallee FR, Goodfriend TL, et al. Fatty acids enhance neurovascular reflex responses by effects on a_1-adrenoceptors. Am J Physiol 1996; 270:R1340–R1346.
25. Steinberg HO, Brechtel G, Johnson A, et al. Insulin-mediated skeletal muscle vasodilation is nitric oxide dependent. A novel action of insulin to increase nitric oxide release. J Clin Invest 1994; 94:1172–1179.
26. Steinberg HO, Paradisi G, Hook G, et al. Free fatty acid elevation impairs insulin-mediated vasodilation and nitric oxide production. Diabetes 2000; 49:1231–1238.
27. Bollheimer LC, Skelly RH, Chester MW, et al. Chronic exposure to free fatty acid reduces pancreatic β cell insulin content by increasing basal insulin secretion that is not compensated for by a corresponding increase in proinsulin biosynthesis translation. J Clin Invest 1998; 101:1094–1101.
28. Mason TM, Goh T, Tchipashvili V, et al. Prolonged elevation of plasma free fatty acids desensitizes the insulin secretory response to glucose in vivo in rats. Diabetes 1999; 48:524–530.
29. Paolisso G, Gambardella A, Amato L, et al. Opposite effects of short- and long-term fatty acid infusion on insulin secretion in healthy subjects. Diabetologia 1995; 38:1295–1299.
30. Randle PJ, Garland PB, Hales CN, et al. The glucose-fatty acid cycle: Its role in insulin sensitivity and the metabolic disturbances of diabetes mellitus. Lancet 1963; 281:785–789.
31. Dresner A, Laurent D, Marcucci M, et al. Effects of free fatty acids on glucose transport and IRS-1-associated phosphatidylinositol 3-kinase activity. J Clin Invest 1999; 103:253–259.
32. Guo Z, Jensen MD. Intramuscular fatty acid metabolism evaluated with stable isotopic tracers. J Appl Physiol 1998; 84:1674–1679.
33. Guo Z, Burguera B, Jensen MD. Kinetics of intramuscular triglyceride fatty acids in exercising humans. J Appl Physiol 2000; 89:2057–2064.

10 Animal Models of Visceral Obesity

Derek M. Huffman and Nir Barzilai
Albert Einstein College of Medicine of Yeshiva University, Jack and Pearl Resnick Campus, Bronx, New York, U.S.A.

BACKGROUND

Obesity has reached epidemic proportions in most of the developed world and is now known to increase the risk for many diseases and shorten life expectancy (1). Among the various fat depots, the accumulation of visceral fat (VF), which is the fat surrounding the viscera, is most strongly related to many health conditions, including insulin resistance and diabetes (2). The mechanism(s) linking VF with the metabolic syndrome is not entirely clear, but it has been suggested to involve its anatomical location, leading to a "portal" effect of greater free fatty acids (FFA) and glycerol released by increased omental fat (3). More recently, evidence has shown that adipose tissue is an active endocrine organ, capable of secreting many peptides that can promote inflammation and insulin resistance (4). Our studies have shown that several genes from adipose tissue, thought to be involved in insulin resistance (PPARγ, leptin) and metabolic syndrome (angiotensinogen, resistin, PAI-1), are more highly expressed in VF, as compared to subcutaneous (SC) fat (5,6).

As obesity, and specifically VF accrual, is strongly associated with disease risk (2), the importance of having good animal models to recapitulate the obesity phenotype is crucial in understanding its pathophysiology. Several strategies exist for generating obesity in animals, which has been reviewed in detail elsewhere (7). Briefly, some of the approaches taken include high-fat feeding in rodents (8) and dogs (9), seasonal models (10), transgenics (11), and spontaneous mutants such as the Lep^{ob}/Lep^{ob} and *db/db* mouse (12). In addition, a common feature of obese animal models is a marked increase in VF and hyperinsulinemia, but similar to human studies, the distinct contribution of body fat distribution in these models cannot be directly elucidated. Since VF is more strongly related with disease risk than other fat depots, this chapter will review work utilizing animal models which confirm this association by demonstrating a causal role for VF, rather than SC fat, in the etiology of insulin resistance, atherosclerosis, and aging in mammalians.

VISCERAL FAT ACCRETION STUDIES

Transgenic Model of Visceral Obesity

Excess glucocorticoids are known to promote VF deposition and insulin resistance in obesity. As glucocorticoids can be produced locally by the enzyme 11 β hydroxysteroid dehydrogenase type 1 (11 β HSD-1), Masuzaki et al. (13) produced transgenic mice overexpressing this enzyme in adipose tissue. These mice were reported to be hyperphagic, despite elevated leptin levels, obese and displayed greater levels of corticosterone in fat. Most important, transgenic mice displayed exaggerated visceral obesity on a high-fat diet as compared to controls. Furthermore, transgenic animals demonstrated greater adipokine levels than controls, hyperlipidemia, glucose intolerance, and hyperinsulinemia.

Fat Transplantation

Using a surgical approach, Ohman et al. (14) determined whether transplanting epididymal fat pads from C57BL/6J mice could affect vascular disease in atherosclerosis-prone apolipoprotein E–deficient ApoE(−/−) mice. Plasma from ApoE(−/−) mice receiving fat transplants displayed elevated levels of leptin, resistin, and monocyte chemoattractant protein-1 (MCP-1) compared with plasma from sham-operated mice. Furthermore, mice transplanted with VF developed significantly more atherosclerosis than controls. In contrast, SC fat transplants did not accelerate

Table 1 Effect of Visceral Fat Removal on Metabolic Parameters in Rodents

Study	Species/strain	Glucose/insulin	Cytokines	Lipids	Insulin action
Barzilai et al. (15)	Male SD rats	↔Glucose ↓Insulin 49%	↓TNF-α 75% and ↓Leptin 60% expression in SC fat	↔FFA ↔Glycerol	↓Insulin infusion rate 53% ↓IGFBP-1 68%
Kim et al. (22)	Female SD rats (MSG treated)	↔Glucose ↔Insulin	NA	↓FFA 66% ↓TG 18% ↔ Cholesterol	NA
Gabriely et al. (18)	Male SD rats	↔Glucose ↓Insulin 39%	NA	↔FFA	↑Glucose infusion rate 80% ↑Glucose uptake 30% ↓Glucose production 50%
Gabriely et al. (18)	Male ZDF rats	↓Insulin 50%	NA	↓FFA 44% during clamp	↑Glucose infusion rate ↔Glucose uptake ↓Glucose production 20%
Borst et al. (17)	Male SD rats	↔Insulin	↓IL-6 53%, ↔TNF-α ↓Adiponectin 30% ↓ Resistin 26% ↔Leptin	↔FFA	↓GTT AUC 15% ↑Insulin-stimulated glucose transport in muscle 24–31%
Pitombo et al. (19)	Male Swiss mice	↓Glucose 35% ↓Insulin 45%,	↓TNF-α 40% ↓IL-6 60% ↑Adiponectin 40%	NA	↑Insulin action 45%
Einstein et al. (16)	Female pregnant SD rats	↔Glucose ↔Insulin	↔IL-6 ↔Adiponectin	↓Hepatic TG 60% ↓FFA 38%	↑GIR 32%, ↓HGP 42% ↔Glucose uptake

atherosclerosis despite a similar degree of inflammation, suggesting that VF, rather than SC fat-related inflammation, accelerates atherosclerosis development in this model.

VISCERAL FAT REMOVAL STUDIES

Improvement in Insulin Action

Using a different surgical approach to demonstrate causality between VF and disease, we and others have selectively removed perinephric and epididymal fat pads from rats and mice and studied its impact on insulin action. Please refer to Table 1 for a summary of the metabolic effects of VF removal in rodents. In an initial study (15) from our lab, moderately obese Sprague-Dawley (SD) rats were randomized either to surgical removal of VF (VF−) or to sham operation (VF+). Since the VF that was removed accounted for only ~10% of total fat mass (FM), there was no difference between groups for body weight or total FM. Nevertheless, VF− rats demonstrated significantly reduced plasma insulin levels, and during a glucose clamp, the rates of insulin infusion required to maintain plasma glucose levels and hepatic glucose production (HGP) were reduced by 50%. More recently, we have shown that VF accretion is an important determinant of hepatic insulin resistance during pregnancy, which can be largely prevented by surgical removal of VF prior to mating (16), providing further evidence that VF directly impacts hepatic insulin action.

Borst et al. (17) studied the impact of VF removal on insulin action and skeletal muscle glucose transport in male SD rats. VF removal in rats tended to improve glucose tolerance (15% reduction in glucose AUC) and significantly lowered some pro-inflammatory adipokines in serum. Most striking, VF− animals displayed increased insulin-stimulated glucose transport in excised soleus and digitorum longus muscle as compared to sham-operated controls. Overall, these studies provide verification that VF is a potent modulator of both hepatic and peripheral insulin action.

Prevention of Diabetes

Our group (18) and others (19) have also demonstrated a protection from type 2 diabetes in rodents with VF removal. In our study, 2-month-old Zucker Diabetic Fatty (ZDF) rats were assigned to receive either a sham operation (ZDVF+) or surgical removal of visceral fat (ZDVF−) (18). Despite no differences in plasma glucose or FFA levels, ZDVF− rats had a marked reduction in fasting insulin levels by ~50%. In addition, during a glucose clamp, ZDVF− rats demonstrated a greater glucose infusion rate and insulin suppression of glucose production than controls. Furthermore, when rats were monitored longitudinally, the development of diabetes, as determined by fasting glucose, was delayed in ZDVF− rats but not in sham-operated rats.

Using a mouse model of diet-induced obesity and diabetes, Pitombo et al. (19) assessed the impact of VF removal on glucose metabolism, insulin signaling, and serum adipokine levels. Control mice became diabetic and hyperinsulinemic, but VF removal partially restored metabolic parameters. In addition, VF removal completely attenuated the impairment of insulin signaling, observed in muscle from control animals, and lowered serum adipokines to near normal levels. Taken together, these studies demonstrate the ability of VF removal to prevent diabetes in both a spontaneous and diet-induced obesity-prone rodent model.

Mediator of Caloric Restriction

Visceral Versus Subcutaneous Fat

Caloric restriction (CR) limits the accumulation of VF with aging, prevents the onset of diabetes, and extends life span in a variety of species (20). As we have shown that CR preserves hepatic insulin action by decreasing VF (21), we suspected that the ability of CR to prevent insulin resistance with aging was due to the attenuation of VF, rather than other fat depots. To directly test this hypothesis, we studied four groups of rats: VF−, SC− (equivalent SC fat removed), SO (sham-operated controls), and CR (CR + sham operated) (18). Post-absorptive plasma insulin levels were nearly 50% greater in the SC− and SO rats as compared to CR and VF− animals. During a glucose clamp, VF− rats had an 80% increase in the rate of glucose infusion, significantly greater glucose uptake, and 50% increase in the ability of insulin to suppress HGP compared to SC− and SO rats. Most striking, the dramatic improvement in insulin action with VF, but not SC fat removal, closely resembled the effects of prolonged CR, suggesting that decreased VF could largely account for the beneficial effects of a reduction in food intake.

In a related study, Kim et al. (22) surgically removed SC (SC−) or VF (VF−) pads from monosodium glutamate–obese (MSG-Ob) rats and assessed markers of the metabolic syndrome. In the VF− group, basal insulin levels were not different, but FFA and HGP were restored to normal levels, while glucose uptake tended to be normalized. In contrast, removal of SC fat only partially normalized FFA and glucose uptake while HGP was unchanged. Overall, these results demonstrate a causal relationship between VF and metabolism, and suggest that VF accrual is more relevant to the metabolic syndrome than SC fat.

Longevity

As previously mentioned, VF accretion is a common hallmark of aging, and we have demonstrated metabolic benefits to VF removal (21), and that decreased VF largely accounts for the improvement in insulin action with CR (18,21). Therefore, it seemed plausible that the beneficial effects of CR on longevity may be due to the attenuation of VF (23). Therefore, we prospectively studied life span in three groups of rats: ad libitum (AL) fed, 40% CR and VF− rats (24). CR rats demonstrated the greatest survival among all experimental groups (Fig. 1). Remarkably, VF removal also resulted in improved survival as compared to AL, albeit to a lesser extent than CR. Furthermore, VF− and CR rats had a greater maximum life span than AL animals, suggesting that the reduction in VF may be an important underlying cause of life span extension with CR. Please refer to Figure 2, which summarizes the shared benefits of VF removal and CR on metabolism and aging.

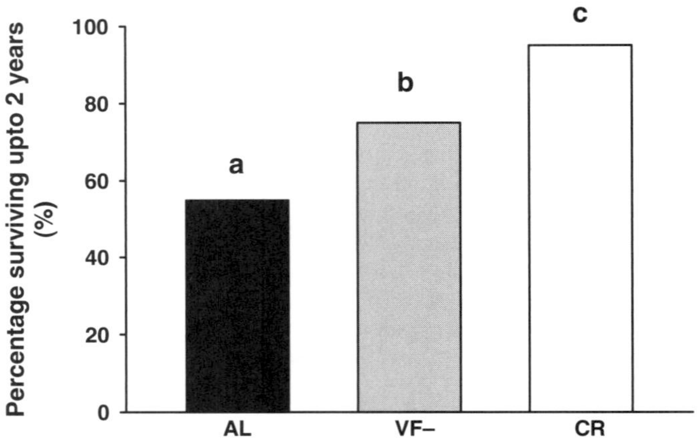

Figure 1 Percentage of rats surviving up to 2 years of age. Rats were either fed ad libitum (AL), had VF removed (VF−), or were caloric restricted (CR). CR rats demonstrated the greatest survival up to 2 years, but VF− also resulted in improved survival as compared to AL controls (24). Different letters denote a significant difference between groups ($p < 0.05$).

TREATMENT STUDIES

Leptin and ß3-Agonist Administration

Our group and others have demonstrated various treatment strategies for VF and/or its complications. In an initial study (25), we administered leptin by osmotic minipumps for 8 days to rats, since this fat-derived peptide had been shown to play an important role in energy homeostasis. Remarkably, we found that leptin administration led to a more dramatic decrease in VF than pair-fed controls, which were moderately food restricted, but body weight and total FM were not different. Furthermore, leptin-treated rats demonstrated the greatest enhancement in hepatic insulin action. Likewise, because the effects of leptin function primarily through the ß3-adrenoreceptor, we performed an analogous experiment designed to decrease VF to a similar extent by ß3-adrenoreceptor agonist or CR (26). Similarly, compared to controls, hepatic insulin sensitivity was increased (~3-fold) in CR and ß3-treated animals, further demonstrating that a pharmacologic reduction in VF can improve insulin action.

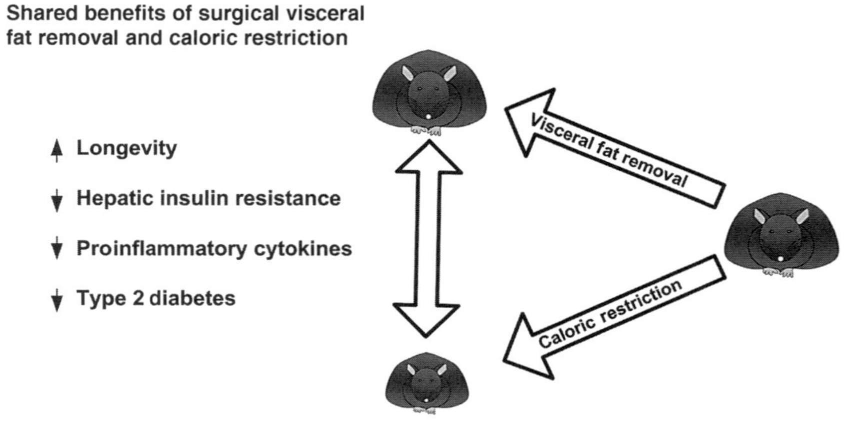

Figure 2 The benefits of VF, rather than SC fat removal, resembles many of the effects of prolonged CR in aging rodents, including improved hepatic insulin action, systemic inflammation, and longevity. Furthermore, the benefits observed in our surgical model are entirely due to a reduction in the epididymal and perinephric fat pads (VF), while the benefits of CR include, reductions in body weight, total fat mass (VF and SC fat), and food intake.

11β-Hydroxysteroid Dehydrogenase Inhibitors

As previously mentioned, the enzyme 11 β HSD-1 type 1 converts inactive cortisone into active cortisol in cells and excess glucocorticoids promote VF deposition. When this enzyme was overexpressed in adipose tissue in mice, animals developed visceral obesity and diabetes (13). Therefore, it seemed intuitive to Hermanowski-Vosatka and colleagues that pharmacologic inhibition of 11 β HSD-1 might serve as a therapeutic target for the metabolic syndrome. When a selective and potent 11 β HSD-1 inhibitor was given to DIO mice, they observed a reduction in body mass, retroperitoneal fat pad weight, as well as serum insulin, glucose, and lipids (26). Similarly, this inhibitor resulted in improved glucose tolerance in a mouse model of type 2 diabetes and attenuated vascular plaque formation in ApoE(−/−) mice (26).

Prevention of Systemic Inflammation

Mounting evidence supports a role for adipose tissue–derived pro-inflammatory cytokines in the pathogenesis of diabetes and atherosclerotic diseases. Therefore, Ohman et al. (14) administered pioglitazone, which has been shown to reduce MCP-1 levels and fat inflammation, to ApoE(−/−) mice that received a VF transplant or sham-operated controls. Pioglitazone treatment lowered MCP-1 levels and macrophage content in the VF transplant and reduced atherosclerosis development in VF-transplant mice, but not in sham-operated mice. Likewise, in obese mice, short-term treatment with a pharmacological antagonist of CCR2 lowered macrophage content in adipose tissue and systemic inflammation, resulting in improved insulin action (28). Therefore, drugs which can interfere with the infiltration of macrophages into fat, and specifically VF, may provide an effective strategy for the prevention of cardiovascular complications and metabolic syndrome due to visceral obesity.

SUMMARY

The accumulation of VF is strongly related to the development of metabolic syndrome. Utilizing novel models of visceral obesity, several studies have demonstrated a cause–effect relationship between VF, insulin action, metabolic syndrome, and longevity in mammalians. In contrast, SC fat does not appear to play an important role in the etiology of disease risk in animal models. Treatment strategies including pharmacologic agents (leptin, ß3-agonists) can improve glucose tolerance by effectively reducing VF. Compelling evidence also supports a role for inhibitors of macrophage infiltration into fat (thiazolidinediones, CCR2 antagonists), and hence systemic inflammation, for the treatment of insulin resistance and vascular disease. Therefore, two lines of investigation worth pursuing include (1) understanding the secretory biology of VF to identify the important mediators of the metabolic syndrome and (2) the development of drugs designed to modulate body fat distribution. In summary, these studies in animals highlight the distinct metabolic capacity of VF, the importance of accounting for body fat distribution in disease risk, and the potential of treating VF-mediated insulin resistance.

REFERENCES

1. Fontaine KR, Redden DT, Wang C, et al. Years of life lost due to obesity. JAMA 2003; 289(2):187–193.
2. Carr DB, Utzschneider KM, Hull RL, et al. Intra-abdominal fat is a major determinant of the National Cholesterol Education Program Adult Treatment Panel III criteria for the metabolic syndrome. Diabetes 2004; 53(8):2087–2094.
3. Bjorntorp P. "Portal" adipose tissue as a generator of risk factors for cardiovascular disease and diabetes. Arteriosclerosis 1990; 10(4):493–496.
4. Trayhurn P, Wood IS. Signalling role of adipose tissue: Adipokines and inflammation in obesity. Biochem Soc Trans 2005; 33(Pt 5):1078–1081.
5. Atzmon G, Yang XM, Muzumdar R, et al. Differential gene expression between visceral and subcutaneous fat depots. Horm Metab Res 2002; 34(11–12):622–628.
6. Einstein FH, Atzmon G, Yang XM, et al. Differential responses of visceral and subcutaneous fat depots to nutrients. Diabetes 2005; 54(3):672–678.
7. Speakman J, Hambly C, Mitchell S, Krol E. Animal models of obesity. Obes Rev 2007; 8(Suppl. 1):55–61.

8. Buettner R, Scholmerich J, Bollheimer LC. High-fat diets: Modeling the metabolic disorders of human obesity in rodents. Obesity (Silver Spring) 2007; 15(4):798–808.
9. Kim SP, Catalano KJ, Hsu IR, et al. Nocturnal free fatty acids are uniquely elevated in the longitudinal development of diet-induced insulin resistance and hyperinsulinemia. Am J Physiol Endocrinol Metab 2007; 292(6):E1590–E1598.
10. Powell CS, Blaylock ML, Wang R, et al. Effects of energy expenditure and Ucp1 on photoperiod-induced weight gain in collard lemmings. Obes Res 2002; 10(6):541–550.
11. Davey RA, MacLean HE. Current and future approaches using genetically modified mice in endocrine research. Am J Physiol Endocrinol Metab 2006; 291(3):E429–E438.
12. Friedman JM, Halaas JL. Leptin and the regulation of body weight in mammals. Nature 1998; 395(6704):763–770.
13. Masuzaki H, Paterson J, Shinyama H, et al. A transgenic model of visceral obesity and the metabolic syndrome. Science 2001; 294(5549):2166–2170.
14. Ohman MK, Shen Y, Obimba CI, et al. Visceral adipose tissue inflammation accelerates atherosclerosis in apolipoprotein E-deficient mice. Circulation 2008; 117(6):798–805.
15. Barzilai N, She L, Liu BQ, et al. Surgical removal of visceral fat reverses hepatic insulin resistance. Diabetes 1999; 48(1):94–98.
16. Einstein FH, Fishman S, Muzumdar RH, et al. Accretion of visceral fat and hepatic insulin resistance in pregnant rats. Am J Physiol Endocrinol Metab 2008; 294(2):E451–455.
17. Borst SE, Conover CF, Bagby GJ. Association of resistin with visceral fat and muscle insulin resistance. Cytokine 2005; 32(1):39–44.
18. Gabriely I, Ma XH, Yang XM, et al. Removal of visceral fat prevents insulin resistance and glucose intolerance of aging: An adipokine-mediated process? Diabetes 2002; 51(10):2951–2958.
19. Pitombo C, Araujo EP, De Souza CT, et al. Amelioration of diet-induced diabetes mellitus by removal of visceral fat. J Endocrinol 2006; 191(3):699–706.
20. Weindruch R. The retardation of aging by caloric restriction: Studies in rodents and primates. Toxicol Pathol 1996; 24(6):742–745.
21. Barzilai N, Banerjee S, Hawkins M, et al. Caloric restriction reverses hepatic insulin resistance in aging rats by decreasing visceral fat. J Clin Invest 1998; 101(7):1353–1361.
22. Kim YW, Kim JY, Lee SK. Surgical removal of visceral fat decreases plasma free fatty acid and increases insulin sensitivity on liver and peripheral tissue in monosodium glutamate (MSG)-obese rats. J Korean Med Sci 1999; 14(5):539–545.
23. Barzilai N, Gupta G. Revisiting the role of fat mass in the life extension induced by caloric restriction. J Gerontol A Biol Sci Med Sci 1999; 54(3):B89–B96; discussion B7–B8.
24. Muzumdar R, Allison DB, Huffman DM, et al. Visceral adipose tissue modulates mammalian longevity. Aging Cell 2008; 7:438–440.
25. Barzilai N, Wang J, Massilon D, et al. Leptin selectively decreases visceral adiposity and enhances insulin action. J Clin Invest 1997; 100(12):3105–3110.
26. Barzilai N, Gabriely I. The role of fat depletion in the biological benefits of caloric restriction. J Nutr 2001; 131(3):903S–906S.
27. Hermanowski-Vosatka A, Balkovec JM, Cheng K, et al. 11beta-HSD1 inhibition ameliorates metabolic syndrome and prevents progression of atherosclerosis in mice. J Exp Med 2005; 202(4):517–527.
28. Weisberg SP, Hunter D, Huber R, et al. CCR2 modulates inflammatory and metabolic effects of high-fat feeding. J Clin Invest 2006; 116(1):115–124.

11 Insulin Sensitivity and Visceral Adiposity: Effects of Rimonabant

Joyce M. Richey, Morvarid Kabir, Orison O. Woolcott, Stella P. Kim, Lisa N. Harrison, Darko Stefanovski, Isabel Hsu, Dan Zheng, Maya Lottati, Cathryn Kolka, Viorica Ionut, Karyn Catalano, Jenny D. Chiu, and Richard N. Bergman

Department of Physiology and Biophysics, University of Southern California, Los Angeles, California, U.S.A.

INTRODUCTION

It is now generally accepted that obesity is increasing in the United States and other "westernized" countries, and that it is becoming epidemic in several parts of the underdeveloped world (1,2). Part and parcel with the increase in obesity are rampant increases in diseases associated with increased body weight, including not just type 2 diabetes mellitus, but also cardiovascular diseases, and cancer (3–5). While the causes of the increased fat deposition are not entirely clear (6), it is widely believed that increased consumption of palatable foods marketed by so-called "fast-food" vendors is an important cause (7,8). Such food intake appears to have increased fat deposition in various depots of the body, including the subcutaneous and visceral fat depots.

Compelling epidemiological evidence exists that visceral fat is particularly problematic as a cause of insulin resistance. Insulin resistance, in turn, is a primary risk factor for type 2 diabetes, although not sufficient as a beta-cell defect is required for most forms of the disease (9). Yet, the mechanisms underlying the "sinister trio" of visceral fat, insulin resistance, and diabetes mellitus remain to be understood. Understanding the trio is an important step in approaches to reduce risk for diabetes and other chronic diseases by reducing visceral fat, in particular.

One potential approach to reduction of visceral adiposity, and therefore risk of diabetes is to exploit our knowledge of the so-called cannabinoid system. Following the understanding that use of marijuana, and consumption of the active factor tetrahydrocannabinoid (THC) increased food consumption, led to a bevy of studies attempting to reduce body weight by blocking THC receptors (CB_1, in particular). There is now extensive evidence that such blockade by a variety of antagonists will lead to a beneficial metabolic profile (10,11). In our laboratory, we also have been studying the effects of CB_1 receptor blockade with the compound rimonabant. In fact, we have exploited a unique canine model of adiposity in which we have validated under a variety of conditions as being a good representation of visceral adiposity as observed in man (12,13). This model has increased our understanding of the linkage between visceral fat and insulin resistance, but has generated new and intriguing questions as well.

THE MODEL

Our studies are performed in animals without a single genetic background. We used magnetic resonance imaging (MRI) to measure with accuracy the amount of fat stored in visceral versus subcutaneous depots of the animals. Because the dog stores most fat in the truncal region, it is possible to obtain accurate measures of stored fat. When arriving in the laboratory, we have found that similar to humans, even animals which are nonobese still have widely varying amounts of fat stored in different depots (Fig. 1).

In a population of 20 animals, for example, we have found that total fat varied from 10% to 40% of body weight, and that the visceral component averaged 17% of the total fat deposits. Likewise, insulin sensitivity is highly varied, but is negatively correlated with the amount of stored fat (Fig. 2).

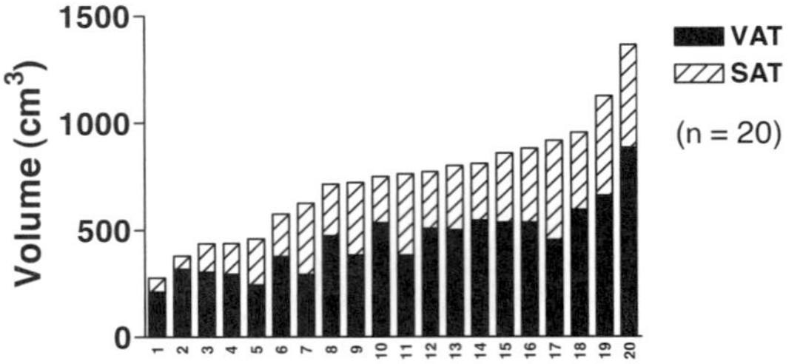

Figure 1 Baseline normal distribution of total fat depots, visceral adipose tissue (VAT), and subcutaneous adipose tissue (SAT) in 20 normal dogs.

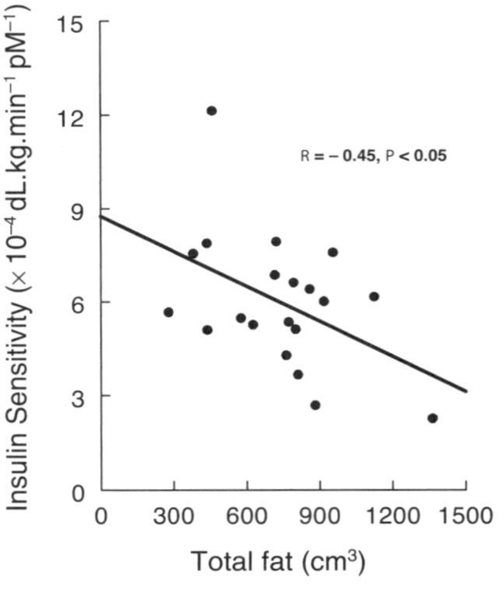

Figure 2 Negative relationship between insulin sensitivity and total body fat in normal dogs.

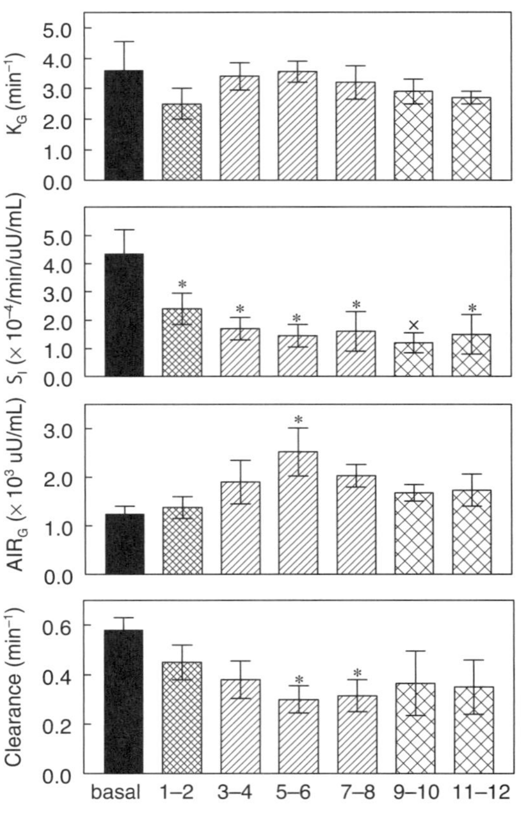

Figure 3 Glucose tolerance (K_G), insulin sensitivity (S_I), acute insulin response (AIR_G), and insulin clearance in dogs maintained on an isocaloric fat diet for 12 weeks.

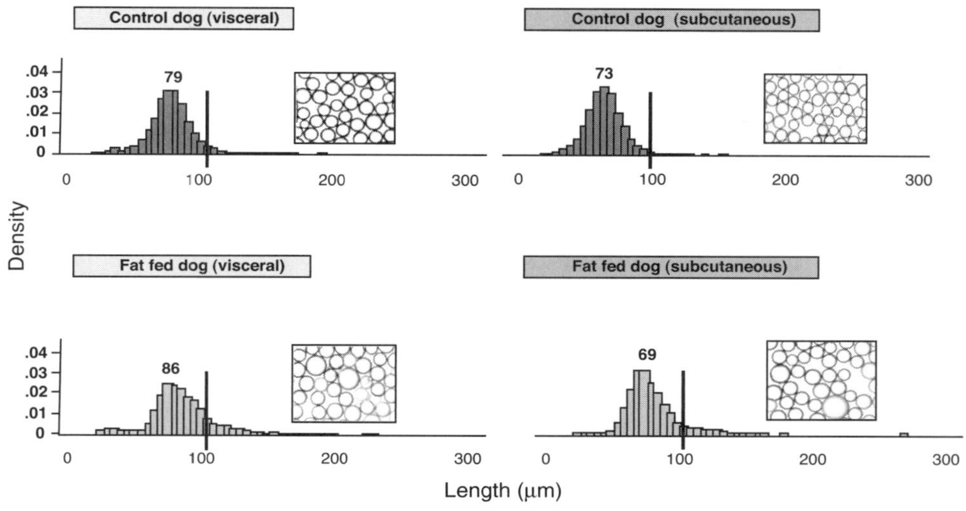

Figure 4 Adipocyte size distribution in control and fat-fed dogs. Cell diameter increased from 79 to 86 in the visceral depot.

Fat Feeding in the Canine Model

We have examined the effects of high-fat feeding in the canine model. The results are very reminiscent to that of fat feeding in normal humans.

In our first study, we found that an isocaloric diet with a modest elevation in fat calories (~10%) caused reduced insulin sensitivity within 1 week, which was maintained for 12 weeks of observation (Fig. 3). Interestingly, despite insulin resistance, there was no change in glucose tolerance, due to a responsive increase in insulin secretion, and a reduction in clearance of insulin by the liver. We have also reported that with elevated fat intake, first-pass clearance of insulin by the liver is reduced over 25%, from 60% to 44% after 12 weeks of isocaloric fat feeding (14). Thus, the canine model, like the human (15), reflects a highly integrated closed-loop feedback system that maintains normal carbohydrate metabolism despite changes in diet. This regulatory system is critical to metabolic health, and it is only with significant dysfunction of the beta cells that overt disease can result after changes in insulin sensitivity (16).

Deposition of Fat

Using MRI, we are able to measure with accuracy the amount of fat in visceral versus subcutaneous fat depots. Figure 1 shows that about 62% of total fat stored is located in the visceral depot in these nonobese animals. After 6 weeks of a hypercaloric diet that consisted of 5386 kcal/day (carbohydrates 28%, fat 53%, proteins 19%), we observed a 26% increase in visceral and a doubling of subcutaneous fat deposition, associated with a reduction in insulin sensitivity of 37%. It is interesting that not all animals store fat in the same pattern. Thus, there was a tendency for some animals to deposit fat specifically in the visceral depot, while others deposited it subcutaneously. In fact, the ratio of fat deposition (visceral:subcutaneous) varied from 0.9 to 5.0 among 20 animals, with a mean of 1.8 ± 0.2.

Adipocytes Distribution and Morphology

In this canine model, we are able to take adipose tissue biopsies of the two major fat depots, as well as that of the liver. Figure 4 represents the distribution of adipocyte size in control and fat-fed dogs. Under control conditions, visceral adipocytes are slightly larger than subcutaneous adipocytes (~8%). After fat feeding, the differences between visceral versus subcutaneous fat become more pronounced. There are more large cells (>100 μm) in the visceral fat depot compared to subcutaneous. In addition, there is a rightward shift in the distribution of cell size in visceral and subcutaneous cell distribution (Fig. 4). An additional contrast between visceral and subcutaneous adipocytes relates to the ability of adrenergic agonists to stimulate lipolysis; lipolysis from the visceral depot has been shown to be more responsive to adrenergic stimulus, more specifically to isoprotenerol. This sensitivity increases the possibility that visceral lipolysis

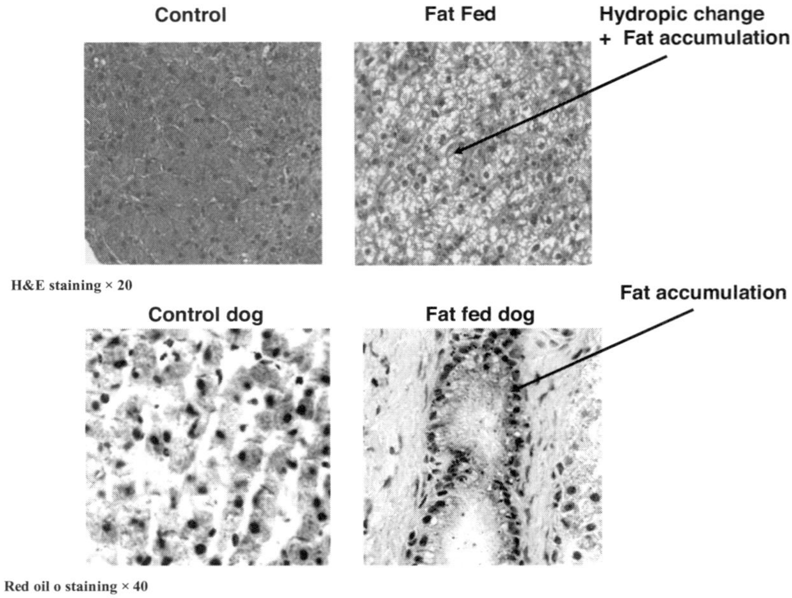

Figure 5 Demonstration of slight fat accumulation and hydropic change in a representative fat-fed dog.

can be stimulated by adrenergic signals. Furthermore, the visceral depot is less sensitive to inhibition by insulin than is the subcutaneous depot. We have reported a 3-fold increase in the ED50 of insulin to suppress lipolysis in visceral tissue (17).

Hepatic Morphology

It is well established that increased fat intake results in deposition of fat in human liver, a condition which can progress to nonalcoholic fatty liver disease (NAFLD). A reminiscent increase in liver fat is observed in the dog model. We have previously reported that after fat intake, there is an increase in triglyceride deposition (18). More recently, we have also observed hydropic changes in combination with slight fat accumulation in liver images, similar to changes observed in man (Fig. 5). Thus, in less than 2 months, increasing the fat content of the diet will cause hepatic changes which may well reflect the earliest signs of hepatic steatosis. Again, this demonstration confirms the appropriate use of the fat-fed dog as a model for insulin resistance in human.

MECHANISMS OF DIET-INDUCED INSULIN RESISTANCE

What is the cause of the insulin resistance observed in the fat-fed dog model? While various mechanisms have been proposed relating changes in diet and insulin resistance, our data is consistent with the so-called "portal theory," that is, the visceral fat is associated with increased flux of free fatty acids (FFA) in the portal vein, resulting in deposition of liver triglycerides and insulin resistance. We have shown that the changes in genes expression and visceral fat and liver are consistent with the portal hypothesis—upregulation of gene expression reflective of visceral fat turnover (hormone sensitivity lipase, lipoprotein lipase, SREBP-1), as well as gluconeogenic genes in liver (PEPCK, glucose-6-phosphatase) (18). We have not observed changes in gene expression for adipose cytokines ("adipokines"), which have been proposed to mediate insulin resistance. Based upon our results, we concur with the views of other investigators (19), which have implicated FFA as an important signal by which visceral fat results in insulin resistance at the liver, and possibly in the peripheral tissues as well.

Why does lipolysis increase in the fat-fed dog model? We have entertained the possibility that the sympathetic nervous system plays an important, if not critical, role in the increase in FFA flux from the visceral depot to the liver. Several years ago, we reported that lipolysis from the visceral fat depot was oscillatory, with a period of about 11 minutes (20). The oscillations could be blocked with a high-affinity β-3 blocking agent—in canine, the most β-3 receptors are in the visceral fat depot (21). Recently, we have demonstrated in our laboratory that pulsatile FFA administration is more potent than constant FFA release in stimulating endogenous (hepatic) glucose production (22). Therefore, it is reasonable to suggest that the sympathetic nervous system plays a role in the pathogenesis of temporal increases in FFA in blood, which in turn may render the liver resistant to insulin. Thus, we suggest that the putative increase in flux of FFA from the visceral fat depot is due, at least in part, to sympathetic signals which presumably stimulate β-3 receptors in the visceral fat depot. This result supports the previous work of Landsberg (18) and others demonstrating increased sympathetic tone in obesity, and may in fact play a role in the negative effects of increased central fat stores.

Effects of Rimonabant

The large animal model provides an excellent platform to examine the metabolic effects of the CB_1 receptor antagonist, rimonabant. While there is abundant evidence that rimonabant acts centrally to control body weight (23), many questions regarding the importance and role of the cannabinoid system in metabolic function still remain. Among the most important are whether CB_1 receptor antagonists work only centrally, or have effects outside the central nervous system, and whether the effects are on food intake per se, or whether they have additional effects on energy utilization? We have examined the effects of rimonabant (RIM), administered orally at a dose of 1.25 mg/kg/day, on many metabolic functions of the fat-fed conscious canine model. We have found the effects of the compound to be profound along with their potential benefit with respect to metabolic regulation.

Body Weight

The design of our study is shown in Figure 6. Animals were put on normal diets (~33% fat calories) for 3 weeks, after which they were switched to a hypercaloric, high-fat diet (~53% fat calories). We observed the animals for 6 weeks, during which they gained weight (+2.2 kg) and deposited fat in the visceral and subcutaneous depots (increased 26% and 50%, respectively). At 6 weeks, about half the animals (11/20) were randomized to RIM, while the remaining others ($n = 9$) were treated as placebo.

As expected, we observed that the placebo animals continued to gain weight throughout the additional 16 weeks of treatment. In contrast, body weight in the RIM animals was stabilized. As expected, rimonabant prevented additional weight *gain* in the face of a high-fat diet. But, we only observed a slight reduction in body weight with RIM, *reducing* by only 2.8% by week 16, while the placebo dogs *increased* their body weight by 6.5%. Reduced food intake could not totally account for the RIM effect on body weight. Figure 7 presents the relationship between the change in food intake versus the change in body weight in the RIM and placebo animals. If food intake were able to explain RIM's effect on body weight, we would expect that RIM versus placebo animals could be represented by a single line. But, overall the RIM animals lost more weight than could be attributed to food intake alone; that is, in Figure 7, the RIM-treated animals were on a lower line, with the difference between the lines attributable to an effect of RIM on energy expenditure. Thus, RIM has a potent effect to change expenditure of energy which explains much of its effect on body weight. Measurements of energy expenditure revealed that the RIM animals "switched" from carbohydrate to fat consumption (24). Metabolically

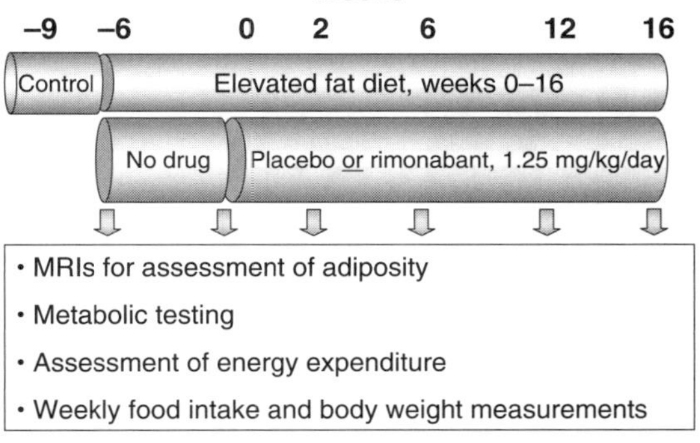

Figure 6 Rimonabant study research design.

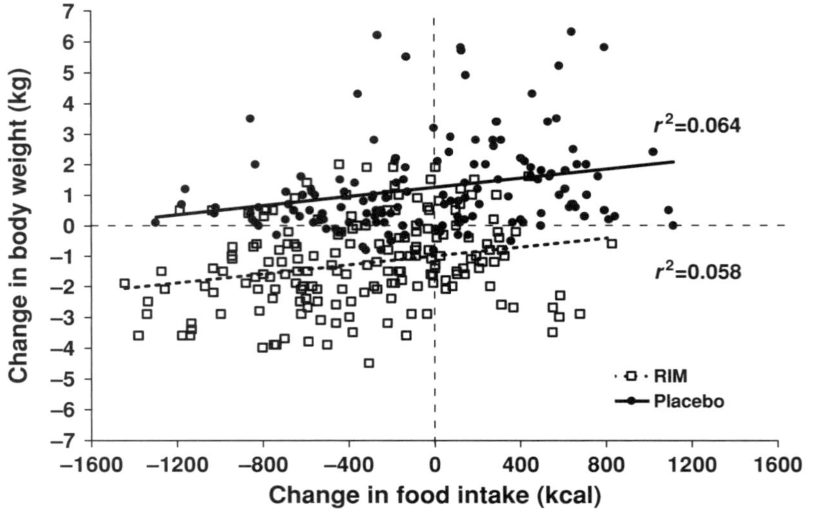

Figure 7 Relationship between the changes in food intake and changes in body weight in rimonabant and placebo treated dogs.

switching from carbohydrate to fat consumption can explain much of the RIM effect on stored calories.

Insulin Action

Figure 8 shows the effect of rimonabant on changes in insulin sensitivity. All animals had reduced insulin sensitivity after 6 weeks of high-fat feeding. During the remaining period,

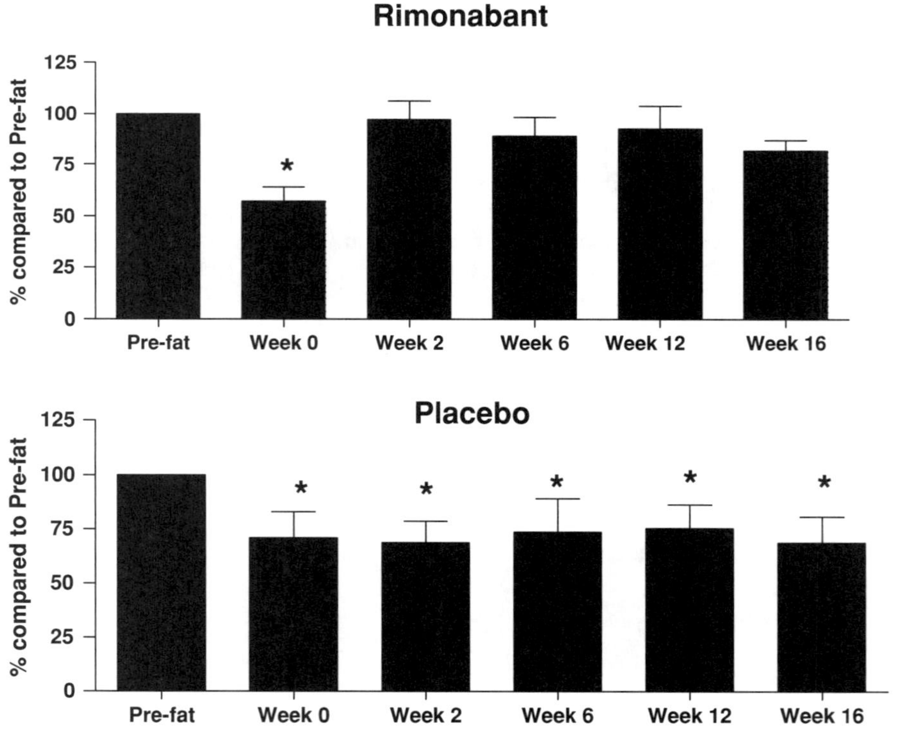

Figure 8 Effect of rimonabant on insulin sensitivity during sustained fat feeding. RIM promptly restores insulin sensitivity.

reduced insulin sensitivity was maintained in placebo animals, whereas the animals treated with RIM demonstrated a reversal, such that insulin sensitivity was returned to pre-fat values. It is likely that the effect of RIM to prevent a further reduction in insulin sensitivity was due, at least in part, to the switch from carbohydrate to fat utilization; it is also possible that adipokines may have played a role. In fact, we observed a significant 2-fold increase in adiponectin in the RIM-treated animals compared to controls. Thus, blockade of the CB_1 receptors resulted in a better metabolic profile due to improved insulin sensitivity, conversion from carbohydrate to fat oxidation, and elevated adiponectin.

Rimonabant Effects on Adipocytes and Liver

CB_1 blockade had remarkable restoration powers with regard to fat deposition in adipose tissue and liver. We were surprised to find that adipocyte size distribution of fat in visceral and subcutaneous depots was virtually restored to the pattern observed under control conditions—that is RIM reversed the rightward shift in visceral and subcutaneous size distribution which was caused by fat feeding, and which was continued with the high-fat diet in the absence of a CB_1 blocker. Similarly, we noted the evidence of reduced fat accumulation in liver tissues with RIM treatment. Further analysis is required to understand whether the positive effects of CB_1 blockade can be explained by increased adiponectin alone, or whether additional mechanisms are involved.

SUMMARY

The canine model serves as an excellent tool in attempting to unravel the complex relationship between obesity and insulin resistance. This animal model develops visceral and subcutaneous fat deposition when the diet is enriched with fat, even without an increase in total calories. The degree of obesity is reminiscent of that seen in humans and consequently associated with increased metabolic risks. Studies from our laboratory have demonstrated that increased fat deposition with fat feeding results in reduced insulin sensitivity as well as adverse morphological changes within adipocytes and the liver. Interestingly, the CB_1 receptor antagonist rimonabant has been shown to reverse diet-induced insulin resistance and also reverse the adverse changes observed in adipocytes and liver. How rimonabant produces these beneficial effects is not clearly understood, but changes in substrate utilization and adipokines may be the critical mediators. However, in light of the recent findings, understanding crosstalk between the endocannabinoid system and metabolism will be the key in attempting to unravel the complexities between obesity and disease risk.

REFERENCES

1. Wild S, Roglic G, Green A, et al. Global prevalence of diabetes: Estimates for the year 2000 and projections for 2030. Diabetes Care 2004; 27;1047–1053.
2. Wild SH, Forouhi NG. What is the scale of the future diabetes epidemic, and how certain are we about it? Diabetologia 2007; 50:903–905.
3. Bergman RN, Kim SP, Hsu IR, et al. Abdominal obesity: Role in the pathophysiology of metabolic disease and cardiovascular risk. Am J Med 2007; 120;S3–S8.
4. Hsu IR, Kim SP, Kabir M, et al. Metabolic syndrome, hyperinsulinemia, and cancer. Am J Clin Nutr 2007; 86:s867–s871.
5. Thygesen LC, Gronbaek M, Johansen C, et al. Prospective weight change and colon cancer risk in male US health professionals. Int J Cancer 2008; 123(5):1160–1165.
6. St Onge MP, Newcomer BR, Buchthal S, et al. Intramyocellular lipid content is lower with a low-fat diet than with high-fat diets, but that may not be relevant for health. Am J Clin Nutr 2007; 86:1316–1322.
7. Frazier DA. The link between fast food and the obesity epidemic. Health Matrix Clevel 2007; 17:291–317.
8. Maddock J. The relationship between obesity and the prevalence of fast food restaurants: State-level analysis. Am J Health Promot 2004; 19:137–143.
9. Kahn SE, Hull RL, Utzschneider KM. Mechanisms linking obesity to insulin resistance and type 2 diabetes. Nature 2006; 444:840–846.

10. Despres JP, Golay A, Sjostrom L. Effects of rimonabant on metabolic risk factors in overweight patients with dyslipidemia. N Engl J Med 2005; 353:2121–2134.
11. Pi-Sunyer FX, Aronne LJ, Heshmati HM, et al. Effect of rimonabant, a cannabinoid-1 receptor blocker, on weight and cardiometabolic risk factors in overweight or obese patients: RIO-North America: A randomized controlled trial. JAMA 2006; 295:761–775.
12. Bray GA, Jablonski KA, Fujimoto WY, et al. Relation of central adiposity and body mass index to the development of diabetes in the Diabetes Prevention Program. Am J Clin Nutr 2008; 87:1212–1218.
13. Haffner SM. Abdominal adiposity and cardiometabolic risk: Do we have all the answers? Am J Med 2007; 120;S10–S16.
14. Kim SP, Ellmerer M, Kirkman EL, et al. Beta-cell "rest" accompanies reduced first-pass hepatic insulin extraction in the insulin-resistant, fat-fed canine model. Am J Physiol Endocrinol Metab 2007; 292:E1581–E1589.
15. Bergman RN, Ader M, Huecking K, et al. Accurate assessment of beta-cell function: The hyperbolic correction. Diabetes 2002; 51(Suppl. 1):S212–S220.
16. Festa A, Williams K, Hanley AJ, et al. Beta-cell dysfunction in subjects with impaired glucose tolerance and early type 2 diabetes: Comparison of surrogate markers with first-phase insulin secretion from an intravenous glucose tolerance test. Diabetes 2008; 57:1638–1644.
17. Mittelman SD, Van Citters GW, Kirkman EL, et al. Extreme insulin resistance of the central adipose depot in vivo. Diabetes 2002; 51:755–761.
18. Kabir M, Catalano KJ, Ananthnarayan S, et al. Molecular evidence supporting the portal theory: A causative link between visceral adiposity and hepatic insulin resistance. Am J Physiol Endocrinol Metab 2005; 288:E454–E461.
19. Lewis GF, Vranic M, Harley P, et al. Fatty acids mediate the acute extrahepatic effects of insulin on hepatic glucose production in humans. Diabetes 1997; 46:1111–1119.
20. Getty L, Panteleon AE, Mittelman SD, et al. Rapid oscillations in omental lipolysis are independent of changing insulin levels in vivo. J Clin Invest 2000; 106;421–430.
21. Hucking K, Hamilton-Wessler M, Ellmerer M, et al. Burst-like control of lipolysis by the sympathetic nervous system in vivo. J Clin Invest 2003; 111;257–264.
22. Hsu IR, Zuniga E, Bergman RN. Importance of pulsatile changes in FFA for the enhancement of glucose output from the liver. Diabetes 2006; 55:A4.
23. Pagotto U, Marsicano G, Cota D, et al. The emerging role of the endocannabinoid system in endocrine regulation and energy balance. Endocr Rev 2006; 27:73–100.
24. Stefanovski D, Richey JM, Kim SP, et al. Rimonabant weight-loss independent effects on insulin action can be attributed to alterations in resting substrate utilization. Diabetes 2008; 57:A402.

12 Physical Activity in the Management of Visceral Obesity and Related Cardiometabolic Risk

Peter M. Janiszewski
School of Kinesiology and Health Studies, Queen's University, Kingston, Ontario, Canada

Robert Ross
School of Kinesiology and Health Studies, Department of Medicine, Division of Endocrinology and Metabolism, Queen's University, Kingston, Ontario, Canada

INTRODUCTION

Physical inactivity is a prominent risk factor for type 2 diabetes (1) and cardiovascular diseases (CVD) (2), and along with poor nutrition, is a leading cause of mortality in North America (3). Numerous health organizations promote the use of physical activity as a therapeutic strategy for the management of metabolic risk (4–6). Unfortunately, although physicians often counsel their at-risk patients regarding physical activity (7), these patients seldom adopt the recommended behavior (8). In fact, current estimates suggest that over half of Americans (51.9%) (9) and a similar proportion of Canadians (51.0%) (10) perform less than the recommended minimum of 30 minutes of moderate-intensity physical activity on most days of the week (11).

While the promotion of physical activity in today's environment remains a challenge, the utility of physical activity in the management of cardiometabolic risk is evident. Indeed, significant improvements in a number of cardiometabolic risk factors are observed after only a single session of moderate-intensity physical activity—improvements, which are further enhanced through chronic physical activity. While weight loss remains the desired outcome of chronic physical activity, mounting evidence also suggests that significant improvements in cardiometabolic risk can be achieved through physical activity in the absence of significant weight change. This chapter outlines the influence of aerobic-type physical activity without caloric restriction on cardiometabolic risk, with specific focus on visceral obesity, insulin resistance, dyslipidemia (triglycerides, HDL cholesterol, LDL cholesterol), elevated blood pressure, thrombosis, and inflammation.

VISCERAL OBESITY

It is suggested that visceral obesity represents a central component of cardiometabolic risk, one that is mechanistically linked to many other individual risk factors (12; see Chapter 1 in this volume). As reviewed here, an expanding literature base suggests that chronic physical activity with or without significant changes in body weight is associated with significant reductions in visceral obesity (13,14).

Chronic Physical Activity

It is reported that as little as 20 minutes of moderate-intensity daily physical activity with an energy expenditure of less than 1500 kcal/wk is generally associated with modest reductions in visceral fat (5–10%) (15,16). Not surprisingly, increasing physical activity to 60 min/day (energy expenditure of 3500–4500 kcal/wk), generally leads to much greater reductions in visceral fat (~30%) (17,18). Evidence from rigorously controlled physical activity studies suggests that the reduction in visceral fat approximates $1/10^{th}$ of the reduction in body weight (17,18). That is, as illustrated in Figure 1, for every 10 kg loss in body weight, visceral fat is reduced by about 1.5 kg in men and 1.0 kg in women (17,18). Since baseline visceral fat values predict the magnitude of reduction ($R^2 = 0.53$, $p < 0.001$; unpublished results), the greater relative reduction in visceral fat among men is likely a consequence of higher baseline values.

As a caveat to the above generalizations, the visceral fat changes reported across physical activity studies have been quite varied and inconsistent (+3.1% to −30.2% change) (18,19). Not surprisingly, attempts to derive a dose–response relationship between physical activity

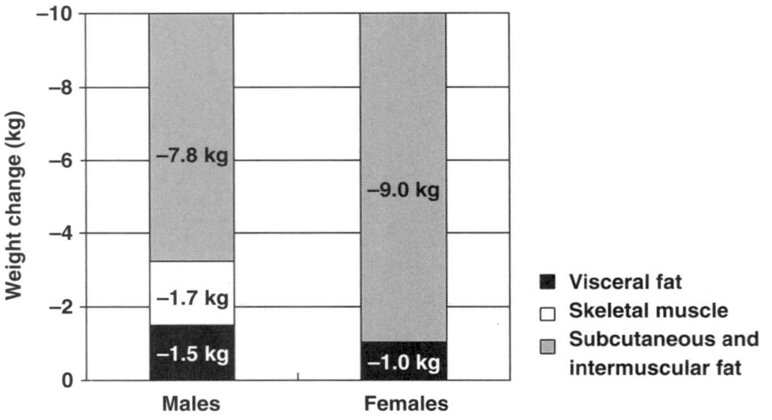

(A)

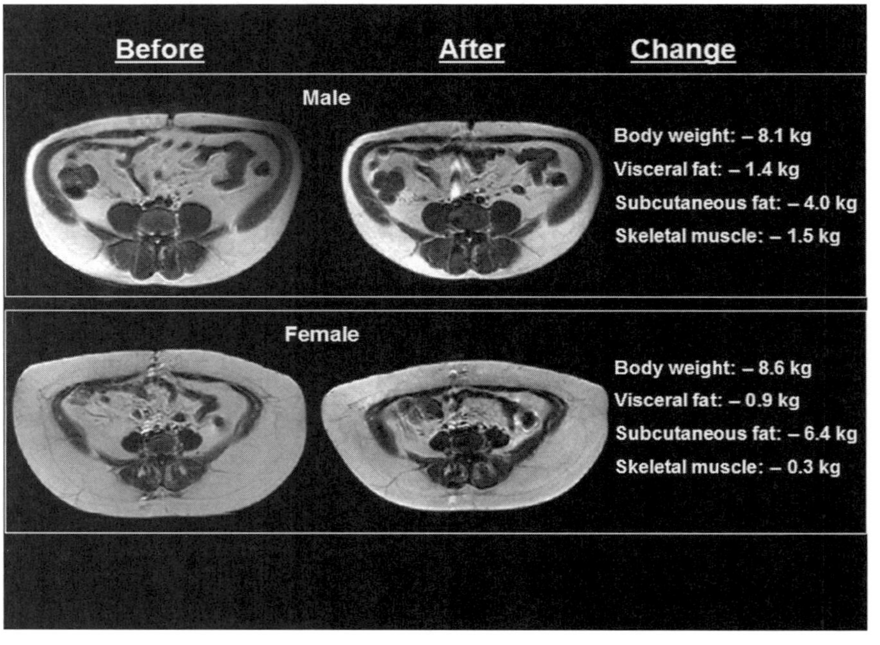

(B)

Figure 1 (A) Average composition of a 10-kg reduction in body weight due to regular physical activity in males and females. (B) An example of typical body composition changes due to a physical activity intervention in a male and female.

and visceral fat reduction have been unsuccessful (14,20). Indeed, the relationships between physical activity energy expenditure, weight loss, and visceral fat reduction are complex. Figure 2(A) documents the relationship between physical activity energy expenditure and consequent weight change derived from numerous intervention studies in nondiseased Caucasian samples conducted over the past 10 years (15,17–19,21–34). Surprisingly, there does not appear to be a significant relationship between physical activity energy expenditure and degree of weight loss across these studies ($R^2 = 0.10$, $p > 0.1$). Furthermore, as Figure 2(B) clearly shows, while those studies which report the greatest mean reduction in body weight generally observe the highest loss of visceral fat, weight change explains less than half (48%) of the variance in visceral fat change. Additionally, the variability noted between studies [Fig. 2(B)] masks the true extent of the variation in visceral fat reduction associated with physical activity–induced weight loss between individuals [Fig. 2(C)].

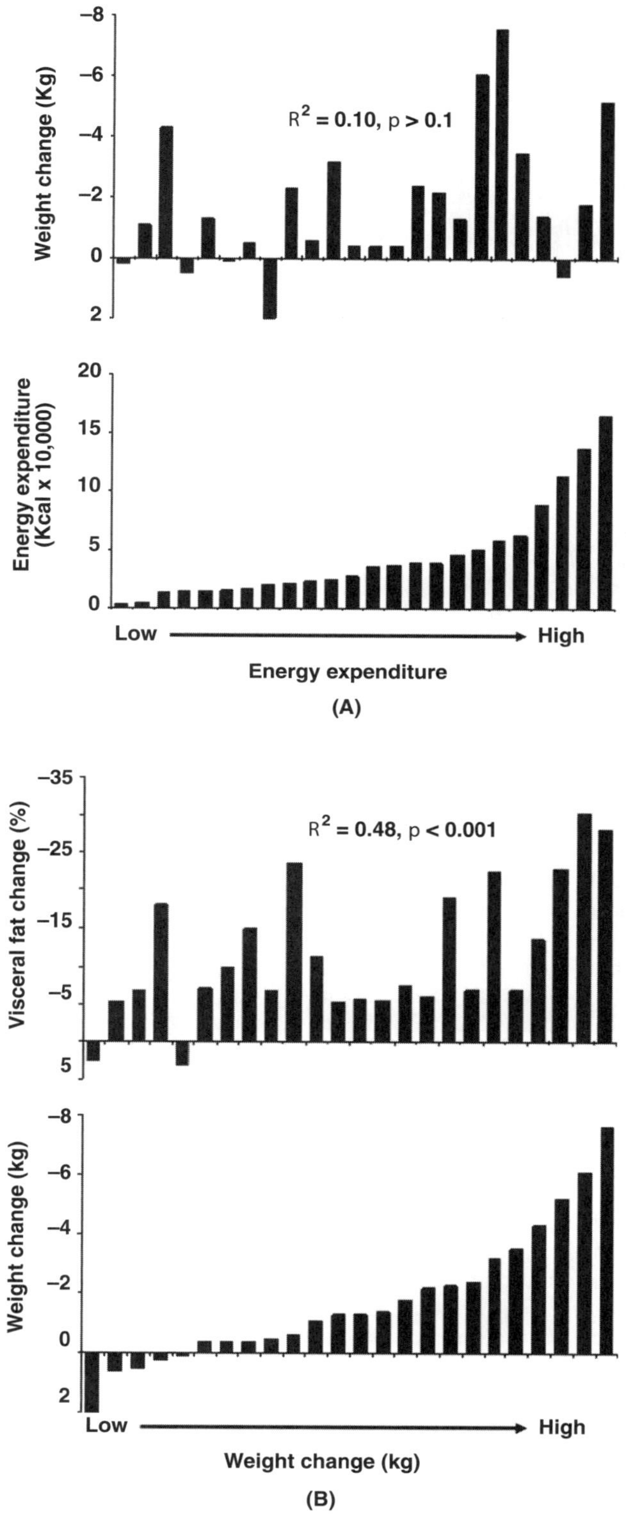

Figure 2 (A) Weight change with increasing energy expenditure across 24 physical activity intervention studies in healthy Caucasians from the past 10 years. (B) Visceral fat change with increasing weight loss across 24 physical activity intervention studies in healthy Caucasians from the past 10 years. (C) Visceral fat change with increasing weight loss in individuals undergoing physical activity intervention.

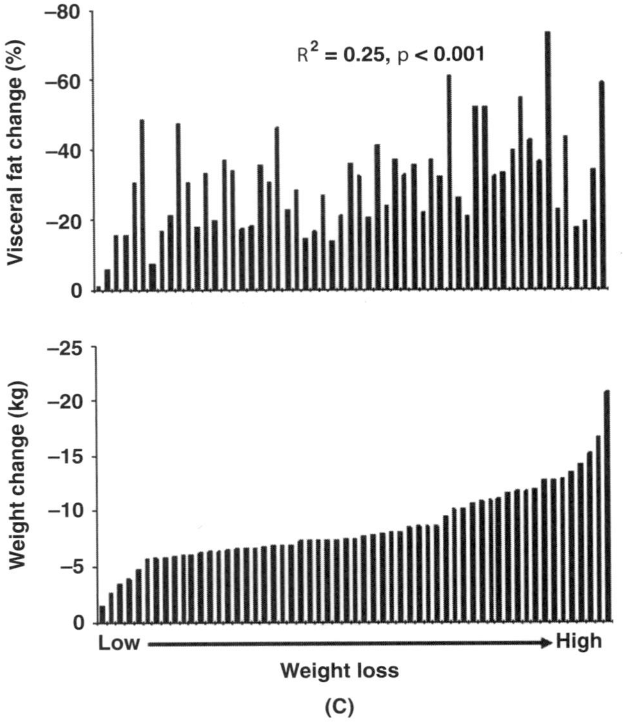

Figure 2 (*Continued*)

Accordingly, regular physical activity can often lead to marked reductions in visceral fat, even when body weight is largely unchanged. Findings from studies in type 2 diabetic subjects suggest that approximately 2 to 3 months of regular moderate-intensity aerobic exercise is associated with substantive reductions in visceral fat (−27% to −45%) despite little or no change in weight (25,35,36). Similar results have been documented in healthy nonobese premenopausal women (27) and middle-aged men (23). Furthermore, several studies have specifically examined the effect of physical activity on visceral obesity, independent of weight loss, by having study participants consume compensatory kilocalories equivalent to the amount expended during physical activity (17,18,25). These results suggest that in Caucasian lean and obese men and women, significant reductions in visceral fat (−10% to −19%) occur through 3–4 months of regular physical activity (40–60 min/day), despite no significant change in body weight.

In unison, the above observations clearly highlight the notion that changes in body composition rather than body weight are more meaningful outcomes in response to physical activity (13). In fact, significant reductions in fat mass, especially visceral fat, often occur concurrent with compensatory increases in lean body mass in response to physical activity (18). These equal but opposite changes in fat mass and lean mass are obviously undetected by alterations in body weight (18). Nevertheless, the reductions in visceral fat in response to physical activity are generally less among those who maintain body weight than those who lose significant amounts (17,18). Thus, while physical activity–induced weight loss is likely to be associated with the greatest reduction in visceral fat, it is equally important to recognize that visceral obesity can be markedly reduced in response to minimal weight loss.

INSULIN RESISTANCE

Insulin resistance has been postulated to represent the common soil for the development of both type 2 diabetes and CVD, and has also been regarded as a central tenet of cardiometabolic risk (37,38). Insulin resistance is well established as the key factor in the pathogenesis of impaired glucose tolerance, impaired fasting glucose and is the earliest detectable abnormality in the development of subsequent type 2 diabetes (39–41). As reviewed here, both an acute bout and/or chronic physical activity with or without significant changes in weight have been shown to significantly improve insulin sensitivity, and thereby reduce risk of diabetes (42).

Acute Physical Activity

Significant improvements in insulin resistance, as measured by the rate of glucose clearance during a euglycemic–hyperinsulinemic clamp, have been achieved after approximately 1 hour of moderate-intensity physical activity in healthy normoglycemic subjects (43,44), insulin-resistant subjects (45), and diabetics (44,46). The enhanced insulin sensitivity is not only present immediately after the acute exercise bout (44), but also appears to persist 20 to 48 hours postexercise (43,45,46). The magnitude of improvement in insulin sensitivity after a single exercise bout ranges from 15% (43) to 24% (44)—improvements, which are equivalent to those achieved through chronic pharmacological intervention (47,48). Although the exact influence of acute physical activity duration and/or intensity on insulin resistance has yet to be established (49), some report shows that higher intensity (70% Vo_{2max}) activity may provide the greatest improvements (50). A potential mechanism underlying the enhanced glucose disposal after an acute bout of physical activity may be the increased translocation of the glucose transporter GLUT-4 into the sarcolemma and the T-tubules of the muscle (51), the main site of insulin-stimulated glucose disposal (52). This enhanced translocation of GLUT-4 may occur due to physical activity–induced muscle contraction (53) and/or tissue hypoxia (54).

Chronic Physical Activity

In addition to the acute effect of exercise, repeated bouts of exercise over an extended period of time result in even greater improvements in insulin sensitivity. Indeed, approximately 3 to 4 months of daily aerobic exercise training inducing 6–8% body weight reduction was shown to improve insulin sensitivity by 32% and 60% in middle-aged women and men, respectively (17,18). It is noteworthy that measurements of insulin sensitivity in these studies were performed 4 days after the last physical activity session (17,18), and thus obviate the acute effects of the last activity session (discussed above). Thus, had insulin sensitivity been measured within 24 hours following the last physical activity bout, the cumulative effects of chronic and acute physical activity would have likely resulted in a greater improvement in insulin sensitivity than reported. Indeed, among sedentary and overweight men and women who underwent exercise interventions of varying volume and intensity, insulin sensitivity improved by as much as 85% when it was assessed 24 hours after the last bout of activity (55).

Several studies have also shown that improvements in insulin sensitivity through chronic exercise can occur in the absence of significant weight reduction (16,17,56,57). For example, 3 months of daily aerobic training in obese men, who consumed compensatory kilocalories equivalent to the amount expended during exercise, resulted in a 30% improvement in insulin sensitivity despite no change in weight (17).

The mechanisms behind the improvements in insulin sensitivity in response to chronic physical activity likely include changes in body composition, in particular reductions in visceral fat (17), an augmented expression of GLUT-4 protein in skeletal muscle (58,59), as well as enhanced metabolic efficiency of muscle (60,61). As described above, while the reduction in visceral fat is not incumbent on a significant reduction in body weight, the magnitude of visceral fat reduction is generally more substantive when body weight is also reduced (17,18). This may explain why reductions in insulin resistance in response to chronic physical activity are generally greater when body weight is significantly reduced.

In all, the beneficial effects of physical activity on insulin resistance may explain the results of a number of large studies (62,63), which report that physical activity can prevent the development of diabetes in predisposed patients. In fact, physical activity may reduce the risk of diabetes to a greater degree than what can be achieved through pharmacological intervention (62).

DYSLIPIDEMIA

The atherogenic lipid profile, consisting of hypertriglyceridemia, low levels of HDL cholesterol, and high levels of LDL cholesterol, in particular small and dense LDL particles, has been tied to abdominal obesity (64), insulin resistance (65), and cardiovascular-related morbidity and mortality (66). Additionally, levels of apolipoprotein B, the apolipoprotein moiety of the atherogenic lipoproteins (VLDL, IDL, and LDL), have been shown to predict CVD and related events, independent of traditional risk factors (67).

Acute Physical Activity

Subsequent to the seminal work of Holloszy et al. (68), numerous studies have reinforced the notion that a single bout of aerobic physical activity can lead to significant reductions in TG and increases in HDL-cholesterol levels (49). These lipid changes are apparent between 24 and 48 hours post acute physical activity in both untrained (69,70) and trained subjects (71) in response to caloric expenditures of 350–500 and 1000 kcal, respectively. Typical reductions in TG levels range in magnitude from about −10% to −25% (69–71), and are greatest among those with the highest baseline TG values (69). In comparison, increases in HDL-cholesterol postacute activity range from approximately 7% to 15% (69–71). These increases are largely due to the increase in the HDL_3-C subfraction among untrained subjects, in contrast to the predominant increase in HDL_2-C among trained subjects (72). While no minimum duration of physical activity appears to exist for inducing improvements in TG or HDL-C, generally, the greater the duration of the physical activity bout, and thus the greater the caloric expenditure, the more pronounced is the improvement in lipid levels (73). On the other hand, the intensity of the acute activity bout has not been shown to have a clear effect on the degree of lipid improvements (69).

Although reductions in LDL-C following extreme feats of physical activity (i.e., following a 42-km marathon) have been reported (74), more modest sessions of aerobic activity (350–500 kcal expenditures) have failed to note a change in LDL-C levels (69,70). Finally, in contrast to the reductions generally reported following chronic physical activity (discussed below), acute aerobic activity (inducing a 350-kcal energy expenditure) in both trained and untrained subjects has been reported to transiently elevate levels of apolipoprotein B by 4% to 9% (69,75).

Chronic Physical Activity

The evidence for beneficial lipid changes due to chronic physical activity is strongest for HDL-C and TG (76–80). A meta-analysis reveals that 30 to 60 minutes of aerobic physical activity, 3–5 times per week, at a moderate intensity results in a mean increase in HDL-cholesterol levels of ~4% (0.05 mmol/L), predominantly as a result of increases in the HDL_2-C subfraction (81,82), and a decrease in triglyceride levels of ~12% (0.21 mmol/L) (79). Others have concluded that physical activity, which induces an energy expenditure of 1200 to 2200 kcal/wk may bring about a 4% to 22% (0.05–0.21 mmol/L) increase in HDL-cholesterol levels, and a 4% to 37% (0.01–0.43 mmol/L) decrease in triglyceride levels (77). Considering that every 0.025 mmol/L increase in HDL-C has been shown to reduce risk of CVD by approximately 5% (83), these findings suggest that only a modest amount of physical activity is required to produce clinically significant improvements in HDL cholesterol and triglycerides. However, a clear dose–response relationship between duration of physical activity and lipid changes has yet to be established (78). Additionally, it is apparent that the relative intensity of the activity and the extent of the improvement in cardiorespiratory fitness in response to training has little, if any influence on lipid changes (84).

In contrast to the consistent findings for HDL-C and TG, the preponderance of available evidence suggests that chronic physical activity does not significantly alter the levels of LDL cholesterol (77,79). However, an elevated proportion of small, dense LDL particles has been shown to predict incidence of CVD independently of total LDL cholesterol levels (85). It is thus noteworthy that irrespective of training intensity and clinically significant weight loss, 25 minutes of daily aerobic activity can increase the mean LDL particle size without altering total LDL-cholesterol levels (84).

Additionally, cross-sectional studies suggest that those who are most active tend to have the lowest apolipoprotein B levels (86,87). A number of exercise intervention studies (88–90) have also shown physical activity to significantly reduce apolipoprotein B levels by a magnitude of 7% to 20%. This reduction appears to be the greatest among those with elevated baseline triglyceride concentrations (91).

It has previously been suggested that physical activity–induced weight loss must be achieved in order to bring about significant improvements in lipid status (76). However, others have concluded that while improvements in HDL-C and TG are generally greater in those who lose weight, these improvements can be seen even when weight remains virtually unchanged (77,79,84). For example, a number of physical activity interventions that do not significantly alter body weight have documented −5% to −35% reductions in TG levels (29,92) and/or 3% to 5% increases in HDL values (27,92). Additionally, others have failed to note a correlation between reductions in body weight and changes in TG, HDL-C, and apolipoprotein B (75). Finally, significant increases in the average LDL-C particle size have also been noted in response to physical activity consequent to clinically insignificant weight changes (<2% reduction) (84).

These lipid improvements, independent of significant weight reduction, may be mediated by improvements in body composition, such as reductions in visceral fat and/or improvements in cardiorespiratory fitness (17,18). Indeed, physical activity–induced reductions in visceral fat have been shown to independently predict improvements in lipid status (93). Additionally, while the improvement in cardiorespiratory fitness in response to training has apparently little influence on TG and HDL-C changes (84), the reduction in apolipoprotein B levels has been reported to correlate with improvement in cardiorespiratory fitness, independent of changes in abdominal obesity (88).

ELEVATED BLOOD PRESSURE

High blood pressure is an established risk factor for stroke, coronary heart disease, and renal disease, and its reduction is associated with a significant decrease in the risk of cardiovascular-related morbidity and mortality (94). Furthermore, the magnitude of blood pressure reduction need not be large in order to see significant decrements in associated health risk (95). Inactivity is a major risk factor for high blood pressure, and sedentary individuals have up to a 50% greater chance of hypertension as compared to more active counterparts (96).

Acute Physical Activity

The lowering effect of blood pressure resulted from a single bout of aerobic physical activity has been long established (97). This effect, termed postexercise hypotension, is especially pronounced among hypertensive individuals with documented maximal reductions in systolic blood pressure (SBP) and diastolic blood pressure (DBP) of −11 and −6 mmHg, respectively (98,99). However, averaged across studies in both normotensive and hypertensive subjects, documented reductions in SBP and DBP following a single activity session tend to be more modest −2.1 and −0.3 mmHg, respectively (49). These rather modest average estimates are largely due to the nonsignificant changes in blood pressure in response to acute activity among studies of normotensive samples (49). The onset of postexercise hypotension is immediate and can persist for up to 22 hours after an acute bout of aerobic physical activity (100). Available evidence suggests that as little as 15 minutes of low intensity (40% of maximal oxygen consumption) aerobic physical activity can induce marked postexercise hypotension that persist throughout the day (101). These encouraging results suggest that independent of any training effects, repeated bouts of aerobic physical activity may be a viable treatment strategy for the treatment of mild hypertension (102).

Chronic Physical Activity

It is well documented that regular aerobic physical activity consistently leads to reductions in blood pressure (103–109). In fact, chronic physical activity has been shown to reduce both SBP and DBP in lean (103,108), obese (103,108), hypertensive (103,106,107), and normotensive (103,104,106) subjects. The results of various reviews and meta-analyses suggest that independent of age and body mass index, 40 minutes of moderate-intensity physical activity performed 3 times per week reduces SBP by a range from −3 to −11 mmHg and DBP by −3 to −8 mmHg (103–109). Further, the blood pressure reductions are significantly greater among hypertensive versus normotensive subjects (−7 and −5 mmHg vs. −2 and −2 mmHg reductions in SBP and DBP, respectively) (109). In contrast to the short duration of postexercise hypotension, the blood pressure reductions of chronic physical activity can take up to 2 weeks of inactivity to fully dissipate (110).

Interestingly, the training-induced blood pressure reductions do not appear to be related to alterations in body weight or abdominal obesity (109). In fact, it is noteworthy that the average weight loss across studies included in the meta-analyses of physical activity and blood pressure (discussed above) was largely inconsequential (−1.2 kg) (109). Nevertheless, some studies report that individuals who become active and also lose a significant amount of weight (−7.9 kg) in comparison to those who lose minimal weight (−1.8 kg) show greater reductions in SBP and DBP (−7 and −5 mmHg vs. −4 and −4 mmHg, respectively) (111). Thus, it is plausible that physical activity and weight loss may have additive effects on blood pressure reduction (111). On the other hand, reductions in blood pressure have been shown to be significantly related to training-induced improvements in cardiorespiratory fitness (109).

Specifically, mean blood pressure is dictated by the product of cardiac output (heart rate and stroke volume) and systemic vascular resistance. It appears that the blood pressure reductions in response to chronic physical activity are the result of reduced systemic vascular resistance but unchanged cardiac output (due to equal but opposite changes in heart rate and stroke volume) (109). The changes in systemic peripheral resistance with physical activity may be attributable to alterations in autonomic nervous system activity, renin–angiotensin system activity, and/or endothelial function (109).

With regard to ideal physical activity training parameters, most reports have suggested that low-to-moderate intensity is ideal for inducing reductions in blood pressure (103,107), but other parameters (duration, frequency) have no clear impact on the level of improvement (103,108,112). Overall, it can be concluded that chronic physical activity of low-to-moderate intensity induces modest reductions in blood pressure, but it rarely decreases to sufficient magnitude to bring about normal blood pressure in previously hypertensive individuals (113). Nevertheless, given that a 2 mmHg reduction in SBP is associated with a 4–6% lower risk of mortality due to stroke and coronary heart disease (114), the blood pressure changes associated with chronic physical activity, while modest, are clinically significant.

THROMBOSIS

Thrombosis, or the formation of a blood clot in an intact blood vessel, is a key antecedent to stroke, myocardial infarction, and other overt symptoms of blood flow obstruction throughout the circulatory system (115). The process of thrombus formation is dependent on the balance between the opposing coagulatory (clot forming) and fibrinolytic (clot dissolving) systems, as well as the influence of blood platelets.

Acute Physical Activity

The notion of acute physical activity acting as a trigger for myocardial infarction is established (116). Indeed, while physical inactivity is a major risk factor for thrombosis, an acute bout of strenuous physical activity among sedentary and at-risk individuals has been reported to lead to a prothrombotic state, and predispose to cardiovascular events (115,117). Interestingly, a single bout of physical activity appears to simultaneously augment both coagulation and fibrinolysis (118,119). However, while increased coagulation persists into the recovery period, the enhanced fibrinolysis quickly dissipates, thus providing an ideal environment for clot formation postactivity (118,119). Additionally, acute physical activity can also increase blood platelet adhesiveness and aggregation (120), changes which may further predispose to a cardiovascular event (121). Nevertheless, numerous potential factors can influence the effect of acute physical activity on thrombosis such as baseline fitness and intensity of the activity (115). For example, a number of studies (122,123) have documented that while acute moderate intensity (55–65% Vo_{2max}) physical activity can lead to improved fibrinolysis and attenuated platelet adhesiveness and aggregation, high intensity (80% Vo_{2max}) exercise can induce the opposite effect resulting in a prothrombotic state.

Chronic Physical Activity

Cross-sectional studies (124,125) regularly document an anti-thrombotic effect of chronic physical activity, in particular lower coaguability along with a higher fibrinolytic capacity. Additionally, numerous intervention studies have documented an enhanced fibrinolytic capacity following physical activity training, as indicated by an increase in tissue plasminogen activator (a fibrolytic stimulator) and a decrease in its inhibitor (plasminogen activator inhibitor-1) (126–128). Further, chronic aerobic physical activity at a moderate intensity also appears to suppress platelet adhesiveness and aggregation at rest and following acute intense physical activity (129,130), and thus may attenuate the cardiovascular risk associated with an acute bout of high-intensity activity. Emerging evidence also suggests that chronic physical activity may increase levels of adiponectin (131), a cytokine released from adipose tissue which may act to decrease thrombosis and platelet aggregation (132). Nevertheless, the effects of chronic exercise on these hemostatic factors are reversed to pre-training values within 4 weeks of cessation of regular physical activity (129,130), and suggest that regular exercise must be maintained for sustained anti-thrombotic effects. Lastly, although weight reduction has been shown to lead to improvement in hemostatic factors (133), the independent effects of chronic physical activity and weight reduction on thrombosis are largely unknown.

SYSTEMIC INFLAMMATION

Systemic inflammation may be a common thread linking various cardiometabolic risk factors including insulin resistance, obesity, and dyslipidemia (134). Chronic low-grade inflammation, as evidenced by the increased concentration of proinflammatory markers such as C-reactive protein (CRP), tumor necrosis factor-α (TNF-α), and interleukin-6 (IL-6) among others, may also be a causal factor in the development of atherosclerosis (135).

Acute Physical Activity

Similar to the evidence for thrombosis, an acute bout of physical activity has been shown to lead to an overall proinflammatory state, as evidenced by significantly elevated (up to 2000%) levels of CRP postactivity (136). The magnitude of the spike in inflammation due to physical activity depends highly on activity intensity, duration, the mass of the muscles recruited, and cardiorespiratory fitness of the participant (137,138). An approximately 100-fold increase of IL-6 is the most immediate and pronounced inflammatory marker response to acute activity (139)—an effect which can directly augment CRP levels by promoting its production by the liver (140). It is thought that the combination of muscle injury and the process of muscle contraction are likely responsible for the rise in IL-6 during acute physical activity (138). Interestingly, acute physical activity is also associated with elevations in numerous anti-inflammatory markers (i.e., IL-10) as well as inhibitors of proinflammatory markers (i.e., IL-1 receptor antagonist) (139). This simultaneous increase in anti-inflammatory mediators may, via counter-regulation, act to limit the extent and duration of the inflammatory response to acute physical activity (136).

Chronic Physical Activity

Counter to the proinflammatory effect of acute physical activity, numerous cross-sectional studies have documented an inverse relationship between levels of chronic exercise and systemic levels of inflammatory markers (141–144). Paradoxically, given that high-intensity acute activity results in the greatest inflammatory response (138), in reference to chronic physical activity, vigorous intensity appears to be superior to low or moderate intensity for the reduction of inflammation (145). Additionally, only a limited number of intervention studies have examined the effect of exercise training on systemic inflammation (143,146–148). Most (143,146,148,149), but not all (147,150), exercise interventions ranging in duration from 3 to 9 months reported significant reductions in inflammatory status postintervention. Chronic physical activity also appears to blunt the acute inflammatory response to a single strenuous bout of activity (151). However, it is suggested that physical activity–induced improvements in inflammatory status may be exclusive to individuals with high levels of inflammatory markers at baseline (148). The magnitude of reduction in the levels of inflammatory markers postexercise intervention appears to be around 25% to 48% (143,146,148,149). In all, the available evidence would support the contention that regular exercise, of sufficient intensity, appears to be anti-inflammatory in nature (152).

A recent systematic review concluded that weight reduction is linearly associated with decrements in CRP, such that for every 1-kg reduction in body weight, CRP levels fell by −0.13 mg/L (153). However, others (154–156) have shown that increases in physical activity and reductions in body weight are independently predictive of improvements in inflammatory status, suggesting that in the absence of body-weight change, chronic physical activity may reduce inflammatory markers. Nonetheless, some have also noted that without significant weight loss, chronic physical activity appears to have no effect on inflammatory status (150,157).

Table 1 Summary of the Effects of Physical Activity on Cardiometabolic Risk

	Visceral obesity	Insulin resistance	Dyslipidemia	Blood pressure	Thrombosis	Inflammation
Acute physical activity	NA	Improvements of 15–24% lasting up to 48hr postactivity	TG reduced by 10–25% HDL increased by 7–15%	Across studies: SBP/DBP = −2.1/−0.3 mmHg Among hypertensives SBP/DBP = −11/−6 mmHg	High intensity: prothrombotic Low-moderate intensity: anti-thrombotic	Stimulation of mainly proin-flammatory but also anti-inflammatory markers Largely mediated by increase in IL-6 production
Chronic physical activity	20min/day = 5–10% reduction 60 min/day = 30% reduction 1–1.5 kg of visceral fat lost for every 1 kg of weight loss	Improvements of 32–85% with modest weight loss	TG reduced by 4–37% HDL increased by 4–22% Increased mean LDL particle size Apolipoprotein B reduced by 7–20%	SBP reduced by 3–11 mmHg DBP reduced by 3–8 mmHg Reductions more pronounced in hypertensives	Anti-thrombotic Enhanced fibrinolytic capacity Suppressed platelet adhesiveness and aggregation	Reduction in inflammatory markers of 25–48% Reduced proinflamma-tory response to acute activity

Thus, it remains unclear whether chronic physical activity independent of significant weight loss has an effect on reducing systemic inflammation.

LIMITATIONS

The preponderance of evidence presented in this chapter is derived from samples of middle-aged Caucasians. Additionally, the evaluation of how gender, race, and age mediates the relationships between physical activity and the cardiometabolic risk factors discussed is beyond the scope of this chapter. Nevertheless, limited evidence suggests that interventions consisting of physical activity appear to be effective in the treatment of cardiometabolic risk irrespective of gender and race (158).

CONCLUSION

An acute bout of physical activity has clear beneficial implications for insulin resistance, elevated blood pressure, and dyslipidemia, while a strenuous activity bout may induce a transiently proinflammatory and prothrombotic state. Further, chronic physical activity is associated with beneficial effects on all cardiometabolic risk factors discussed, including thrombosis and inflammation. Although the improvements in cardiometabolic risk factors with chronic physical activity tend to be more pronounced when a modest reduction in body weight is achieved; significant reductions in visceral obesity, insulin resistance, dyslipidemia, and blood pressure are also observed in the absence of significant weight change. These observations (summarized in Table 1) reinforce the recommendation that regular, moderate-intensity physical activity be used as a therapeutic strategy for the reduction of global cardiometabolic risk.

REFERENCES

1. Helmrich SP, Ragland DR, Leung RW, et al. Physical activity and reduced occurrence of non-insulin-dependent diabetes mellitus. N Engl J Med 1991; 325(3):147–152.

2. Paffenbarger RS, Jr., Wing AL, Hyde RT. Physical activity as an index of heart attack risk in college alumni, 1978. Am J Epidemiol 1995; 142(9):889–903; discussion 887–888.
3. Mokdad AH, Marks JS, Stroup DF, et al. Actual causes of death in the United States, 2000. JAMA 2004; 291(10):1238–1245.
4. Executive summary of the third report of the National Cholesterol Education Program (NCEP) Expert Panel on detection, evaluation, and treatment of high blood cholesterol in adults (Adult Treatment Panel III). JAMA 2001; 285(19):2486–2497.
5. Grundy SM, Brewer HB, Jr., Cleeman JI, et al. Definition of metabolic syndrome: Report of the National Heart, Lung, and Blood Institute/American Heart Association conference on scientific issues related to definition. Circulation 2004; 109(3):433–438.
6. Grundy SM, Hansen B, Smith SC, Jr., et al. Clinical management of metabolic syndrome: Report of the American Heart Association/National Heart, Lung, and Blood Institute/American Diabetes Association conference on scientific issues related to management. Circulation 2004; 109(4):551–556.
7. Petrella RJ, Lattanzio CN, Overend TJ. Physical activity counseling and prescription among canadian primary care physicians. Arch Intern Med 2007; 167(16):1774–1781.
8. Effects of physical activity counseling in primary care: The activity counseling trial: a randomized controlled trial. JAMA 2001; 286(6):677–687.
9. U.S. Physical Activity Statistics. Department of Health and Human Services, 2005. (Accessed May 17, 2007, at http://apps.nccd. cdc.gov/PASurveillance/StateSumResultV.asp?CI=&Year=2005&State=0#data.)
10. Canadian Fitness and Lifestyle Research Institutes. Physical activity among Canadians: The current situation 2005.
11. Pate RR, Pratt M, Blair SN, et al. Physical activity and public health. A recommendation from the Centers for Disease Control and Prevention and the American College of Sports Medicine. JAMA 1995; 273(5):402–407.
12. Despres JP. Abdominal obesity: The most prevalent cause of the metabolic syndrome and related cardiometabolic risk. Eur Heart J Suppl 2006; 8(Suppl. B):B4–B12.
13. Janiszewski PM, Ross R. Physical activity in the treatment of obesity: Beyond body weight reduction. Applied physiology, nutrition, and metabolism. Physiologie appliquee, nutrition et metabolisme 2007; 32(3):512–522.
14. Ross R, Janssen I. Physical activity, total and regional obesity: Dose–response considerations. Med Sci Sports Exerc 2001; 33(6 Suppl.):S521–S527; discussion S8–S9.
15. Irwin ML, Yasui Y, Ulrich CM, et al. Effect of exercise on total and intra-abdominal body fat in postmenopausal women: A randomized controlled trial. JAMA 2003; 289(3):323–330.
16. Giannopoulou I, Ploutz-Snyder LL, Carhart R, et al. Exercise is required for visceral fat loss in postmenopausal women with type 2 diabetes. J Clin Endocrinol Metab 2005; 90(3):1511–1518.
17. Ross R, Dagnone D, Jones PJ, et al. Reduction in obesity and related comorbid conditions after diet-induced weight loss or exercise-induced weight loss in men. A randomized, controlled trial. Ann Intern Med 2000; 133(2):92–103.
18. Ross R, Janssen I, Dawson J, et al. Exercise-induced reduction in obesity and insulin resistance in women: A randomized controlled trial. Obes Res 2004; 12(5):789–798.
19. Green JS, Stanforth PR, Rankinen T, et al. The effects of exercise training on abdominal visceral fat, body composition, and indicators of the metabolic syndrome in postmenopausal women with and without estrogen replacement therapy: The HERITAGE family study. Metabolism 2004; 53(9):1192–1196.
20. Ohkawara K, Tanaka S, Miyachi M, et al. A dose–response relation between aerobic exercise and visceral fat reduction: Systematic review of clinical trials. Int J Obes (Lond) 2007; 31(12):1786–1797.
21. Poehlman ET, Dvorak RV, DeNino WF, et al. Effects of resistance training and endurance training on insulin sensitivity in nonobese, young women: A controlled randomized trial. J Clin Endocrinol Metab 2000; 85(7):2463–2468.
22. Donnelly JE, Hill JO, Jacobsen DJ, et al. Effects of a 16-month randomized controlled exercise trial on body weight and composition in young, overweight men and women: The Midwest Exercise Trial. Arch Intern Med 2003; 163(11):1343–1350.
23. Shojaee-Moradie F, Baynes KC, Pentecost C, et al. Exercise training reduces fatty acid availability and improves the insulin sensitivity of glucose metabolism. Diabetologia 2007; 50(2):404–413.
24. Wilmore JH, Despres JP, Stanforth PR, et al. Alterations in body weight and composition consequent to 20 wk of endurance training: The HERITAGE Family Study. Am J Clin Nutr 1999; 70(3):346–352.
25. Lee S, Kuk JL, Davidson LE, et al. Exercise without weight loss is an effective strategy for obesity reduction in obese individuals with and without type 2 diabetes. J Appl Physiol 2005; 99(3):1220–1225.
26. Short KR, Vittone JL, Bigelow ML, et al. Impact of aerobic exercise training on age-related changes in insulin sensitivity and muscle oxidative capacity. Diabetes 2003; 52(8):1888–1896.
27. Thomas EL, Brynes AE, McCarthy J, et al. Preferential loss of visceral fat following aerobic exercise, measured by magnetic resonance imaging. Lipids 2000; 35(7):769–776.

28. Halverstadt A, Phares DA, Ferrell RE, et al. High-density lipoprotein-cholesterol, its subfractions, and responses to exercise training are dependent on endothelial lipase genotype. Metabolism 2003; 52(11):1505–1511.
29. Gan SK, Kriketos AD, Ellis BA, et al. Changes in aerobic capacity and visceral fat but not myocyte lipid levels predict increased insulin action after exercise in overweight and obese men. Diabetes Care 2003; 26(6):1706–1713.
30. Hays NP, Starling RD, Sullivan DH, et al. Effects of an ad libitum, high carbohydrate diet and aerobic exercise training on insulin action and muscle metabolism in older men and women. J Gerontol A Biol Sci Med Sci 2006; 61(3):299–304.
31. Slentz CA, Duscha BD, Johnson JL, et al. Effects of the amount of exercise on body weight, body composition, and measures of central obesity: STRRIDE—A randomized controlled study. Arch Intern Med 2004; 164(1):31–39.
32. Stewart KJ, Bacher AC, Turner K, et al. Exercise and risk factors associated with metabolic syndrome in older adults. Am J Prev Med 2005; 28(1):9–18.
33. O'Leary VB, Marchetti CM, Krishnan RK, et al. Exercise-induced reversal of insulin resistance in obese elderly is associated with reduced visceral fat. J Appl Physiol 2006; 100(5):1584–1589.
34. McTiernan A, Sorensen B, Irwin ML, et al. Exercise effect on weight and body fat in men and women. Obesity (Silver Spring) 2007; 15(6):1496–1512.
35. Boudou P, Sobngwi E, Mauvais-Jarvis F, et al. Absence of exercise-induced variations in adiponectin levels despite decreased abdominal adiposity and improved insulin sensitivity in type 2 diabetic men. Eur J Endocrinol 2003; 149(5):421–424.
36. Mourier A, Gautier JF, De Kerviler E, et al. Mobilization of visceral adipose tissue related to the improvement in insulin sensitivity in response to physical training in NIDDM. Effects of branched-chain amino acid supplements. Diabetes Care 1997; 20(3):385–391.
37. Reaven GM. Banting lecture 1988. Role of insulin resistance in human disease. Diabetes 1988; 37(12):1595–1607.
38. DeFronzo RA. Insulin resistance, hyperinsulinemia, and coronary artery disease: A complex metabolic web. J Cardiovasc Pharmacol 1992; 20(Suppl. 11):S1–S16.
39. DeFronzo RA, Bonadonna RC, Ferrannini E. Pathogenesis of NIDDM. A balanced overview. Diabetes Care 1992; 15(3):318–368.
40. Lillioja S, Mott DM, Spraul M, et al. Insulin resistance and insulin secretory dysfunction as precursors of non-insulin-dependent diabetes mellitus. Prospective studies of Pima Indians. N Engl J Med 1993; 329(27):1988–1992.
41. Report of the expert committee on the diagnosis and classification of diabetes mellitus. Diabetes Care 2003; 26(Suppl. 1):S5–S20.
42. Henriksen EJ. Invited review: Effects of acute exercise and exercise training on insulin resistance. J Appl Physiol 2002; 93(2):788–796.
43. Mikines KJ, Sonne B, Farrell PA, et al. Effect of physical exercise on sensitivity and responsiveness to insulin in humans. Am J Physiol 1988; 254(3 Pt 1):E248–E259.
44. Burstein R, Epstein Y, Shapiro Y, et al. Effect of an acute bout of exercise on glucose disposal in human obesity. J Appl Physiol 1990; 69(1):299–304.
45. Perseghin G, Price TB, Petersen KF, et al. Increased glucose transport-phosphorylation and muscle glycogen synthesis after exercise training in insulin-resistant subjects. N Engl J Med 1996; 335(18):1357–1362.
46. Devlin JT, Hirshman M, Horton ED, et al. Enhanced peripheral and splanchnic insulin sensitivity in NIDDM men after single bout of exercise. Diabetes 1987; 36(4):434–439.
47. Widen EI, Eriksson JG, Groop LC. Metformin normalizes nonoxidative glucose metabolism in insulin-resistant normoglycemic first-degree relatives of patients with NIDDM. Diabetes 1992; 41(3):354–358.
48. Nolan JJ, Ludvik B, Beerdsen P, et al. Improvement in glucose tolerance and insulin resistance in obese subjects treated with troglitazone. N Engl J Med 1994; 331(18):1188–1193.
49. Thompson PD, Crouse SF, Goodpaster B, et al. The acute versus the chronic response to exercise. Med Sci Sports Exerc 2001; 33(6 Suppl.):S438–S445; discussion S52–S53.
50. Kang J, Robertson RJ, Hagberg JM, et al. Effect of exercise intensity on glucose and insulin metabolism in obese individuals and obese NIDDM patients. Diabetes Care 1996; 19(4):341–349.
51. Kennedy JW, Hirshman MF, Gervino EV, et al. Acute exercise induces GLUT4 translocation in skeletal muscle of normal human subjects and subjects with type 2 diabetes. Diabetes 1999; 48(5):1192–1197.
52. Baron AD, Brechtel G, Wallace P, Edelman SV. Rates and tissue sites of non-insulin- and insulin-mediated glucose uptake in humans. Am J Physiol 1988; 255(6 Pt 1):E769–E774.
53. Gao J, Ren J, Gulve EA, et al. Additive effect of contractions and insulin on GLUT-4 translocation into the sarcolemma. J Appl Physiol 1994; 77(4):1597–1601.
54. Cartee GD, Douen AG, Ramlal T, et al. Stimulation of glucose transport in skeletal muscle by hypoxia. J Appl Physiol 1991; 70(4):1593–1600.

55. Houmard JA, Tanner CJ, Slentz CA, et al. Effect of the volume and intensity of exercise training on insulin sensitivity. J Appl Physiol 2004; 96(1):101–106.
56. Boudou P, De Kerviler E, Vexiau P, et al. Effects of a single bout of exercise and exercise training on steroid levels in middle-aged type 2 diabetic men: Relationship to abdominal adipose tissue distribution and metabolic status. Diabetes Metab 2000; 26(6):450–457.
57. Dengel DR, Pratley RE, Hagberg JM, et al. Distinct effects of aerobic exercise training and weight loss on glucose homeostasis in obese sedentary men. J Appl Physiol 1996; 81(1):318–325.
58. Houmard JA, Shinebarger MH, Dolan PL, et al. Exercise training increases GLUT-4 protein concentration in previously sedentary middle-aged men. Am J Physiol 1993; 264(6 Pt 1):E896–E901.
59. Hughes VA, Fiatarone MA, Fielding RA, et al. Exercise increases muscle GLUT-4 levels and insulin action in subjects with impaired glucose tolerance. Am J Physiol 1993; 264(6 Pt 1):E855–E862.
60. Menshikova EV, Ritov VB, Toledo FG, et al. Effects of weight loss and physical activity on skeletal muscle mitochondrial function in obesity. Am J Physiol Endocrinol Metab 2005; 288(4):E818–E825.
61. Toledo FG, Menshikova EV, Ritov VB, et al. Effects of physical activity and weight loss on skeletal muscle mitochondria and relationship with glucose control in type 2 diabetes. Diabetes 2007; 56(8):2142–2147.
62. Knowler WC, Barrett-Connor E, Fowler SE, et al. Reduction in the incidence of type 2 diabetes with lifestyle intervention or metformin. N Engl J Med 2002; 346(6):393–403.
63. Tuomilehto J, Lindstrom J, Eriksson JG, et al. Prevention of type 2 diabetes mellitus by changes in lifestyle among subjects with impaired glucose tolerance. N Engl J Med 2001; 344(18):1343–1350.
64. Sattar N, Tan CE, Han TS, et al. Associations of indices of adiposity with atherogenic lipoprotein subfractions. Int J Obes Relat Metab Disord 1998; 22(5):432–439.
65. Howard BV, Mayer-Davis EJ, Goff D, et al. Relationships between insulin resistance and lipoproteins in nondiabetic African Americans, Hispanics, and non-Hispanic whites: The insulin resistance atherosclerosis study. Metabolism 1998; 47(10):1174–1179.
66. Lehto S, Ronnemaa T, Haffner SM, et al. Dyslipidemia and hyperglycemia predict coronary heart disease events in middle-aged patients with NIDDM. Diabetes 1997; 46(8):1354–1359.
67. Lamarche B, Moorjani S, Lupien PJ, et al. Apolipoprotein A-I and B levels and the risk of ischemic heart disease during a five-year follow-up of men in the Quebec cardiovascular study. Circulation 1996; 94(3):273–278.
68. Holloszy JO, Skinner JS, Toro G, et al. Effects of a six month program of endurance exercise on the serum lipids of middle-aged man. Am J Cardiol 1964; 14:753–760.
69. Crouse SF, O'Brien BC, Rohack JJ, et al. Changes in serum lipids and apolipoproteins after exercise in men with high cholesterol: Influence of intensity. J Appl Physiol 1995; 79(1):279–286.
70. Grandjean PW, Crouse SF, Rohack JJ. Influence of cholesterol status on blood lipid and lipoprotein enzyme responses to aerobic exercise. J Appl Physiol 2000; 89(2):472–480.
71. Bounds RG, Grandjean PW, O'Brien BC, et al. Diet and short term plasma lipoprotein-lipid changes after exercise in trained men. Int J Sport Nutr Exer Metab 2000; 10(2):114–127.
72. Kantor MA, Cullinane EM, Sady SP, et al. Exercise acutely increases high density lipoprotein-cholesterol and lipoprotein lipase activity in trained and untrained men. Metabolism 1987; 36(2):188–192.
73. Cullinane E, Siconolfi S, Saritelli A, et al. Acute decrease in serum triglycerides with exercise: Is there a threshold for an exercise effect? Metabolism 1982; 31(8):844–847.
74. Goodyear LJ, Van Houten DR, Fronsoe MS, et al. Immediate and delayed effects of marathon running on lipids and lipoproteins in women. Med Sci Sports Exerc 1990; 22(5):588–592.
75. Crouse SF, O'Brien BC, Grandjean PW, et al. Effects of training and a single session of exercise on lipids and apolipoproteins in hypercholesterolemic men. J Appl Physiol 1997; 83(6):2019–2028.
76. Stefanick ML. Physical activity for preventing and treating obesity-related dyslipoproteinemias. Med Sci Sports Exerc 1999; 31(11 Suppl.):S609–S618.
77. Durstine JL, Grandjean PW, Davis PG, et al. Blood lipid and lipoprotein adaptations to exercise: A quantitative analysis. Sports Med (Auckland, NZ) 2001; 31(15):1033–1062.
78. Leon AS, Sanchez OA. Response of blood lipids to exercise training alone or combined with dietary intervention. Med Sci Sports Exerc 2001; 33(6 Suppl.):S502–S515; discussion S28–S29.
79. Carroll S, Dudfield M. What is the relationship between exercise and metabolic abnormalities? A review of the metabolic syndrome. Sports Med (Auckland, NZ) 2004; 34(6):371–418.
80. Halbert JA, Silagy CA, Finucane P, et al. Exercise training and blood lipids in hyperlipidemic and normolipidemic adults: A meta-analysis of randomized, controlled trials. Eur J Clin Nutr 1999; 53(7):514–522.
81. Ballantyne FC, Clark RS, Simpson HS, et al. The effect of moderate physical exercise on the plasma lipoprotein subfractions of male survivors of myocardial infarction. Circulation 1982; 65(5):913–918.
82. Stubbe I, Hansson P, Gustafson A, et al. Plasma lipoproteins and lipolytic enzyme activities during endurance training in sedentary men: Changes in high-density lipoprotein subfractions and composition. Metabolism 1983; 32(12):1120–1128.

83. Gordon DJ, Knoke J, Probstfield JL, et al. High-density lipoprotein cholesterol and coronary heart disease in hypercholesterolemic men: The lipid research clinics coronary primary prevention trial. Circulation 1986; 74(6):1217–1225.
84. Kraus WE, Houmard JA, Duscha BD, et al. Effects of the amount and intensity of exercise on plasma lipoproteins. N Engl J Med 2002; 347(19):1483–1492.
85. Lamarche B, Tchernof A, Moorjani S, et al. Small, dense low-density lipoprotein particles as a predictor of the risk of ischemic heart disease in men. Prospective results from the Quebec Cardiovascular Study. Circulation 1997; 95(1):69–75.
86. Ziogas GG, Thomas TR, Harris WS. Exercise training, postprandial hypertriglyceridemia, and LDL subfraction distribution. Med Sci Sports Exerc 1997; 29(8):986–991.
87. Mora S, Lee IM, Buring JE, et al. Association of physical activity and body mass index with novel and traditional cardiovascular biomarkers in women. JAMA 2006; 295(12):1412–1419.
88. Holme I, Hostmark AT, Anderssen SA. ApoB but not LDL-cholesterol is reduced by exercise training in overweight healthy men. Results from the 1-year randomized Oslo Diet and Exercise Study. J Intern Med 2007; 262(2):235–243.
89. Alam S, Stolinski M, Pentecost C, et al. The effect of a six-month exercise program on very low-density lipoprotein apolipoprotein B secretion in type 2 diabetes. J Clin Endocrinol Metab 2004; 89(2):688–694.
90. Ring-Dimitriou S, von Duvillard SP, Paulweber B, et al. Nine months aerobic fitness induced changes on blood lipids and lipoproteins in untrained subjects versus controls. Eur J Appl Physiol 2007; 99(3):291–299.
91. Couillard C, Despres JP, Lamarche B, et al. Effects of endurance exercise training on plasma HDL cholesterol levels depend on levels of triglycerides: Evidence from men of the Health, Risk Factors, Exercise Training and Genetics (HERITAGE) Family Study. Arterioscler Thromb Vasc Biol 2001; 21(7):1226–1232.
92. Leon AS, Rice T, Mandel S, et al. Blood lipid response to 20 weeks of supervised exercise in a large biracial population: The HERITAGE Family Study. Metabolism 2000; 49(4):513–520.
93. Fujioka S, Matsuzawa Y, Tokunaga K, et al. Improvement of glucose and lipid metabolism associated with selective reduction of intra-abdominal visceral fat in premenopausal women with visceral fat obesity. Int J Obes 1991; 15(12):853–859.
94. He J, Whelton PK. Elevated systolic blood pressure and risk of cardiovascular and renal disease: Overview of evidence from observational epidemiologic studies and randomized controlled trials. Am Heart J 1999; 138(3 Pt 2):211–219.
95. Cook NR, Cohen J, Hebert PR, et al. Implications of small reductions in diastolic blood pressure for primary prevention. Arch Intern Med 1995; 155(7):701–709.
96. Paffenbarger RS, Jr., Wing AL, Hyde RT, et al. Physical activity and incidence of hypertension in college alumni. Am J Epidemiol 1983; 117(3):245–257.
97. Kenney MJ, Seals DR. Postexercise hypotension. Key features, mechanisms, and clinical significance. Hypertension 1993; 22(5):653–664.
98. Rueckert PA, Slane PR, Lillis DL, Hanson P. Hemodynamic patterns and duration of post-dynamic exercise hypotension in hypertensive humans. Med Sci Sports Exerc 1996; 28(1):24–32.
99. Pescatello LS, Miller B, Danias PG, et al. Dynamic exercise normalizes resting blood pressure in mildly hypertensive premenopausal women. Am Heart J 1999; 138(5 Pt 1):916–921.
100. Brandao Rondon MU, Alves MJ, Braga AM, et al. Postexercise blood pressure reduction in elderly hypertensive patients. J Am Coll Cardiol 2002; 39(4):676–682.
101. Guidry MA, Blanchard BE, Thompson PD, et al. The influence of short and long duration on the blood pressure response to an acute bout of dynamic exercise. Am Heart J 2006; 151(6):1322e5–e12.
102. Cornelissen VA, Fagard RH. Exercise intensity and postexercise hypotension. J Hypertens 2004; 22(10):1859–1861.
103. Whelton SP, Chin A, Xin X, et al. Effect of aerobic exercise on blood pressure: A meta-analysis of randomized, controlled trials. Ann Intern Med 2002; 136(7):493–503.
104. Kelley GA. Effects of aerobic exercise in normotensive adults: A brief meta-analytic review of controlled clinical trials. South Med J 1995; 88(1):42–46.
105. Kelley GA. Aerobic exercise and resting blood pressure among women: A meta-analysis. Prev Med 1999; 28(3):264–275.
106. Arroll B, Beaglehole R. Does physical activity lower blood pressure: A critical review of the clinical trials. J Clin Epidemiol 1992; 45(5):439–447.
107. Hagberg JM, Park JJ, Brown MD. The role of exercise training in the treatment of hypertension: An update. Sports Med (Auckland, NZ) 2000; 30(3):193–206.
108. Fagard RH. Physical activity in the prevention and treatment of hypertension in the obese. Med Sci Sports Exerc 1999; 31(11 Suppl.):S624–S630.
109. Cornelissen VA, Fagard RH. Effects of endurance training on blood pressure, blood pressure-regulating mechanisms, and cardiovascular risk factors. Hypertension 2005; 46(4):667–675.

110. Meredith IT, Jennings GL, Esler MD, et al. Time-course of the antihypertensive and autonomic effects of regular endurance exercise in human subjects. J Hypertens 1990; 8(9):859–866.
111. Blumenthal JA, Sherwood A, Gullette EC, et al. Exercise and weight loss reduce blood pressure in men and women with mild hypertension: Effects on cardiovascular, metabolic, and hemodynamic functioning. Arch Intern Med 2000; 160(13):1947–1958.
112. Church TS, Earnest CP, Skinner JS, et al. Effects of different doses of physical activity on cardiorespiratory fitness among sedentary, overweight or obese postmenopausal women with elevated blood pressure: A randomized controlled trial. JAMA 2007; 297(19):2081–2091.
113. Eriksson J, Taimela S, Koivisto VA. Exercise and the metabolic syndrome. Diabetologia 1997; 40(2):125–135.
114. Chobanian AV, Bakris GL, Black HR, et al. Seventh report of the Joint National Committee on Prevention, Detection, Evaluation, and Treatment of High Blood Pressure. Hypertension 2003; 42(6):1206–1252.
115. Lee KW, Lip GY. Effects of lifestyle on hemostasis, fibrinolysis, and platelet reactivity: A systematic review. Arch Intern Med 2003;163(19):2368–2392.
116. Tofler GH, Stone PH, Maclure M, et al. Analysis of possible triggers of acute myocardial infarction (the MILIS study). Am J Cardiol 1990; 66(1):22–27.
117. Koenig W, Ernst E. Exercise and thrombosis. Coron Artery Dis 2000; 11(2):123–127.
118. Hegde SS, Goldfarb AH, Hegde S. Clotting and fibrinolytic activity change during the 1h after a submaximal run. Med Sci Sports Exerc 2001; 33(6):887–892.
119. Lin X, El-Sayed MS, Waterhouse J, Reilly T. Activation and disturbance of blood haemostasis following strenuous physical exercise. Int J Sports Med 1999; 20(3):149–153.
120. El-Sayed MS, Ali N, El-Sayed Ali Z. Aggregation and activation of blood platelets in exercise and training. Sports Med (Auckland, NZ) 2005; 35(1):11–22.
121. Fitzgerald DJ, Roy L, Catella F, et al. Platelet activation in unstable coronary disease. N Engl J Med 1986; 315(16):983–989.
122. Weiss C, Welsch B, Albert M, et al. Coagulation and thrombomodulin in response to exercise of different type and duration. Med Sci Sports Exerc 1998; 30(8):1205–1210.
123. Wang JS, Jen CJ, Kung HC, et al. Different effects of strenuous exercise and moderate exercise on platelet function in men. Circulation 1994; 90(6):2877–2885.
124. El-Sayed MS. Effects of exercise on blood coagulation, fibrinolysis and platelet aggregation. Sports Med (Auckland, NZ) 1996; 22(5):282–298.
125. Eliasson M, Asplund K, Evrin PE. Regular leisure time physical activity predicts high activity of tissue plasminogen activator: The Northern Sweden MONICA Study. Int J Epidemiol 1996; 25(6):1182–1188.
126. De Paz JA, Lasierra J, Villa JG, et al. Effects of aerobic and anaerobic physical conditioning on fibrinolysis. J Sports Med Phys Fitness 1995; 35(4):263–267.
127. Lindahl B, Nilsson TK, Jansson JH, et al. Improved fibrinolysis by intense lifestyle intervention. A randomized trial in subjects with impaired glucose tolerance. J Intern Med 1999; 246(1):105–112.
128. Coppola L, Grassia A, Coppola A, et al. Effects of a moderate-intensity aerobic program on blood viscosity, platelet aggregation and fibrinolytic balance in young and middle-aged sedentary subjects. Blood Coagul Fibrinolysis 2004; 15(1):31–37.
129. Wang JS, Jen CJ, Chen HI. Effects of exercise training and deconditioning on platelet function in men. Arterioscler Thromb Vasc Biol 1995; 15(10):1668–1674.
130. Wang JS, Jen CJ, Chen HI. Effects of chronic exercise and deconditioning on platelet function in women. J Appl Physiol 1997; 83(6):2080–2085.
131. Simpson KA, Singh MA. Effects of exercise on adiponectin: A systematic review. Obesity (Silver Spring) 2008; 16(2):241–256.
132. Kato H, Kashiwagi H, Shiraga M, et al. Adiponectin acts as an endogenous antithrombotic factor. Arterioscler Thromb Vasc Biol 2006; 26(1):224–230.
133. Rissanen P, Vahtera E, Krusius T, et al. Weight change and blood coagulability and fibrinolysis in healthy obese women. Int J Obes Relat Metab Disord 2001; 25(2):212–218.
134. Das UN. Obesity, metabolic syndrome X, and inflammation. Nutrition 2002; 18(5):430–432.
135. Ross R. Atherosclerosis—An inflammatory disease. N Engl J Med 1999; 340(2):115–126.
136. Kasapis C, Thompson PD. The effects of physical activity on serum C-reactive protein and inflammatory markers: A systematic review. J Am Coll Cardiol 2005; 45(10):1563–1569.
137. Petersen AM, Pedersen BK. The anti-inflammatory effect of exercise. J Appl Physiol 2005; 98(4):1154–1162.
138. Febbraio MA, Pedersen BK. Muscle-derived interleukin-6: Mechanisms for activation and possible biological roles. Faseb J 2002; 16(11):1335–1347.
139. Ostrowski K, Rohde T, Asp S, et al. Pro- and anti-inflammatory cytokine balance in strenuous exercise in humans. J Physiol 1999; 515(Pt 1):287–291.
140. Heinrich PC, Castell JV, Andus T. Interleukin-6 and the acute phase response. Biochem J 1990; 265(3):621–636.

141. Abramson JL, Vaccarino V. Relationship between physical activity and inflammation among apparently healthy middle-aged and older US adults. Arch Intern Med 2002; 162(11):1286–1292.
142. Geffken DF, Cushman M, Burke GL, et al. Association between physical activity and markers of inflammation in a healthy elderly population. Am J Epidemiol 2001; 153(3):242–250.
143. Mattusch F, Dufaux B, Heine O, et al. Reduction of the plasma concentration of C-reactive protein following nine months of endurance training. Int J Sports Med 2000; 21(1):21–24.
144. Wannamethee SG, Lowe GD, Whincup PH, et al. Physical activity and hemostatic and inflammatory variables in elderly men. Circulation 2002; 105(15):1785–1790.
145. Ford ES. Does exercise reduce inflammation? Physical activity and C-reactive protein among U. S. adults. Epidemiology (Cambridge, Massachusetts) 2002; 13(5):561–568.
146. Tisi PV, Hulse M, Chulakadabba A, et al. Exercise training for intermittent claudication: Does it adversely affect biochemical markers of the exercise-induced inflammatory response? Eur J Vasc Endovasc Surg 1997; 14(5):344–350.
147. Smith JK, Dykes R, Douglas JE, et al. Long-term exercise and atherogenic activity of blood mononuclear cells in persons at risk of developing ischemic heart disease. JAMA 1999; 281(18):1722–1727.
148. Lakka TA, Lakka HM, Rankinen T, et al. Effect of exercise training on plasma levels of C-reactive protein in healthy adults: The HERITAGE Family Study. Eur Heart J 2005; 26(19):2018–2025.
149. Goldhammer E, Tanchilevitch A, Maor I, et al. Exercise training modulates cytokines activity in coronary heart disease patients. Int J Cardiol 2005; 100(1):93–99.
150. Hammett CJ, Prapavessis H, Baldi JC, et al. Effects of exercise training on 5 inflammatory markers associated with cardiovascular risk. Am Heart J 2006; 151(2):367 e7–e16.
151. Liesen H, Dufaux B, Hollmann W. Modifications of serum glycoproteins the days following a prolonged physical exercise and the influence of physical training. Eur J Appl Physiol Occup Physiol 1977; 37(4):243–254.
152. Das UN. Anti-inflammatory nature of exercise. Nutrition 2004; 20(3):323–326.
153. Selvin E, Paynter NP, Erlinger TP. The effect of weight loss on C-reactive protein: A systematic review. Arch Intern Med 2007; 167(1):31–39.
154. Esposito K, Marfella R, Giugliano D. Fitness versus fatness: The debate continues. Arterioscler Thromb Vasc Biol 2005; 25(3):e20–e21; author reply e-1.
155. Esposito K, Pontillo A, Di Palo C, et al. Effect of weight loss and lifestyle changes on vascular inflammatory markers in obese women: A randomized trial. JAMA 2003; 289(14):1799–1804.
156. Esposito K, Giugliano F, Di Palo C, et al. Effect of lifestyle changes on erectile dysfunction in obese men: A randomized controlled trial. JAMA 2004; 291(24):2978–2984.
157. Kelly AS, Steinberger J, Olson TP, et al. In the absence of weight loss, exercise training does not improve adipokines or oxidative stress in overweight children. Metabolism 2007; 56(7):1005–1009.
158. Katzmarzyk PT, Leon AS, Wilmore JH, et al. Targeting the metabolic syndrome with exercise: Evidence from the HERITAGE Family Study. Med Sci Sports Exerc 2003; 35(10):1703–1719.

13 Can We Change the Lifestyle of High-Risk Patients? Lessons from the Prevention of Diabetes Trials

Jaakko Tuomilehto

Department of Public Health, University of Helsinki and
Diabetes Unit, Department of Health Promotion and Chronic Disease Prevention, National Public Health Institute, Helsinki, Finland and
South Ostrobothnia Central Hospital, Seinäjoki, Finland

Jaana Lindström

Department of Public Health, University of Helsinki and
Diabetes Unit, Department of Health Promotion and Chronic Disease Prevention, National Public Health Institute, Helsinki, Finland

INTRODUCTION

Type 2 diabetes (T2D) develops as a result of complex multifactorial process having both lifestyle and genetic origins. The main risk factors for T2D are obesity and sedentary lifestyle (1). A "Westernized" dietary pattern with low fiber (2–4) and high saturated (5) and trans fats (6), refined carbohydrates (7), sweetened beverages (8), sodium (9), and red meat (10,11) intake has been shown to be associated with increased T2D risk. Another feature of modern lifestyle, voluntary sleep deprivation, also increases diabetes risk (12,13). Fortunately, there are also protective lifestyle-related factors such as physical activity (14). The data are also accumulating on decreased T2D risk associated with coffee (15–17) and moderate alcohol, particularly wine consumption (18).

There are some "natural" experiments available in which ethnic groups have experienced rapid westernization and with it a rapid increase in the rates of obesity and T2D (19). Therefore, it is logical to assume that by reversing these lifestyle changes it would be possible to prevent the development of the disease. Such a potential for the reversibility has been shown among Australian Aboriginals by O'Dea (20). In these experiments, hyperglycaemic people returned back to nature living in traditional hunter-gatherer way of life. As a result hyperglycaemia reversed.

MAJOR LIFESTYLE TRIALS IN PREVENTION OF T2D

The Malmö Feasibility Study

The feasibility of diet and exercise intervention in 217 men with IGT was assessed in the Malmö feasibility study (21). The effect of exercise and diet ($n = 161$) was compared to a reference group ($n = 56$) with no intervention. The reference group consisted of men who themselves decided not to join the intervention program. Thus, the groups were not assigned at random. The lifestyle intervention was delivered in group sessions, aiming at reduction in the intake of refined sugar, simple carbohydrates, fat, saturated fat, energy, and alcohol (if relevant) and increase in the intake of complex carbohydrates and vegetables. Physical activity training consisted of two weekly 60-minute sessions with various dynamic activities.

By the end of the 5-year study period, 11% of the intervention group and 29% of the reference group had developed diabetes. This study is important in demonstrating the feasibility of carrying out a diet–exercise program for 5 years among the volunteers, and it furthermore suggests that the incidence of T2D might be reduced by approximately 50%. Overall, the progression to diabetes in these Swedish men was relatively low even in the reference group compared with the data from the observational studies (22). Among the men who did not want to join the intervention program, some may have changed their lifestyle as a result of the screening program. Thus, these results based on intention-to-treat analysis may underestimate the true effect of lifestyle changes. This intervention resulted in significant changes in lifestyle and physiological parameters. While the results on diabetes risk in the Malmö feasibility study are likely to be due to the effects on diet and exercise, the nonrandomized study design limits the generalizability of the results.

The Da-Qing Study

Data on the preventive effect of a diet and exercise intervention have been reported in a cluster-randomized clinical trial in Da-Qing, China (23). Altogether 577 subjects (mean age, 45.0 years; mean BMI 25.8) with IGT were assigned either to the control, exercise alone, diet alone, or exercise and diet group. In clinics assigned to dietary intervention, the participants were encouraged to reduce weight if BMI was $\geq$25 kg/m^2 (61% of all participants) aiming at 23 kg/m^2, otherwise high-carbohydrate (55–65% of energy) and moderate-fat (25–30% of energy) diet was recommended. Counselling was done individually by physicians, and also group sessions were organized weekly for the first month, monthly for 3 months, and every 3 months thereafter. In clinics assigned to physical exercise, counselling sessions were arranged at a similar frequency. The participants were encouraged to increase their level of leisure-time physical activity by at least 1 to 2 "units" per day. One unit would correspond, for instance, 30-minute slow walking, 10-minute slow running or 5-minute swimming.

The cumulative 6-year incidence of T2D was lower in each of the three intervention groups (41–46%) compared with the control group (68%). In this study, the relative risk reduction was approximately 40% while the absolute risk reduction was 22% to 26% during the 6-year period. The progression from IGT to diabetes was high, more than 10% per year in the control group, which is more than usually reported in observational studies.

The study did not apply an individual allocation of study subjects to the intervention and control groups, but the participating clinics were assigned. Furthermore, the study subjects were relatively lean making inferences, for instance, to European obese IGT subjects difficult. Body weight did not change in lean subjects, and there was a modest ($\sim$1 kg/m^2) reduction in subjects with baseline BMI>25 kg/m^2.

The Finnish Diabetes Prevention Study (DPS)

The results of the DPS conducted in Finland provided the first convincing evidence from a proper randomized controlled trial (RCT) that T2D can be prevented by lifestyle modification (24,25). A total of 522 persons (mean age, 55 years; all with IGT) were randomized to either an intensive lifestyle or a control intervention. During an average of 3.2 years of follow-up, T2D incidence was reduced by 58% in the lifestyle group compared to the control group. The subjects in the intervention group had frequent consultation visits with a nutritionist (7-times during the first year and every 3 months thereafter). They received individual advice about how to achieve the intervention goals. These goals were 1) reduction in weight of $\geq$5%, 2) total fat intake less than 30% of energy consumed, 3) saturated fat intake less than 10% of energy consumed, 4) fiber intake of at least 15 g/1000 kcal, and 5) moderate exercise for 30 min/day or more. During the first year of the study, body weight decreased on average 4.5 kg in the intervention group and 1.0 kg in the control group subjects ($p < 0.0001$). Indicators of central adiposity and fasting glucose and insulin, 2-hour postchallenge glucose and insulin, and HbA1c reduced significantly more in the intervention group compared with the control group at 1-year examination.

The Diabetes Prevention Program (DPP)

The United States DPP (26) was completed 1 year after the DPS. In the DPP, 3234 individuals (mean age, 51; mean BMI, 34.0; all with IGT and fasting glucose $\geq$95 mg/dL) were randomized to receive intensive dietary and exercise counselling, metformin, or placebo. The lifestyle intervention included a 16-session (individual and/or group) core curriculum for 24 weeks and a maintenance period thereafter, with monthly contacts between the case manager and participant (27). Furthermore, many different exercise activities were offered. The main aims of the intervention were 7% weight reduction and 150 minutes of moderate physical activity in a week. The relative risk reduction after 2.8 years of follow-up in the lifestyle intervention group compared with the placebo control group was exactly as in the DPS, that is, 58%. The effect of lifestyle was higher than the effect of metformin, which showed 35% relative risk reduction compared with the placebo control group. During the first year of the intervention, weight reduction was 5.6 kg (~6%), with slight, gradual regain to the end of the study at year 4 (26).

Indian Diabetes Prevention Program (IDPP)

The IDPP (28) recruited 531 subjects with IGT (mean age, 45.9 ± 5.7 years; BMI, 25.8 ± 3.5 kg/m^2) who were randomized into four groups (control, lifestyle modification, metformin, and combined lifestyle modification and metformin). Lifestyle modification included advice on physical activity (30 minutes of brisk walking per day) and reduction in total calories, refined carbohydrates and fats, avoidance of sugar, and inclusion of fiber-rich foods. The intervention included personal sessions at baseline and 6-monthly, and monthly telephonic contacts. The intensity of the intervention was thus lower than those in the DPP and DPS. After median follow-up of 30 months, the relative risk reduction was 28.5% with lifestyle modification, 26.4% with metformin, and 28.2% with lifestyle modification and metformin, as compared with the control group. Thus, there was no added benefit from combining the drug and lifestyle interventions. In the control group, diabetes incidence was high (55.0% in 3 years) and comparable to the findings from the Chinese study (23). These populations apparently have high rates of insulin resistance and IGT, and lower thresholds for the risk factors for diabetes (29).

Japanese Prevention Trial

The Japanese trial with IGT males (30) included 458 men who were diagnosed with IGT in health screening and allocated randomly to receive either intensive lifestyle intervention ($n = 102$) or standard intervention ($n = 356$). The participants in the intensive intervention group visited hospital every 3 to 4 months where they were given detailed, repeated advise to reduce body weight, if their BMI was ≥22 kg/m^2 (otherwise, to maintain present weight), by consuming large amount of vegetables and reducing the total amount of other foods by 10%, for example, by using a smaller rice bowl. Intake of fat (<50 g/day) and alcohol (<50 g/day) were limited, as was eating out (no more than once a day) and physical activity recommended (30–40 min/day of walking, etc.). The participants in the control group visited hospital every 6 months and were given standard adviced to eat smaller meals and increase physical activity.

The cumulative 4-year incidence of diabetes was 3% in the intervention group and 9.3% in the control group, with 67.4% risk reduction ($p < 0.001$). BMI at baseline was 23.8 ± 2.1 in the intervention group and 24.0 ± 2.3 in the control group. Body weight decreased by 2.18 kg in the intervention group and 0.39 kg in the control group during these 4 years ($p < 0.001$). Thus, there was a remarkable reduction in diabetes risk despite the relatively modest weight reduction. Post hoc analyses in the control group revealed that diabetes incidence was positively correlated with change in body weight in this population, however, weight loss apparently was not the sole explanator of diabetes risk reduction.

EFFECT OF LIFESTYLE INTERVENTION ON THE METABOLIC SYNDROME (METS)

The DPP research group has recently reported that the intensive lifestyle intervention they applied reduced CVD risk factors (31) and also the prevalence of the MetS (32). In the DPS, at baseline the prevalence of the MetS was 74%, in both the groups. After the first year, the prevalence was 57.3 versus 66.8% ($p = 0.020$) and at the end of the trial 60.2 versus 68.9% ($p = 0.026$) in the intervention and control group, respectively (33). This corresponds to an odds ratio of 0.62 (95%CI 0.41;0.95). At the end of the study, 26.7% versus 17.6% ($p = 0.026$) of those fulfilling the criteria for the MetS at baseline in the intervention and control group no longer met the criteria. In participants who had the MetS at baseline, the mean weight loss was 4.7 kg (95%CI 4.0;5.5) versus 0.8 kg (0.4;1.4) at year 1 and 2.4 kg (1.6;3.1) versus 0.3 kg (−0.4;1.1) at the end of the trial in the intervention and control group, respectively. The corresponding mean reduction in waist circumference was 4.7 cm (3.9;5.4) versus 1.4 cm (0.7;2.0) at year 1 and 2.3 cm (1.6;3.1) versus 0.5 cm (−0.3;1.3) at the end of the trial. Thus, intensive lifestyle counseling resulted in a significant long-term decrease in the prevalence of the MetS, body weight and abdominal obesity in this high-risk group participating in the DPS. At the end of the trial, the participants of the intervention group showed a significantly larger decrease in weight, BMI, waist circumference, fasting, and 2-hour insulin levels, the $HOMA_{IR}$ index, and a larger increase in HDL-cholesterol.

LONG-TERM EFFECTIVENESS OF LIFESTYLE PREVENTION OF T2D

The 12-year follow-up of the Malmö study (21,34) revealed that the mortality rate among men in the former IGT intervention group was lower than among the men in the nonrandomized IGT group who received "routine care" only (6.5 vs. 14.0 per 1000 person years, $p = 0.009$). The findings suggest that a long-term intervention program including dietary counselling and physical exercise will reduce mortality in subjects with IGT who are at an increased risk of premature death due to IHD and other causes.

In an analysis using the data collected during the extended follow-up of the DPS, we were able to show that after a median of 7 years total follow-up, a marked reduction in the cumulative incidence of diabetes was sustained (35). The relative risk reduction during the total follow-up was 43%. More importantly, the effect of intervention on diabetes risk was maintained among those who after the intervention period were without diabetes: after median postintervention follow-up time of 3 years, the number of incident new cases of T2D was 31 in the intervention group among 221 people at risk, and 38 in the control group among 185 people at risk. The corresponding incidence rates were 4.6 and 7.2 per 100 person years, respectively (log-rank test $p = 0.0401$), that is, 36% relative risk reduction. Thus, the absolute risk difference between the groups increased slightly during the postintervention period. There is an important message from the public-health point of view: An intensive lifestyle intervention lasting for a limited time can yield long-term benefits in reducing the risk of T2D in high-risk individuals.

EVIDENCE OF THE EFFECT OF LIFESTYLE FACTORS ON T2D RISK

In most of the published prevention trials, the main aim was to see if comprehensive lifestyle intervention reduces T2D risk. In the Chinese prevention study (23), an attempt to determine whether a diet or exercise intervention is more effective by randomizing the perticipating centres to diet only, physical activity only, or diet plus physical activity intervention, revealed no difference in outcome between the two interventions.

In the DPS, the risk of being diagnosed with diabetes was strongly associated with the number of lifestyle goals achieved (35). Success in achieving the intervention goals in the DPS was estimated from the food records and exercise questionnaires. The success score (from 0 to 5) was calculated as the sum of achieved lifestyle goals. There was a strong inverse correlation between the success score and the incidence of diabetes during the total follow-up. This was especially apparent when the success in achieving the goals was assessed at year 3, which probably reflects the importance of sustained lifestyle changes. The hazard ratios were 1.00, 0.87, 0.67, 0.70, and 0.23, for success score from 0 to 4–5, respectively (p for trend <0.001).

Because the question about the effects of different components of intervention is interesting, we did complete some post hoc analyses related to this issue. The independent effects of achieving the success score components at 3-year examination was assessed by including each of the five lifestyle goal variables individually in a Cox model. Univariate hazard ratios for diabetes incidence (95%CI) were 0.45 (0.31–0.64) for weight reduction from baseline, 0.65 (0.45–0.95) for intake of fat, 0.59 (0.31–1.13) for intake of saturated fat, 0.69 (0.49–0.96) for intake of fiber, and 0.62 (0.46–0.84) for physical activity, comparing those who did or did not achieve the respective goal. When all the five success score components were simultaneously included in the Cox model, the multivariate-adjusted hazard ratios for diabetes (95%CI) were 0.43 (0.30–0.61) for weight reduction, 0.80 (0.48–1.34) for intake of fat, 0.55 (0.26–1.16) for intake of saturated fat, 0.97 (0.63–1.51) for intake of fiber, and 0.80 (0.57–1.12) for physical activity. Furthermore, weight change was significantly associated with the achievement of each of the other four lifestyle goals, and consequently, success score was strongly and inversely correlated with weight reduction (35).

Correspondingly, the reduction in body weight was reported to be the main determinant of risk reduction in the US DPP (36). After adjusment for other components of the intervention, there was a 16% reduction in diabetes risk per 1 kg weight lost during the first year of the intervention. Furthermore, lower percent of calories from fat and increased physical activity predicted weight loss, and increased physical activity was important to help sustain weight loss. Achieving the physical activity goal of 150 min/wk reduced diabetes risk especially among those participants who did not achieve the weight reduction goal of 7%, with risk reduction of

44% compared with those who achieved neither the weight reduction nor the physical activity goal.

The findings suggest that dietary composition and physical activity are important in diabetes prevention but their effect on diabetes risk is in large part, although not entirely, mediated through resulting weight reduction. Nevertheless, due to multicolinearity, the interpretation of the results should be done cautiously. Also, it should be noted that in the IDPP (28) and Chinese prevention study (23), the participants were relatively lean and there was no large change in body weight, but in spite of that a remarkable reduction in diabetes risk was apparent. Thus, in these studies other components of the intervention than weight control were responsible for the beneficial effects on diabetes risk.

CONCLUSIONS

The DPS and other prevention trials have shown that with intensive lifestyle intervention, it is possible to influence high-risk individuals' lifestyle, and that T2D can be prevented. Most importantly, lifestyle changes do not have to be extreme: If people would adopt the lifestyle including physical activity and balanced diet advocated to healthy population, the diabetes trend could at least be leveled out.

Behavior change is a process, and we should not assume that significant lifestyle changes could be achieved after one brief counselling session. Information must be personalized, and the implementation must be very practical; people eat food, not nutrients. Few people are willing and/or able to make extreme changes in their food-intake pattern. Permanent lifestyle changes can only be achieved through small, concrete steps towards specific goals. Obesity and susceptibility to weight gain is a chronic condition. Continuous care is required especially after intensive weight loss. Lifestyle goals must be realistic, practical, and individualized.

While it is now firmly established that T2D is preventable in high-risk individuals with lifestyle intervention in a clinical trial setting, it remains to be seen how this strategy can be implemented at the population level, and what the effectiveness of such a strategy will be. Most importantly, obesogenic environment is to some extent a political issue. Walking and bicycling to work, school, and shops should be made easy and appealing. Kindergartens, schools, and staff canteens are in an excellent position to guide children, adolescents, and adults to healthy diet.

REFERENCES

1. WHO Study Group. Diabetes Mellitus—Technical Report Series No. 727. Geneva, 1985.
2. Salmeron J, Manson JE, Stampfer MJ, et al. Dietary fiber, glycemic load, and risk of non-insulin-dependent diabetes mellitus in women. JAMA 1997; 277:472–477.
3. Schulze MB, Liu S, Rimm EB, et al. Glycemic index, glycemic load, and dietary fiber intake and incidence of type 2 diabetes in younger and middle-aged women. Am J Clin Nutr 2004; 80:348–356.
4. Montonen J, Knekt P, Järvinen R, et al. Whole-grain and fiber intake and the incidence of type 2 diabetes. Am J Clin Nutr 2003; 77:622–629.
5. Feskens EJ, Virtanen SM, Räsänen L, et al. Dietary factors determining diabetes and impaired glucose tolerance. A 20-year follow-up of the Finnish and Dutch cohorts of the Seven Countries Study. Diabetes Care 1995; 18:1104–1112.
6. Salmeron J, Hu FB, Manson JE, et al. Dietary fat intake and risk of type 2 diabetes in women. Am J Clin Nutr 2001; 73:1019–1026.
7. Hodge AM, English DR, O'Dea K, et al. Glycemic index and dietary fiber and the risk of type 2 diabetes. Diabetes Care 2004; 27:2701–2706.
8. Schulze MB, Manson JE, Ludwig DS, et al. Sugar-sweetened beverages, weight gain, and incidence of type 2 diabetes in young and middle-aged women. JAMA 2004; 292:927–934.
9. Hu G, Jousilahti P, Peltonen M, et al. Urinary sodium and potassium excretion and the risk of type 2 diabetes: A prospective study in Finland. Diabetologia 2005; 48:1477–1483.
10. Fung TT, Schulze M, Manson JE, et al. Dietary patterns, meat intake, and the risk of type 2 diabetes in women. Arch Intern Med 2004; 164:2235–2240.
11. Song Y, Manson JE, Buring JE, et al. A prospective study of red meat consumption and type 2 diabetes in middle-aged and elderly women: The women's health study. Diabetes Care 2004; 27:2108–2115.

12. Ayas NT, White DP, Al-Delaimy WK, et al. A prospective study of self-reported sleep duration and incident diabetes in women. Diabetes Care 2003; 26:380–384.
13. Mallon L, Broman J-E, Hetta J. High incidence of diabetes in men with sleep complaints or short sleep duration: A 12-year follow-up study of a middle-aged population. Diabetes Care 2005; 28:2762–2767.
14. Hu G, Lakka TA, Kilpelainen TO, et al. Epidemiological studies of exercise in diabetes prevention. Appl Physiol Nutr Metab 2007; 32:583–595.
15. Salazar-Martinez E, Willett WC, Ascherio A, et al. Coffee consumption and risk for type 2 diabetes mellitus. Ann Intern Med 2004; 140:1–8.
16. Tuomilehto J, Hu G, Bidel S, et al. Coffee consumption and risk of type 2 diabetes mellitus among middle-aged Finnish men and women. JAMA 2004; 291:1213–1219.
17. van Dam RM, Willett WC, Manson JE, et al. Coffee, caffeine, and risk of type 2 diabetes: A prospective cohort study in younger and middle-aged U.S. women. Diabetes Care 2006; 29:398–403.
18. Hodge AM, English DR, O'Dea K, et al. Alcohol intake, consumption pattern and beverage type, and the risk of Type 2 diabetes. Diabetic Medicine 2006; 23:690–697.
19. Zimmet P, Alberti KG, Shaw J. Global and societal implications of the diabetes epidemic. Nature 2001; 414:782–787.
20. O'Dea K. Marked improvement in carbohydrate and lipid metabolism in diabetic Australian Aborigines after temporary reversion to traditional lifestyle. Diabetes 1980; 33:596–603.
21. Eriksson KF, Lindgärde F. Prevention of type 2 (non-insulin-dependent) diabetes mellitus by diet and physical exercise. The 6-year Malmö feasibility study. Diabetologia 1991; 34:891–898.
22. Knowler W, Narayan K, Hanson R, et al. Perspectives in diabetes. Preventing non-insulin-dependent diabetes. Diabetes 1995; 44:483–488.
23. Pan XR, Li GW, Hu YH, et al. Effects of diet and exercise in preventing NIDDM in people with impaired glucose tolerance. The Da Qing IGT and Diabetes Study. Diabetes Care 1997; 20:537–544.
24. Lindström J, Louheranta A, Mannelin M, et al. The Finnish Diabetes Prevention Study (DPS): Lifestyle intervention and 3-year results on diet and physical activity. Diabetes Care 2003; 26:3230–3236.
25. Tuomilehto J, Lindström J, Eriksson JG, et al. Prevention of type 2 diabetes mellitus by changes in lifestyle among subjects with impaired glucose tolerance. N Engl J Med 2001; 344:1343–1350.
26. The Diabetes Prevention Program Research Group. Reduction in the incidence of type 2 diabetes with lifestyle intervention or metformin. N Engl J Med 2002; 346:393–403.
27. The Diabetes Prevention Program Research Group. The Diabetes Prevention Program (DPP): Description of lifestyle intervention. Diabetes Care 2002; 25:2165–2171.
28. Ramachandran A, Snehalatha C, Mary S, et al. The Indian Diabetes Prevention Programme shows that lifestyle modification and metformin prevent type 2 diabetes in Asian Indian subjects with impaired glucose tolerance (IDPP-1). Diabetologia 2006; 49:289–297.
29. Ramachandran A, Snehalatha C, Vijay V. Low risk threshold for acquired diabetogenic factors in Asian Indians. Diabetes Res Clin Pract 2004; 65:189–195.
30. Kosaka K, Noda M, Kuzuya T. Prevention of type 2 diabetes by lifestyle intervention: A Japanese trial in IGT males. Diabetes Res Clin Pract 2005; 67:152–162.
31. The Diabetes Prevention Program Research Group. Impact of intensive lifestyle and metformin therapy on cardiovascular disease risk factors in the diabetes prevention program. Diabetes Care 2005; 28:888–894.
32. Orchard TJ, Temprosa M, Goldberg R, et al. The effect of metformin and intensive lifestyle intervention on the metabolic syndrome: The diabetes prevention program randomized trial. Ann Intern Med 2005; 142:611–619.
33. Ilanne-Parikka P, Eriksson JG, Lindstrom J, et al. Effect of lifestyle intervention on the occurrence of metabolic syndrome and its components in the Finnish Diabetes Prevention Study. Diabetes Care 2008; 31:805–807.
34. Eriksson KF, Lindgarde F. No excess 12-year mortality in men with impaired glucose tolerance who participated in the Malmo Preventive Trial with diet and exercise. Diabetologia 1998; 41:1010–1016.
35. Lindström J, Ilanne-Parikka P, Peltonen M, et al. Sustained reduction in the incidence of type 2 diabetes by lifestyle intervention: The follow-up results of the Finnish Diabetes Prevention Study. Lancet 2006; 368:1673–1679.
36. Hamman RF, Wing RR, Edelstein SL, et al. Effect of weight loss with lifestyle intervention on risk of diabetes. Diabetes Care 2006; 29:2102–2107.

14 Can We Change the Body Fat Distribution Phenotype? Lessons from PPARγ Agonists

Zubin Punthakee

Department of Medicine, McMaster University and Hamilton Health Sciences, Hamilton, Ontario, Canada

Hertzel C. Gerstein

Department of Medicine and Population Health Research Institute, McMaster University and Hamilton Health Sciences, Hamilton, Ontario, Canada

PPARγ AND THIAZOLIDINEDIONES

Peroxisome proliferator–activated receptor gamma (PPARγ) is a member of a subfamily of nuclear receptor transcription factors with primary roles in fat metabolism. PPARγ is expressed most abundantly not only in adipose tissue adipocytes and macrophages, but also in muscle and liver and to lesser degrees in other tissues (1). The thiazolidinediones (TZDs) are synthetic agonists of PPARγ. Thiazolidinediones act primarily in adipose tissue, where they have regenerative, lipometabolic, endocrine, and anti-inflammatory effects. These effects directly and indirectly promote insulin-mediated glucose uptake in muscle and fat, insulin-mediated suppression of hepatic glucose production (2), and pancreatic insulin secretion (3). Clinically, the increase in insulin sensitivity promotes lower glucose levels in people with diabetes, impaired fasting glucose (IFG), and impaired glucose tolerance (IGT). To date, the TZDs that have been used to treat diabetes include pioglitazone, rosiglitazone, and troglitazone. Of these, troglitazone was removed from the market due to idiosyncratic liver toxicity (not seen with the other two).

Research with PPARγ agonists has contributed significantly to the understanding of adipose tissue biology and the relationships between obesity and glucometabolic abnormalities, and has suggested that TZDs increase the capacity to safely store excess energy as fat in healthy subcutaneous (sc) adipose tissue, and prevent "toxic" accumulation of fat in visceral adipose tissue, muscle, liver, and pancreas where it may cause metabolic derangements.

TZD ACTIONS ON UNHEALTHY ADIPOSE TISSUE

Excess energy intake overwhelms the normal storage capacity in obesity leading to morphologically and metabolically unhealthy and inflamed fat (Fig. 1). Compared to nonobese individuals, the adipose tissue of those who are obese: (a) contains larger adipocytes, (b) has a lesser ability to take up and retain free fatty acids (FFAs) in response to insulin, (c) is more prone to macrophage infiltration and secretion of inflammatory adipokines (4), and (d) has a lesser ability to secrete adipokines that maintain glucometabolic and vascular health (5). For example, obesity leads to increased production of TNF-α, PAI-1, and angiotensinogen, and decreased production of adiponectin which is an insulin sensitizer that may reduce ectopic fat deposition in muscle and liver, and suppresses inflammation (2).

Thiazolidinediones restore adipose tissue health (Fig. 1). By promoting preadipocyte differentiation and large adipocyte apoptosis, they remodel adipose tissue into an organ with smaller adipocytes that are less susceptible to the abnormalities listed above (6).

DEPOT-SPECIFICITY

As PPARγ expression is greater in sc fat than visceral fat (7), the TZDs have a greater potential to act on sc tissues. Indeed, it is only in sc fat that PPARγ activation induces differentiation of preadipocytes into mature adipocytes (8). In addition, PPARγ upregulates key lipogenic enzymes like lipoprotein lipase (important for lipid uptake), enzymes promoting esterification of FFAs (9) and perilipin (essential for enlargement of lipid droplets) (10) in sc fat but not in

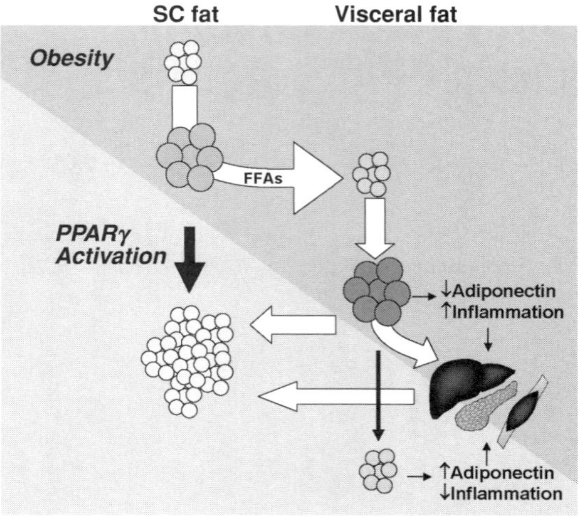

Figure 1 Effects of obesity and PPARγ activation on fat distribution and metabolism. In obesity, excess energy intake leads to hypertrophy of sc adipocytes and overflow of FFAs to visceral fat promoting abnormal adipokine secretion and macrophage infiltration, which along with ectopic fat deposition in liver, pancreas, and muscle lead to diabetogenic and atherogenic abnormalities. PPARγ activation promotes differentiation and expansion of subcutaneous fat to absorb more FFAs and siphon them away from visceral fat and other ectopic sites, restoring these organs to health.

visceral fat. Thus, FFA uptake is increased 14-fold in sc fat after TZD treatment compared to only a 4-fold increase in visceral fat (9). By increasing the capacity of sc fat to store triglycerides, there is less of a burden on visceral adipose tissue which is more prone to obesity-induced macrophage infiltration and adipokine dysregulation (11,12). This may partly explain why TZD treatment leads to reduced macrophage infiltration (13) and increased adiponectin secretion (12) particularly in visceral fat. These effects may minimize excessive lipid release into the portal circulation by lipolysis, which may lead to reduced deposition of ectopic fat in visceral organs.

EFFECT ON TOTAL BODY WEIGHT

It is well established that on average, body weight increases with TZD therapy. Mean weight gain is reportedly 1 to 5.5 kg but ranges in individuals from −30 to 30 kg. Weight gain is progressive over the first year of therapy, but appears to plateau to some degree over time, and is proportionate to TZD dose (14). More interesting is that greater TZD-induced weight gain is associated with better glycemic control; a 2 to 3 kg weight gain is associated with about a 1% reduction in A1 C (1). Moreover, rosiglitazone reduced the risk of diabetes by more than 60% in high-risk people, despite a weight gain of ~0.6 kg/year in the DREAM trial (15). Although some weight gain is due to fluid retention (16), which is known to occur with TZDs, most weight gain is due to increased body fat. The seemingly paradoxical relationship between weight gain and glycemic control with TZDs can be explained by the distribution of body fat deposition induced by these drugs.

WAIST AND HIP CIRCUMFERENCE

Although total body weight and BMI are surrogates for abnormal fat deposition, they are poor markers of risk of cardiovascular disease, whereas waist circumference and waist-to-hip ratio (WHR) are better predictors of cardiovascular disease (17). Large clinical trials in people with IFG or IGT (15) or early diabetes (18) indicate that while long-term treatment with TZDs causes weight gain, they increase hip circumference to a greater degree than waist circumference leading to a lower WHR (Table 1). Thus, TZDs lead to a more favorable fat distribution associated with prevention of diabetes (15) and better long-term diabetes control (18).

SC AND VISCERAL FAT

Reduction of WHR is consistent with redistribution of fat from visceral to sc fat. The effects of TZDs on specific body fat depots has been assessed more accurately in small, short-term studies

Table 1 Effect of Rosiglitazone on Anthropometric Measures in Large Clinical Trials

Trial	Duration (yr)	Compared to	Weight (kg)	Waist circumference (cm)	Hip circumference (cm)	Waist-to-hip ratio
DREAM (15)	3	Placebo	+2.2	0	+1.8	−0.012
ADOPT (18)	4	Metformin	+6.9	+4.1	+5.3	−0.008
		Glyburide	+2.5	+0.8	+2.4	−0.010

measuring sc versus visceral abdominal fat using imaging techniques, such as CT and MRI in people with type 2 diabetes, obesity, and HIV-related lipodystrophy (Table 2).

In people with diabetes, these studies show that TZDs increase total body fat; in most cases, this is due to an increase in sc abdominal fat and in some studies TZDs also decreased visceral abdominal fat, thus leading to a lower visceral to sc fat ratio. Several studies also showed that this redistribution of abdominal fat from visceral to sc depots was associated with improved glucose and lipid metabolism.

Studies of the effects of TZDs on visceral and sc fat in nondiabetic people with obesity and/or insulin resistance are limited (Table 2). However, three small, short-term randomized studies in heterogeneous nondiabetic populations did not show a consistent effect on abdominal fat distribution.

In people with lipodystrophy, abnormal fat distribution leads to metabolic consequences similar to those seen in obesity. HIV lipodystrophy, which may be related to HIV infection itself or to its treatment, manifests as loss of sc fat and an increase in visceral fat. In vitro studies indicate that rosiglitazone prevents the block in adipocyte differentiation induced by protease inhibitors (19). However, randomized studies summarized in Table 2 suggest that in this condition TZDs may not have the same ability to redistribute fat or to increase sc fat

Table 2 Effects of TZDs on Fat Distribution Measured by CT or MRI in Randomized Controlled Trials

Reference	TZD	Control	*N*	Duration (wk)	Effect of TZD on fat: Total body	SAT (cm^2)	VAT	Liver	Other effects
Studies in type 2 diabetes									
(25)	Tro	Placebo	21	12	0	0	−0.47 kg	–	↓FPI, ↓TG
(22)	Tro	Placebo	78	24	–	+7.6	−26.6 cm^2	+7 HU	↓A1c, ↓FPI
(26)	Pio	Placebo	42	24	+4 kg	+44	0	0	↓A1c, ↑HDL
(16)	Pio	Glipizide	19	12	0	−35	−35 cm^2	–	0
(27)	Pio	Metformin	36	26	+4.1 kg	+52	0	–	0
(21)	Rosi	Placebo	33	16	+1.4 kg	+25	0	−45%	↓A1c
(28)	Rosi	Placebo	28	26	0	0	−1.3 kg	–	–
(29)	Rosi	Placebo	19	26	0	0	0	–	↓FPI
(30)	Rosi	Metformin	20	16	–	0	0	−51%	0
Studies in nondiabetic obese individuals									
(31)	Tro	Placebo	29	12	–	0	0	–	↓A1c, ↓TG
(32)	Pio	Diet/exercise	39	19	+10.6 kg	+63	+80 cm^2	–	↓FPG, FPI
(23)	Pio	Metformin	23	10	0	0	0	–	↓VAT/SAT
Studies in HIV lipodystrophy									
(33)	Rosi	Placebo	30	24	0	0	0	−41%	↓FPI, ↑TG
(34)	Rosi	Placebo	28	12	+2.2%	0	0	–	↑Leg fat 2.2 cm^2
(35)	Rosi	Placebo	108	48	0	0	0	–	↓FPI, ↑TG
(36)	Rosi	Metformin	37	26	+4 kg	+27	+24 cm^2	–	↓HDL, ↑TG
(37)	Rosi	Placebo	54	16	−0.4 kg	0	0	–	0

Abbreviations: A1c, glycated hemoglobin; FPG, fasting plasma glucose; FPI, fasting plasma insulin; HU, hounsfield units (higher HU = less liver fat); Pio, pioglitazone; Rosi, rosiglitazone; SAT, subcutaneous abdominal adipose tissue; TG, triglycerides; Tro, trogitazone; TZD, thiazolidinedione; VAT, visceral abdominal adipose tissue; 0, no effect; –, not measured.

mass, and may therefore not have the same metabolic benefit that they have in type 2 diabetes. Conversely, primary forms of lipodystrophy, which are variably associated with loss of sc and visceral fat, and metabolic consequences, did respond in a small study to troglitazone with a 2.4% increase in body fat, increased sc fat, reduced liver size, and improved glucometabolic and lipid parameters (20).

Thus, TZDs increase sc fat and decrease visceral fat; however, their ability to change the body fat distribution phenotype seems to depend on the degree or type of adipose tissue disorder.

ECTOPIC FAT

By increasing storage of fat in sc adipose tissue, TZDs reduce the ectopic deposition of lipid. Liver fat, which is associated with insulin resistance, type 2 diabetes, dyslipidemia, and cardiovascular disease is reduced by TZDs concomitantly with the increase in sc fat (21,22). Furthermore, large clinical trials of TZDs have shown small but significant reductions in alanine aminotransferase (ALT) (15,18), which is a marker of nonalcoholic fatty liver disease. In addition, accumulation of intramyocellular lipid (a factor associated with peripheral insulin resistance) is also reduced by pioglitazone as a result of diversion of lipid from ectopic sites to sc adipose tissue (23). The pancreas is another site where ectopic lipid deposition is associated with impaired function (24), and it has been shown that TZD treatment reduces islet triglyceride content while improving glucose-stimulated insulin secretion in mice (3).

SUMMARY

PPARγ is an important adipose tissue transcription factor with effects on adipocyte differentiation, fatty acid metabolism, adipokine secretion, and inflammation. Activation of these pathways with PPARγ agonists leads to increased sc fat accumulation while shunting lipid away from visceral fat and other ectopic sites including muscle, liver, and pancreas. Thus, while TZDs increase total body fat, the pattern of body fat accumulation and redistribution leads to a phenotype associated with improvements in glucose and lipid metabolism.

REFERENCE

1. Yki-Jarvinen H. Thiazolidinediones. N Engl J Med 2004; 351(11):1106–1118.
2. Sharma AM, Staels B. Review: Peroxisome proliferator-activated receptor gamma and adipose tissue—understanding obesity-related changes in regulation of lipid and glucose metabolism. J Clin Endocrinol Metab 2007; 92(2):386–395.
3. Matsui J, Terauchi Y, Kubota N, et al. Pioglitazone reduces islet triglyceride content and restores impaired glucose-stimulated insulin secretion in heterozygous peroxisome proliferator-activated receptor-gamma-deficient mice on a high-fat diet. Diabetes 2004; 53(11):2844–2854.
4. Fantuzzi G. Adipose tissue, adipokines, and inflammation. J Allergy Clin Immunol 2005; 115(5):911–919.
5. Heilbronn L, Smith SR, Ravussin E. Failure of fat cell proliferation, mitochondrial function and fat oxidation results in ectopic fat storage, insulin resistance and type II diabetes mellitus. Int J Obes Relat Metab Disord 2004; 28 (Suppl. 4):S12–S21.
6. Okuno A, Tamemoto H, Tobe K, et al. Troglitazone increases the number of small adipocytes without the change of white adipose tissue mass in obese Zucker rats. J Clin Invest 1998; 101(6):1354–1361.
7. Giusti V, Verdumo C, Suter M, et al. Expression of peroxisome proliferator-activated receptor-gamma1 and peroxisome proliferator-activated receptor-gamma2 in visceral and subcutaneous adipose tissue of obese women. Diabetes 2003; 52(7):1673–1676.
8. Adams M, Montague CT, Prins JB, et al. Activators of peroxisome proliferator-activated receptor gamma have depot-specific effects on human preadipocyte differentiation. J Clin Invest 1997; 100(12):3149–3153.
9. Laplante M, Festuccia WT, Soucy G, et al. Mechanisms of the depot specificity of peroxisome proliferator-activated receptor gamma action on adipose tissue metabolism. Diabetes 2006; 55(10):2771–2778.

10. Kim HJ, Jung TW, Kang ES, et al. Depot-specific regulation of perilipin by rosiglitazone in a diabetic animal model. Metabolism 2007; 56(5):676–685.
11. Tchoukalova YD, Sarr MG, Jensen MD. Measuring committed preadipocytes in human adipose tissue from severely obese patients by using adipocyte fatty acid binding protein. Am J Physiol Regul Integr Comp Physiol 2004; 287(5):R1132–R1140.
12. Motoshima H, Wu X, Sinha MK, et al. Differential regulation of adiponectin secretion from cultured human omental and subcutaneous adipocytes: Effects of insulin and rosiglitazone. J Clin Endocrinol Metab 2002; 87(12):5662–5667.
13. Okamoto Y, Higashiyama H, Rong JX, et al. Comparison of mitochondrial and macrophage content between subcutaneous and visceral fat in db/db mice. Exp Mol Pathol 2007; 83(1):73–83.
14. Larsen TM, Toubro S, Astrup A. PPARgamma agonists in the treatment of type II diabetes: Is increased fatness commensurate with long-term efficacy? Int J Obes Relat Metab Disord 2003; 27(2):147–161.
15. Gerstein HC, Yusuf S, Bosch J, et al. Effect of rosiglitazone on the frequency of diabetes in patients with impaired glucose tolerance or impaired fasting glucose: A randomised controlled trial. Lancet 2006; 368(9541):1096–1105.
16. Basu A, Jensen MD, McCann F, et al. Effects of pioglitazone versus glipizide on body fat distribution, body water content, and hemodynamics in type 2 diabetes. Diabetes Care 2006; 29(3):510–514.
17. Yusuf S, Hawken S, Ounpuu S, et al. Obesity and the risk of myocardial infarction in 27,000 participants from 52 countries: A case-control study. Lancet 2005; 366(9497):1640–1649.
18. Kahn SE, Haffner SM, Heise MA, et al. Glycemic durability of rosiglitazone, metformin, or glyburide monotherapy. N Engl J Med 2006; 355(23):2427–2443.
19. Caron M, Auclair M, Vigouroux C, et al. The HIV protease inhibitor indinavir impairs sterol regulatory element-binding protein-1 intranuclear localization, inhibits preadipocyte differentiation, and induces insulin resistance. Diabetes 2001; 50(6):1378–1388.
20. Oral EA. Lipoatrophic diabetes and other related syndromes. Rev Endocr Metab Disord 2003; 4(1):61–77.
21. Carey DG, Cowin GJ, Galloway GJ, et al. Effect of rosiglitazone on insulin sensitivity and body composition in type 2 diabetic patients [corrected]. Obes Res 2002; 10(10):1008–1015.
22. Katoh S, Hata S, Matsushima M, et al. Troglitazone prevents the rise in visceral adiposity and improves fatty liver associated with sulfonylurea therapy—A randomized controlled trial. Metabolism 2001; 50(4):414–417.
23. Rasouli N, Raue U, Miles LM, et al. Pioglitazone improves insulin sensitivity through reduction in muscle lipid and redistribution of lipid into adipose tissue. Am J Physiol Endocrinol Metab 2005; 288(5):E930–E934.
24. Lewis GF, Carpentier A, Adeli K, et al. Disordered fat storage and mobilization in the pathogenesis of insulin resistance and type 2 diabetes. Endocr Rev 2002; 23(2):201–229.
25. Kelly IE, Han TS, Walsh K, et al. Effects of a thiazolidinedione compound on body fat and fat distribution of patients with type 2 diabetes. Diabetes Care 1999; 22(2):288–293.
26. Smith SR, De JL, Volaufova J, et al. Effect of pioglitazone on body composition and energy expenditure: A randomized controlled trial. Metabolism 2005; 54(1):24–32.
27. Jacob AN, Salinas K, ms-Huet B,et al. Weight gain in type 2 diabetes mellitus. Diabetes Obes Metab 2007; 9(3):386–393.
28. Virtanen KA, Hallsten K, Parkkola R, et al. Differential effects of rosiglitazone and metformin on adipose tissue distribution and glucose uptake in type 2 diabetic subjects. Diabetes 2003; 52(2):283–290.
29. Iozzo P, Hallsten K, Oikonen V, et al. Effects of metformin and rosiglitazone monotherapy on insulin-mediated hepatic glucose uptake and their relation to visceral fat in type 2 diabetes. Diabetes Care 2003; 26(7):2069–2074.
30. Tiikkainen M, Hakkinen AM, Korsheninnikova E, et al. Effects of rosiglitazone and metformin on liver fat content, hepatic insulin resistance, insulin clearance, and gene expression in adipose tissue in patients with type 2 diabetes. Diabetes 2004; 53(8):2169–2176.
31. Nakamura T, Funahashi T, Yamashita S, et al. Thiazolidinedione derivative improves fat distribution and multiple risk factors in subjects with visceral fat accumulation—Double-blind placebo-controlled trial. Diabetes Res Clin Pract 2001; 54(3):181–190.
32. Shadid S, Jensen MD. Effects of pioglitazone versus diet and exercise on metabolic health and fat distribution in upper body obesity. Diabetes Care 2003; 26(11):3148–3152.
33. Sutinen J, Hakkinen AM, Westerbacka J, et al. Rosiglitazone in the treatment of HAART-associated lipodystrophy—A randomized double-blind placebo-controlled study. Antivir Ther 2003; 8(3):199–207.
34. Hadigan C, Yawetz S, Thomas A, et al. Metabolic effects of rosiglitazone in HIV lipodystrophy: A randomized, controlled trial. Ann Intern Med 2004; 140(10):786–794.

35. Carr A, Workman C, Carey D, et al. No effect of rosiglitazone for treatment of HIV-1 lipoatrophy: Randomised, double-blind, placebo-controlled trial. Lancet 2004; 363(9407):429–438.
36. van Wijk JP, de Koning EJ, Cabezas MC, et al. Comparison of rosiglitazone and metformin for treating HIV lipodystrophy: A randomized trial. Ann Intern Med 2005; 143(5):337–346.
37. Mulligan K, Yang Y, Wininger DA, et al. Effects of metformin and rosiglitazone in HIV-infected patients with hyperinsulinemia and elevated waist/hip ratio. AIDS 2007; 21(1):47–57.

15 Is There an Optimal Diet for the Management of Abdominal Obesity and Related Cardiometabolic Risk

Benoît Lamarche and Caroline Richard

Institute of Nutraceuticals and Functional Foods, Laval University, Québec, Canada

INTRODUCTION

Abdominal obesity has been associated with several metabolic irregularities that increase the risk of cardiovascular disease (CVD) and diabetes, as discussed in previous chapters of this book. Effective management of patients with abdominal obesity and the metabolic syndrome through dietary approaches is considered crucial because it targets key pathophysiological mechanisms responsible for the development of the disease (1). The objective of this short chapter is to review the evidence supporting the role of nutrition in managing abdominal obesity and related cardiometabolic risk.

CALORIC RESTRICTION

An extensive review of the abundant literature pertaining to the impact of weight/visceral fat loss through caloric restriction on cardiometabolic risk factors is beyond the scope of this chapter. Only a brief summary will be provided since we have opted to focus primarily on diet quality rather than on energy intake per se.

Several studies have shown that weight loss as small as 5% of initial body weight, achieved through different hypocaloric regimens, markedly improves almost all aspects of the cardiometabolic risk profile associated with abdominal obesity (2). Indeed, body weight reduction in various studies has been associated with reduced plasma TG and apolipoprotein B (apoB) levels, with a lowered preponderance of small dense LDL particles and with a more efficient postprandial lipid metabolism. Kinetic studies have shown that weight loss reduces VLDL–apoB secretion and reciprocally up regulates LDL–apoB catabolism in viscerally obese patients, probably owing to reduced visceral fat mass, enhanced insulin sensitivity, and decreased hepatic lipogenesis (3). The HDL raising effect of weight loss through caloric restriction has been less consistent with both conclusive and inconclusive studies. Reductions in plasma CRP concentrations have consistently been observed following different weight loss regimens, particularly rigorous dietary restrictions, leading to >10% body weight reductions (4). Data suggest that the magnitude of the response of various lipid and inflammation risk factors to dietary restriction and weight loss may be dependent upon the baseline phenotype of the patient, with metabolically abnormal patients showing more significant improvements than metabolically normal obese subjects (5). Finally, the odds of successful long-term body weight reduction through caloric restriction alone are generally small. On the other hand, there is now overwhelming evidence emphasizing that the importance of modifying the quality of the diet, rather than focussing on energy restriction only, should no longer be overlooked.

LOW-FAT VERSUS LOW-CARBOHYDRATE DIETS

For many years, several health agencies have prescribed low-fat diets (<30% of daily calories as fat) for the management of obesity and its associated comorbidities based on the fact that

[1] Benoît Lamarche is a Canada Research Chair in Nutrition and Cardiovascular Health.

[2] Caroline Richard is a recipient of a Studentship from the Fonds de la recherche en Santé du Québec.

(1) low-fat diets effectively lower blood cholesterol concentrations and (2) dietary fat intake has been considered one of the key etiological factors responsible for the contemporary rise in the obesity epidemic. While the favorable impact of a low-fat diet on plasma cholesterol concentration is beyond debate, its effects on other features of the cardiometabolic risk profile have been controversial. Indeed, low-fat diets when consumed under isoenergetic (weight stable) condition tend to deteriorate plasma triglyceride and HDL-C concentrations and lead to a greater prevalence of the atherogenic small dense LDL phenotype. Small reductions in body weight tend to attenuate these undesirable effects. We have shown that ad libitum consumption of a relatively low-fat diet (27% of calories as fat) in the presence of moderate weight loss led to a parallel reduction in the levels of visceral fat in overweight individuals (6). However, diet-induced reduction in visceral fat did not correlate with the parallel improvements in cardiometabolic risk factors, suggesting that changes in macronutrient quality may alter risk factors through mechanisms that are independent of diet-induced changes in the levels of abdominal obesity.

The controversies surrounding low-fat diets have been further propelled by the recent popular hype for low-carbohydrate/high-fat diets, for which there is growing scientific evidence supporting their efficacy for body weight and cardiovascular risk management (7). In general terms, low-carbohydrate diets have been associated with greater reductions in body weight than low-fat diets, at least in relatively short-term studies (8). In a study of obese diabetic patients consuming energy-restricted diets, the reduction in visceral fat area measured by computed tomography was greater (−40 cm2 vs. −10 cm2) in the low-carbohydrate diet group (protein:carbohydrate:fat = 25%:40%:35%) than in the high-carbohydrate/low-fat diet group (protein:carbohydrate:fat = 25%:65%:10%), despite comparable reductions in body weight between the two groups. The low-calorie/low-carbohydrate diet was also more effective in improving insulin sensitivity and in increasing plasma HDL-C levels than the low-calorie/high-carbohydrate diet in obese patients with type 2 diabetes (9). Krauss et al. have suggested that moderate carbohydrate restriction and weight loss may represent equivalent but nonadditive approaches to improve cardiometabolic risk factors (10).

Although there is convincing evidence supporting the fact that low- to very low-carbohydrate diets are effective in promoting weight loss and modifying the cardiometabolic risk profile; concerns regarding such diets have also been raised. First, a diet with less than 20% of calories as carbohydrates should be seen as extreme and restrictive. Adherence to such diets may result in unwanted behavioral changes in populations, such as obese patients, who already have fragile if not disrupted behaviors toward foods. Risk of potential deficiencies in essential nutrients, minerals, and vitamins, resulting from the restricted consumption of fruits, vegetables, and whole grain products, is also a concern. Long-term applicability has not been established to date. Finally, the efficacy of low-carbohydrate diets in reducing the risk of chronic disease, such as diabetes and CVD, has yet to be shown in large-scale population studies. It should be stressed that the impact of low-fat diets on the risk of diabetes and CVD has also not been convincingly demonstrated so far (11).

THE DASH DIET

The Dietary Approach to Stop Hypertension (DASH) is a carbohydrate-rich diet that emphasizes the consumption of fruits, vegetables, fibers, and low-fat dairy products. It is also reduced in dietary saturated fat, total fat, and cholesterol. Several studies have repeatedly demonstrated that DASH can substantially lower blood pressure, a hallmark of the cardiometabolic risk profile of abdominally obese patients with the metabolic syndrome. DASH can also favorably alter several other cardiovascular risk factors, such as plasma TG, LDL-C, and HDL-C levels, as well as indices of insulin sensitivity (12). Yet, DASH is not known as a weight-reducing diet, thus further exemplifying the importance of nutrient quality as a key determinant of the cardiometabolic risk profile, independent for the most part of variations in body weight (13). The palatability and the applicability of DASH over longer time periods is not a concern. This makes DASH an interesting choice as a primary dietary tool for the management of the cardiometabolic risk associated with abdominal obesity, although further studies are clearly needed to further support this hypothesis.

THE PORTFOLIO DIET

The portfolio diet was devised to comprise four dietary elements that have been granted cholesterol-lowering health, claimed by the Food and Drug Administration in the United States, namely, viscous fibers (10g/1000 kcal), plant sterols (1g/1000 kcal), soy protein (25g/1000 kcal), and almonds (23g/1000 kcal). In a series of metabolically controlled and longer term free-living studies, it has been shown that the combination of these four dietary components was very effective in reducing plasma LDL-C levels (14). The portfolio diet has also been shown to reduce plasma apoB and TG concentrations and the total/HDL-C ratio, and to increase LDL particle size, independent of body weight change, which is generally small with this dietary regimen. The portfolio diet has also been shown to reduce plasma CRP in subjects with moderate concentrations at baseline (15). However, because this diet has been formulated to target patients with elevated plasma cholesterol concentrations, its efficacy in obese patients with abdominal obesity and with the metabolic syndrome has not been demonstrated yet.

THE MEDITERRANEAN DIET (MEDDIET)

A typical Mediterranean-style diet is characterized by a high consumption of fruits, vegetables, legumes, grains and nuts, whole grain products, olive oil, and foods with a high monounsaturated to saturated fatty acid ratio, a moderate consumption of dairy products and alcohol (mostly wine), and a low intake of red meat and meat products in general (16).

Several studies (17,18) have confirmed the early observations from the Seven Countries Study, which first documented in the early 1960s the cardioprotective properties and health benefits attributable to the MedDiet (19). The overall pattern of the MedDiet has been shown to be a stronger correlate of mortality rates than the individual elements of the MedDiet (20) and mechanisms through which the MedDiet exerts its cardioprotective effects are just beginning to being unravelled.

The "Indo-MedDiet Heart Study" involving 1000 subjects who were randomly assigned to the MedDiet ($n = 499$) or a prudent diet ($n = 501$) reported significant reductions in mortality and CVD rates with the MedDiet. The authors observed a significant reduction in serum concentration of total cholesterol (−12%), LDL-C (−18%), and TG (−20%) in the MedDiet group. Plasma HDL-C increased by 2.6% but no change in the fasting blood glucose, blood pressure, and body mass index (BMI) were noticed between the two groups (18). The MedDiet was also associated with marked reductions in CVD rates in the Lyon Heart Study, despite having had no effect on total plasma cholesterol and HDL-C levels, blood pressure, and fasting blood glucose (17). Thus, the cardioprotective properties of the MedDiet cannot be entirely attributable to changes in traditional risk factors, but could also be ascribed to changes in nontraditional risk factors.

The MedDiet has been associated with a 48% net reduction in the prevalence of the metabolic syndrome after 2 years and with greater reductions in body weight and in waist circumference compared with a cardiac-prudent diet (21). Patients on the MedDiet have also shown significant reductions in serum concentrations of several inflammatory markers including CRP and IL-6, in insulin resistance as well as in endothelial function score (21). Finally, the MedDiet may beneficially alter the atherogenic small dense LDL phenotype (22) and reduce LDL oxidation (23). No study has yet examined the extent to which the MedDiet alters the cardiometabolic risk profile independent of concurrent variations in abdominal/visceral fat accumulation.

CONCLUSIONS

In summary, it is clear that there will be no "one size fits all" diet for the management and treatment of abdominal obesity and its associated cardiometabolic risk. However, the MedDiet shows great promises because it is readily applicable and simple, is acceptable from a global nutrition perspective, and there is now sound science supporting its effects. Unlike many other dietary plans, the MedDiet exerts positive effects on almost all components of the metabolic syndrome, including inflammation, insulin resistance, and endothelial dysfunction. Although further research is needed to better understand how this dietary pattern modulates the cardiometabolic risk associated with abdominal and visceral obesity, there is now convincing evidence that the MedDiet could help fighting diseases that are related to chronic inflammation, including abdominal obesity (24).

REFERENCES

1. Grundy SM, Hansen B, Smith SC, Jr., et al. Clinical management of metabolic syndrome: Report of the American Heart/National Heart, Lung, and Blood Institute/American Diabetes Association conference on scientific issues related to management. Circulation 2004; 109(4):551–556.
2. Case CC, Jones PH, Nelson K, et al. Impact of weight loss on the metabolic syndrome. Diabetes Obes Metab 2002; 4(6):407–414.
3. Chan DC, Barrett HP, Watts GF. Dyslipidemia in visceral obesity: Mechanisms, implications, and therapy. Am J Cardiovasc Drugs 2004; 4(4):227–246.
4. Tchernof A, Nolan A, Sites CK, et al. Weight loss reduces C-reactive protein levels in obese postmenopausal women. Circulation 2002; 105:564–569.
5. Shin MJ, Hyun YJ, Kim OY, et al. Weight loss effect on inflammation and LDL oxidation in metabolically healthy but obese (MHO) individuals: Low inflammation and LDL oxidation in MHO women. Int J Obes (Lond) 2006; 30(10):1529–1534.
6. Archer WR, Lamarche B, Deriaz O, et al. Variations in body composition and plasma lipids in response to a high-carbohydrate diet. Obes Res 2003; 11(8):978–986.
7. Klein S. Clinical trial experience with fat-restricted vs. carbohydrate-restricted weight-loss diets. Obes Res 2004; 12(Suppl. 2):141S–144S.
8. Yancy WS, Jr., Olsen MK, Guyton JR, et al. A low-carbohydrate, ketogenic diet versus a low-fat diet to treat obesity and hyperlipidemia: A randomized, controlled trial. Ann Intern Med 2004; 140(10):769–777.
9. Miyashita Y, Koide N, Ohtsuka M, et al. Beneficial effect of low carbohydrate in low calorie diets on visceral fat reduction in type 2 diabetic patients with obesity. Diabetes Res Clin Pract 2004; 65(3):235–241.
10. Krauss RM, Blanche PJ, Rawlings RS, et al. Separate effects of reduced carbohydrate intake and weight loss on atherogenic dyslipidemia. Am J Clin Nutr 2006; 83(5):1025–1031.
11. Howard BV, Van Horn L, Hsia J, et al. Low-fat dietary pattern and risk of cardiovascular disease: The women's health initiative randomized controlled dietary modification trial. JAMA 2006; 295(6):655–666.
12. Miller ER, III, Erlinger TP, Appel LJ. The effects of macronutrients on blood pressure and lipids: An overview of the dash and omniheart trials. Curr Atheroscler Rep 2006; 8(6):460–465.
13. Davy BM, Melby CL. The effect of fiber-rich carbohydrates on features of syndrome X. J Am Diet Assoc 2003; 103(1):86–96.
14. Jenkins DJ, Josse AR, Wong JM, et al. The portfolio diet for cardiovascular risk reduction. Curr Atheroscler Rep 2007; 9(6):501–507.
15. Jenkins DJ, Kendall CW, Marchie A, et al. Direct comparison of dietary portfolio vs statin on C-reactive protein. Eur J Clin Nutr 2005; 59(7):851–860.
16. Willett WC, Sacks F, Trichopoulou A, et al. Mediterranean diet pyramid a cultural model for healthy eating. Am J Clin Nutr 1995; 61(6 Suppl.):1402S–1406S.
17. de Lorgeril M, Salen P, Martin JL, et al. Mediterranean diet, traditional risk factors, and the rate of cardiovascular complications after myocardial infarction: Final report of the lyon diet heart study. Circulation 1999; 99(6):779–785.
18. Singh RB, Dubnov G, Niaz MA, et al. Effect of an Indo-Mediterranean diet on progression of coronary artery disease in high risk patients (Indo-Mediterranean Diet Heart Study): A randomised single-blind trial. Lancet 2002; 360(9344):1455–1461.
19. Keys A, Menotti A, Karvonen MJ, et al. The diet and 15-year death rate in the seven countries study. Am J Epidemiol 1986; 124(6):903–915.
20. Trichopoulou A, Kouris-Blazos A, Wahlqvist ML, et al. Diet and overall survival in elderly people. BMJ 1995; 311(7018):1457–1460.
21. Esposito K, Marfella R, Ciotola M, et al. Effect of a Mediterranean-style diet on endothelial dysfunction and markers of vascular inflammation in the metabolic syndrome: A randomized trial. JAMA 2004; 292(12):1440–1446.

22. Goulet J, Lamarche B, Charest A, et al. Effect of a nutritional intervention promoting the Mediterranean food pattern on electrophoretic characteristics of low-density lipoprotein particles in healthy women from the Quebec City metropolitan area. Br J Nutr 2004; 92(2):285–293.
23. Lapointe A, Goulet J, Couillard C, et al. A nutritional intervention promoting the Mediterranean food pattern is associated with a decrease in circulating oxidized LDL particles in healthy women from the Quebec city metropolitan area. J Nutr 2005; 135(3):410–415.
24. Giugliano D, Esposito K. Mediterranean diet and metabolic diseases. Curr Opin Lipidol 2008; 19(1):63–68.

16 The EC System and Central Control of Energy Balance—The Hypothalamus

Vincenzo Di Marzo

Endocannabinoid Research Group, Institute of Biomolecular Chemistry, National Research Council, Pozzuoli, Naples, Italy

INTRODUCTION: THE ENDOCANNABINOID SYSTEM AND THE HYPOTHALAMUS

All components of the endocannabinoid system are expressed in the hypothalamus, although data on their distribution are still largely incomplete. Cannabinoid CB_1 receptors are expressed in all hypothalamic nuclei except, perhaps, for the suprachiasmatic and lateral mammillary nuclei, and they are mostly (1), but not uniquely (2), found at the presynaptic level. The two major endogenous agonists of cannabinoid CB_1 receptors (or endocannabinoids), anandamide, and 2-arachidonoylglycerol (2-AG), are also present in the hypothalamus (3), and so are the enzymes that catalyze their biosynthesis, the diacylglycerol lipase-α (DAGL-α) for 2-AG and the *N*-acyl-phosphatidylethanolamine–selective phospholipase D (NAPE-PLD) for anandamide (V. Di Marzo and L. Cristino, unpublished results). The endocannabinoid (mostly anandamide)-degrading enzyme, fatty acid amide hydrolase (FAAH), is also known to be expressed in several nuclei of the hypothalamus (4). Anandamide levels in the hypothalamus have been found to peak before puberty and to fluctuate during the oestrus cycle in female rats (3,5), whereas hypothalamic 2-AG levels are modified by stress in various ways (6), thus suggesting a role of the endocannabinoid system in this brain area, at least for what concerns the control of reproductive and emotional function [see (7) for review]. However, as reviewed in this chapter, perhaps the most important function played by the endocannabinoid system in the hypothalamus has to do with the regulation of food-intake (7).

HYPOTHALAMIC CONTROL OF FOOD INTAKE BY THE ENDOCANNABINOID SYSTEM

It has been known for centuries that marijuana induces food intake (8). The stimulatory effects of Δ^9-THC on body weight, as well as its anti-emetic actions, have been exploited for the treatment of cachexia in cancer patients undergoing chemotherapy, and of wasting in AIDS patients, even before the cloning of cannabinoid CB_1 receptors (9). The development of potent, metabolically stable and selective agonists and antagonists/inverse agonists of CB_1 receptors, and of transgenic CB_1 receptor–null mice, made it possible to demonstrate that activation of these receptors is responsible for the appetite-inducing actions of Δ^9-THC and, more importantly, also of anandamide and 2-AG (10–11). In fact, pharmacological or genetic blockade of CB_1 causes reduction of food intake in rodents (12), and this is particularly noticeable either when the animals have been deprived of food for a few hours or in obese animals (13–14). However, the anorectic effect of CB_1 antagonists administered per se seems to undergo to tolerance after a few days of treatment (15). Nevertheless, chronic blockade of CB_1 receptors leads to sustained and significant weight loss, especially in obese rodents (13–14). Since one expects antagonists/inverse agonists to be more efficacious in the presence of an increased endogenous tone of the receptors they target, these data suggest that endocannabinoid levels in the brain centers controlling food intake are elevated following food deprivation and during obesity.

It is now known that CB_1 receptor activation strongly contributes to the intake of "normal" food mostly after brief food deprivation, whereas the consumption of palatable foods and drinks can be stimulated by CB_1 agonists, and blocked by CB_1 antagonists, even in satiated animals (16–18). These observations suggested a potential role of the endocannabinoid system in the control of both motivational and appetitive aspects of food intake. Accordingly, CB_1 receptors have been detected not only in the hypothalamus (19), but also in other brain nuclei involved in the control of energy intake, including the nucleus accumbens (20) and the vagus nerve and its termination at the level of the nodose ganglion (21), as well as in other brainstem areas controlling satiety and emesis, such as the nucleus tractus solitarius and area postrema (22). Although the contribution of the limbic and brainstem endocannabinoid system to food intake is discussed in other chapters, I shall review here the major mechanisms underlying the role of hypothalamic endocannabinoids in stimulating appetite.

Regulation and Dysregulation of Hypothalamic Endocannabinoids

In agreement with data obtained using CB_1 receptor antagonists, rat hypothalamic endocannabinoid, and in particular 2-AG, levels were shown to vary during food consumption and deprivation, being maximal following food deprivation and minimal during food consumption (11). This is similar to what observed for both anandamide and 2-AG in the limbic forebrain (11). In the brainstem nodose ganglion, which controls satiety, CB_1 receptor expression increases during food deprivation, possibly because of the action of ghrelin, the levels of which increase under these conditions; CB_1 expression, instead, decreases following food intake, probably because under the control of cholecystokinin, the levels of which increase following food consumption (21–23). The higher hypothalamic levels of endocannabinoids observed in rats following brief food deprivation (11), and of anandamide during the "lights-on" phase of the day (when the animals are sleeping and food-deprived) (24), might be due to the fact that leptin, whose levels are increased following food consumption and decreased following food deprivation, tonically limits the levels of anandamide and 2-AG in the rat hypothalamus (13), much in the same way it reduces the levels of hypothalamic orexigenic mediators and increases those of anorectic ones. As a consequence, in the hypothalamus of obese rodents that cannot produce leptin (ob/ob mice), or that are characterized by impaired leptin receptor signaling (db/db mice and Zucker rats), permanently elevated endocannabinoid levels were detected (13). This suggests that also in obese humans, who rapidly develop leptin resistance, the hypothalamic levels of endocannabinoids might be increased, and possibly contribute to hyperphagia. Leptin also decreases endocannabinoid levels in other cells or tissues that express the leptin receptors, such as T lymphocytes (25) and the uterus (26), and a negative correlation between blood leptin and anandamide levels was found in normoweight and anorexic women (27).

Ghrelin is another important peripheral hormone involved in food intake and, as mentioned above, is released into the bloodstream from the stomach during food deprivation to stimulate energy intake. This peptide was recently shown to elevate 2-AG levels in the hypothalamus (28), and this effect clearly contributes to its orexigenic actions, as pharmacological and genetic blockade of CB_1 receptors strongly reduces the orexigenic action of the hormone (29) as well as its activation of the AMP kinase (28), which, in the hypothalamus, also causes orexigenic effects. Ghrelin levels are known to be chronically elevated in obese individuals, and this phenomenon, together with leptin resistance, might again lead to elevation of hypothalamic endocannabinoid levels in obesity. Accordingly, unpublished work carried out in the author's laboratory has shown that the expression of the major enzyme involved in 2-AG biosynthesis, the DAGL-α, is significantly upregulated in the hypothalamus (namely, the arcuate nucleus and lateral hypothalamus) of ob/ob mice and of mice with diet-induced obesity.

Glucocorticoids are another likely candidate for the regulation of hypothalamic endocannabinoids. In fact, activation of "fast" glucocorticoid receptors, likely localized in the neuronal plasma membrane, was found to stimulate the biosynthesis of endocannabinoids in this brain area (30), whereas the circulating levels of corticosterone are known to increase after food deprivation and decrease immediately after food consumption. Unlike leptin, ghrelin and glucocorticoids, intracerebral or intra-hypothalamic infusions of α-melanin stimulating hormone and insulin, under conditions in which these hormones cause anorectic and metabolic effects, do not appear to affect the levels of the two major endocannabinoids (31). Conversely, indirect evidence exists suggesting a positive regulation by orexin A on endocannabinoid levels, since sub-effective doses of the CB_1 antagonist rimonabant were recently shown to attenuate the orexigenic actions of the neuropeptide (32).

Effects of Hypothalamic CB_1 Receptor Activation

Activation of hypothalamic CB_1 receptors can, in principle, cause two general types of effects depending on CB_1 distribution in neurons. When the endocannabinoids act as retrograde signals on presynaptic CB_1 receptors (33), they normally lead to rapid modulation of glutamate or GABA release, with subsequent tuning of the activity of either orexigenic or anorectic postsynaptic neurons. Conversely, when postsynaptic CB_1 receptors are stimulated, they might lead to long-term regulation of the expression of genes encoding for orexigenic or anorectic neuropeptides.

Short-Term/Presynaptic Effects

Electrophysiological data support the involvement of endocannabinoids, under the negative control of leptin, as modulators of short-term synaptic plasticity in the hypothalamus (34). The activation of presynaptic CB_1 receptors, located on GABA terminals, decreases GABA release onto orexigenic melanin concentrating hormone (MCH)-releasing neurons of the lateral hypothalamus, and this effect is consistent with increased feeding behavior. The activation of leptin receptors on these neurons inhibits calcium currents, and the consequent decrease in calcium results in reduced endocannabinoid biosynthesis. Leptin-deficient obese mice (ob/ob) are characterized by both an increase in steady-state voltage-gated calcium currents in lateral hypothalamic neurons and a CB_1 receptor–mediated depolarization-induced suppression of inhibition that is 6-fold stronger than that in littermate controls, in agreement with previous data showing elevated endocannabinoid levels in the hypothalamus of these mice (13). Subsequently, perifornical lateral hypothalamic neurons in ob/ob mice have larger calcium currents, which is consistent with upregulated endocannabinoid signaling, enhanced excitability and MCH release, and consequent hyperphagia (34).

Hentges and coworkers recently suggested that the activity of anorectic pre-opiomelanocortin (POMC)–expressing neurons in the arcuate nucleus are also either stimulated or inhibited by presynaptic CB_1 receptors (35), via inhibition of GABAergic or glutamatergic inputs on these neurons, respectively. These two retrograde actions of endocannabinoids might produce opposing effects on melanocortin release, that is, stimulation or inhibition, respectively, only the latter of which would be consistent with the orexigenic actions of CB_1 receptors (35). It is possible that following food deprivation or during obesity, when hypothalamic levels of endocannabinoids increase, the population of CB_1 expressed on glutamatergic neurons is activated preferentially, thus leading to inhibition of POMC neurons and stimulation of food intake. A similar mechanism might also occur with orexigenic orexin A–expressing neurons of the lateral hypothalamus, where it was reported that retrograde endocannabinoids produced from these neurons act on presynaptic CB_1 receptors to inhibit glutamate release and thus cause inhibition of orexin A release (36). On the other hand, unpublished data from the author's laboratory show that CB_1 receptors are also expressed on GABAergic terminals innervating orexin A–expressing neurons in this hypothalamic nucleus, thus raising the possibility that retrograde endocannabinoids might also disinhibit the activity of these neurons.

Finally, it was recently shown that endocannabinoids, acting retrogradely on CB_1-expressing parvocellular neurons of the paraventricular nucleus (PVN) and produced following activation of ghrelin receptors in postsynaptic PVN neurons, inhibit glutamatergic signaling and subsequently the activity of these anorectic neurons (28).

Long-Term/Postsynaptic Effects

By using in situ hybridization techniques, Cota and coworkers demonstrated that CB_1 mRNA is expressed in neurons producing several of the neuropeptides that regulate food intake (37), such as the orexigenic agouti–related protein (AgRP), orexins and MCH, or the anorectic POMC and the cocaine- and amphetamine-regulated transcript (CART). MCH co-localizes with CB_1 in the lateral hypothalamic area and both corticotropin-releasing hormone (CRH) and CART co-localize with CB_1 in the PVN. Importantly, hypothalamic CRH mRNA levels in the PVN, but not in other extrahypothalamic areas, such as the amygdala and piriform cortex, are higher in CB_1-deficient mice, thus indicating that CB_1 receptors tonically downregulate CRH expression (37–38). Accordingly, blood corticosterone levels are increased following CB_1 antagonism in obese Zucker rats (39), which contain high hypothalamic levels of endocannabinoids (13).

It has also been shown that elevation of endogenous anandamide levels, obtained by knocking out the FAAH enzyme, is accompanied by reduced CART release in several hypothalamic regions, an effect antagonized by a CB_1 antagonist (4,40). Based on the finding that stimulation of hypothalamic CB_1 receptors increases the levels of neuropeptide Y (NPY) (41), it was suggested that the orexigenic effects of endocannabinoids could be in part mediated by this neuropeptide. However, no co-localization of CB_1 receptors with NPY was observed by Cota and colleagues in hypothalamic neurons (37), which would indicate that multisynaptic

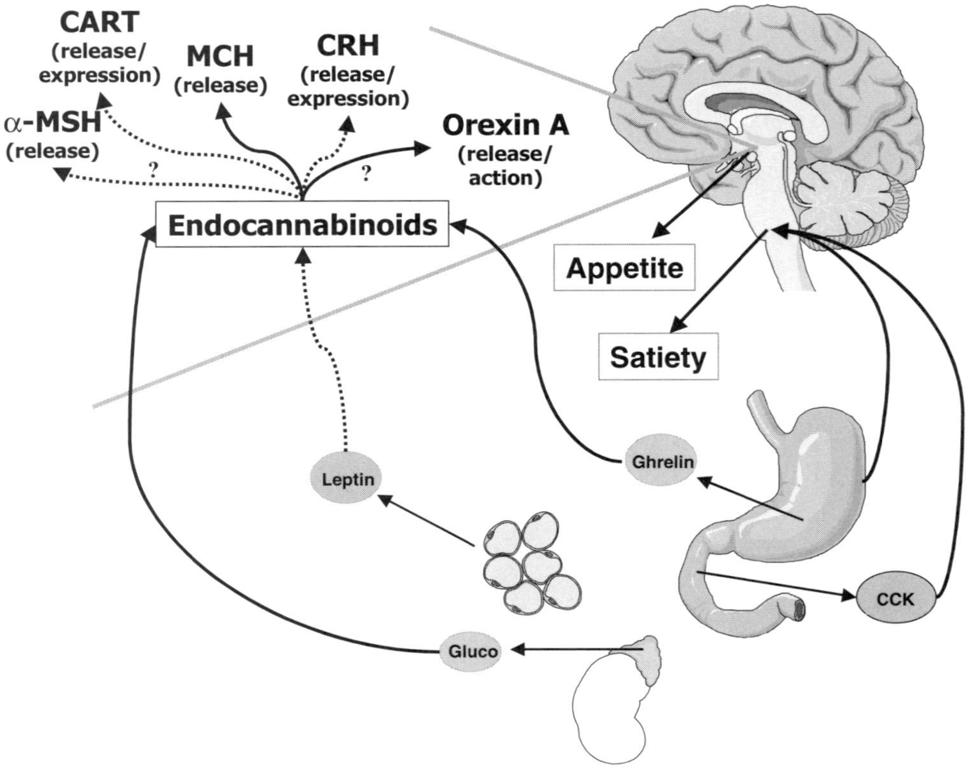

Figure 1 Regulation of hypothalamic endocannabinoids by peripheral hormones and their effects on hypothalamic orexigenic and anorectic mediators. *Abbreviations*: α-MSH, α-melanocyte stimulating hormone; CART, cocaine and amphetamine-regulated transcript; CCK, colecystokinin; CRH, corticotropin-stimulating hormone; Gluco, glucocorticoids; MCH, melanin-concentrating hormone. Continuous arrows denote activation, broken arrows denote inhibition.

mechanisms are required for CB_1 to stimulate NPY release. Furthermore, pharmacological CB_1 blockade reduces food intake in NPY knockout mice as efficaciously as in wild-type mice (13), suggesting that NPY signaling is not necessary for CB_1-mediated food intake. If anything, it is the activation of CB_1 receptors that is down-stream of NPY since the orexigenic effects of this peptide are lost in CB_1 null mice (42).

Finally, another type of effect by postsynaptic CB_1 receptors might be to enhance orexin A signaling. In fact, it has been shown that orexin A receptors can be sensitized by CB_1 receptors co-expressed in the same cells (43–44), and unpublished immunohistochemical work carried out in the author's laboratory showed that, in the mouse hypothalamus, CB_1 and orexin A receptors are indeed strongly co-localized in the arcuate nucleus and PVN, at both the presynaptic and postsynaptic level.

CONCLUSIONS

As reviewed in this chapter, the endocannabinoid system plays a major role in the hypothalamus by stimulating food intake after food deprivation or during obesity. Hypothalamic endocannabinoids are under the positive or negative control of several key players in food intake, and in turn possess several ways to affect the levels and release of orexigenic and anorectic neuropeptides, by acting via pre and postsynaptic mechanisms and with short- and long-term effects (Fig. 1). Although we now know that the central control of food intake and satiety is not the only way through which the endocannabinoid system contributes to body weight (see other chapters in this book), certainly the hypothalamus, with its neural connections to the mesolimbic system and the brainstem, is one of the favorite sites of action for endocannabinoids. There is evidence, in fact, that even activation of CB_1 receptors in the nucleus accumbens, and the subsequent induction of food intake, is accompanied by the activation of several hypothalamic nuclei (45). Importantly, and like in other organs controlling energy homeostasis, the hypothalamic endocannabinoid system, possibly because of the dysregulation of hormones controlling its outputs, is also characterized by aberrant activity during obesity, and this alteration is likely to underlie at least in part the anti-obesity effects of CB_1 receptor antagonists.

REFERENCES

1. Wittmann G, Deli L, Kalló I, et al. Distribution of type 1 cannabinoid receptor (CB1)-immunoreactive axons in the mouse hypothalamus. J Comp Neurol 2007; 503:270–279.
2. Cristino L, de Petrocellis L, Pryce G, et al. Immunohistochemical localization of cannabinoid type 1 and vanilloid transient receptor potential vanilloid type 1 receptors in the mouse brain. Neuroscience 2006; 139:1405–1415.
3. Wenger T, Gerendai I, Fezza F, et al. The hypothalamic levels of the endocannabinoid, anandamide, peak immediately before the onset of puberty in female rats. Life Sci 2002; 70:1407–1414.
4. Osei-Hyiaman D, Depetrillo M, Harvey-White J, et al. Cocaine and amphetamine-related transcript is involved in the orexigenic effect of endogenous anandamide. Neuroendocrinology 2005; 81:273–282.
5. González S, Bisogno T, Wenger T, et al. Sex steroid influence on cannabinoid CB(1) receptor mRNA and endocannabinoid levels in the anterior pituitary gland. Biochem Biophys Res Commun 2000; 270:260–266.
6. Patel S, Roelke CT, Rademacher DJ, et al. Endocannabinoid signaling negatively modulates stress-induced activation of the hypothalamic–pituitary–adrenal axis. Endocrinology 2004; 145:5431–5438.
7. Pagotto U, Marsicano G, Cota D,et al. The emerging role of the endocannabinoid system in endocrine regulation and energy balance. Endocr Rev 2006; 27:73–100.
8. Foltin RW, Fischman MW, Byrne MF. Effects of smoked marijuana on food intake and body weight of humans living in a residential laboratory. Appetite 1988; 11:1–14.
9. Di Marzo V, De Petrocellis L. Plant, synthetic, and endogenous cannabinoids in medicine. Annu Rev Med 2006; 57:553–574.
10. Williams CM, Kirkham TC. Anandamide induces overeating: Mediation by central cannabinoid (CB1) receptors. Psychopharmacology (Berl) 1999; 143:315–317.
11. Kirkham TC, Williams CM, Fezza F, et al. Endocannabinoid levels in rat limbic forebrain and hypothalamus in relation to fasting, feeding, and satiation: Stimulation of eating by 2-arachidonoyl glycerol. Br J Pharmacol 2002; 136:550–557.
12. Colombo G, Agabio R, Diaz G, et al. Appetite suppression and weight loss after the cannabinoid antagonist SR 141716 A. Life Sci 1998; 63:113–117.
13. Di Marzo V, Goparaju SK, Wang L,et al. Leptin-regulated endocannabinoids are involved in maintaining food intake. Nature 2001; 410:822–825.
14. Vickers SP, Webster LJ, Wyatt A, et al. Preferential effects of the cannabinoid CB1 receptor antagonist, SR 141716, on food intake and body weight gain of obese (fa/fa) compared to lean Zucker rats. Psychopharmacology (Berl) 2003; 167:103–111.
15. Rigamonti AE, Giordani C, Bonomo SM, et al. Early tolerance to the hypophagic effect of the cannabinoid receptor antagonist SR141716 does not impede blockade of an orexigenic stimulus. Eur J Pharmacol 2006; 542:116–120.
16. Gallate JE, Saharov T, Mallet PE, et al. Increased motivation for beer in rats following administration of a cannabinoid CB1 receptor agonist. Eur J Pharmacol 1999; 370:233–240.
17. Williams CM, Rogers PJ, Kirkham TC. Hyperphagia in pre-fed rats following oral delta^9-THC. Physiol Behav 1998; 65:343–346.
18. Simiand J, Keane M, Keane PE, et al. SR 141716, a CB1 cannabinoid receptor antagonist, selectively reduces sweet food intake in marmoset. Behav Pharmacol 1998; 9:179–181.
19. Gonzalez S, Manzanares J, Berrendero F, et al. Identification of endocannabinoids and cannabinoid CB(1) receptor mRNA in the pituitary gland. Neuroendocrinology 1999; 70:137–145.
20. Robbe D, Kopf M, Remaury A, et al. Endogenous cannabinoids mediate long-term synaptic depression in the nucleus accumbens. Proc Natl Acad Sci USA 2002; 99:8384–8388.
21. Burdyga G, Lal S, Varro A, et al. Expression of cannabinoid CB1 receptors by vagal afferent neurons is inhibited by cholecystokinin. J Neurosci 2004; 24:2708–2715.
22. Partosoedarso ER, Abrahams TP, Scullion RT, et al. Cannabinoid1 receptor in the dorsal vagal complex modulates lower oesophageal sphincter relaxation in ferrets. J Physiol 2003; 550:149–158.
23. Burdyga G, Varro A, Dimaline R, et al. Ghrelin receptors in rat and human nodose ganglia: Putative role in regulating CB-1 and MCH receptor abundance. Am J Physiol Gastrointest Liver Physiol 2006; 290:G1289–G1297.

24. Murillo-Rodriguez E, Desarnaud F, Prospero-Garcia O. Diurnal variation of arachidonoylethanolamine, palmitoylethanolamide and oleoylethanolamide in the brain of the rat. Life Sci 2006
25. Maccarrone M, Di Rienzo M, Finazzi-Agro A, et al. Leptin activates the anandamide hydrolase promoter in human T lymphocytes through STAT3. J Biol Chem 2003; 278:13318–13324.
26. Maccarrone M, Fride E, Bisogno T, et al. Up-regulation of the endocannabinoid system in the uterus of leptin knockout (ob/ob) mice and implications for fertility. Mol Hum Reprod 2005; 11:21–28.
27. Monteleone P, Matias I, Martiadis V, et al. Blood levels of the endocannabinoid anandamide are increased in anorexia nervosa and in binge-eating disorder, but not in bulimia nervosa. Neuropsychopharmacology 2005; 30:1216–1221.
28. Kola B, Farkas I, Christ-Crain M, et al. The orexigenic effect of ghrelin is mediated through central activation of the endogenous cannabinoid system. Plos One 2008; 3:e1797.
29. Tucci SA, Rogers EK, Korbonits M, et al. The cannabinoid CB1 receptor antagonist SR141716 blocks the orexigenic effects of intrahypothalamic ghrelin. Br J Pharmacol 2004; 143:520–533.
30. Malcher-Lopes R, Di S, Marcheselli VS, et al. Opposing crosstalk between leptin and glucocorticoids rapidly modulates synaptic excitation via endocannabinoid release. J Neurosci 2006; 26:6643–6650.
31. Matias I, Vergoni AV, Petrosino S, et al. Regulation of hypothalamic endocannabinoid levels by neuropeptides and hormones involved in food intake and metabolism: Insulin and melanocortins. Neuropharmacology 2008; 54:206–212.
32. Crespo I, Gómez de Heras R, Rodríguez de Fonseca F, et al. Pretreatment with subeffective doses of Rimonabant attenuates orexigenic actions of orexin A-hypocretin 1. Neuropharmacology 2008; 54:219–225.
33. Wilson RI, Nicoll RA. Endocannabinoid signaling in the brain. Science 2002; 296:678–682.
34. Jo YH, Chen YJ, Chua SC Jr., et al. Integration of endocannabinoid and leptin signaling in an appetite-related neural circuit. Neuron 2005; 48:1055–1066.
35. Hentges ST, Low MJ, Williams JT. Differential regulation of synaptic inputs by constitutively released endocannabinoids and exogenous cannabinoids. J Neurosci 2005; 25:9746–9751.
36. Huang H, Acuna-Goycolea C, Li Y, et al. Cannabinoids excite hypothalamic melanin-concentrating hormone but inhibit hypocretin/orexin neurons: Implications for cannabinoid actions on food intake and cognitive arousal. J Neurosci 2007; 27:4870–4881.
37. Cota D, Marsicano G, Tschöp M, et al. The endogenous cannabinoid system affects energy balance via central orexigenic drive and peripheral lipogenesis. J Clin Invest 2003; 112:423–431.
38. Cota D, Steiner MA, Marsicano G, et al. Requirement of cannabinoid receptor type 1 for the basal modulation of hypothalamic–pituitary–adrenal axis function. Endocrinology 2007; 148:1574–1581.
39. Doyon C, Denis RG, Baraboi ED, et al. Effects of rimonabant (SR141716) on fasting-induced hypothalamic–pituitary–adrenal axis and neuronal activation in lean and obese Zucker rats. Diabetes 2006; 55:3403–3410.
40. Verty AN, McGregor IS, Mallet PE, et al. The impact of cannabinoid receptor (CB1) antagonists on the central neural circuitry mediating energy balance. 36th Neuroscience Annual Meeting, Washington, USA, 2006, Poster number 456.3/BB3.
41. Gamber KM, Macarthur H, Westfall TC. Cannabinoids augment the release of neuropeptide Y in the rat hypothalamus. Neuropharmacology 2005; 49:646–652.
42. Poncelet M, Maruani J, Calassi R, et al. Overeating, alcohol and sucrose consumption decrease in CB1 receptor deleted mice. Neurosci Lett 2003; 343:216–218.
43. Hilairet S, Bouaboula M, Carrière D, et al. Hypersensitization of the Orexin 1 receptor by the CB1 receptor: Evidence for cross-talk blocked by the specific CB1 antagonist, SR141716. J Biol Chem 2003; 278:23731–23737.
44. Ellis J, Pediani JD, Canals M, et al. Orexin-1 receptor–cannabinoid CB1 receptor heterodimerization results in both ligand-dependent and independent coordinated alterations of receptor localization and function. J Biol Chem 2006;281:38812–38824.
45. Soria-Gómez E, Matias I, Rueda-Orozco PE, et al. Pharmacological enhancement of the endocannabinoid system in the nucleus accumbens shell stimulates food intake and increases c-Fos expression in the hypothalamus. Br J Pharmacol 2007; 151:1109–1116.

17 The EC System and Central Control of Energy Balance: The Nucleus Accumbens

Tim C. Kirkham

School of Psychology, University of Liverpool, Eleanor Rathbone Building, Bedford Street South, Liverpool, England, U.K.

INTRODUCTION

The appetite-stimulating actions of *Cannabis sativa* and its extracts have long been recognized and are documented in the most ancient of medicinal texts. These actions are now attributed to phytocannabinoid actions at brain CB_1 cannabinoid receptors (1–2), and are considered to reflect a crucial biological role of endocannabinoids in appetite processes. Indeed, as will be outlined below, endogenous CB_1 agonists have been shown to induce eating via actions at key, appetite-related, brain nuclei, and levels of brain endocannabinoids fluctuate in relation to fasting and food consumption. Recent empirical evidence strongly supports a role for the ECS in the normal controls of appetite, and CB_1 antagonists/inverse agonists—with their established anorectic actions—have been intensively researched as a potential new class of anti-obesity agents. However, there is still much to be learned about the actual mechanisms through which cannabinoids promote appetite and eating, quite apart from ECS involvement in nonbehavioral aspects of energy regulation. More specifically, there is an urgent need to define the precise behavioral and motivational actions of central endocannabinoids, and to characterize the possibly distinct roles that each endocannabinoid may play in these processes. The principal sources of evidence that currently shape our hypotheses regarding the role of the ECS in the psychological aspects of appetite are briefly summarized below.

CANNABINOID EFFECTS ON HUMAN APPETITE

Apart from anecdotal reports obtained from cannabis users, there are very few laboratory-based, empirical studies of phytocannabinoid effects on human appetite (1–4), and only a handful of clinical trials assessing THC (dronabinol) efficacy in the treatment of wasting and appetite loss in cancer cachexia and AIDS patients (5–8). The critical findings are that acute or chronic doses of smoked or orally administered THC or cannabis can stimulate hunger and food craving, and enhance food appreciation (9–12). These effects are associated with substantial increases in caloric intake (typically, but not exclusively, derived from snack foods) and an increased frequency of eating episodes (13–18). We have recently obtained data to show that THC administered by means of an oromucosal spray dose dependently stimulates appetite, accelerating the normal rise in pre-prandial hunger ratings, and increases consumption of a variety of sweet and non-sweet foods (Jones and Kirkham, unpublished observations).

It is probable that the above-described actions of phytocannabinoids are CB_1 receptor–mediated, since the broader psychopharmacological actions of cannabis in people are reversed by the selective CB_1 antagonist rimonabant (19,20). However, no specific antagonist challenge of cannabinoid hyperphagia has been reported. Moreover, although CB_1 antagonists obviously provide a valuable tool to explore the normal role of ECS in appetite processes, and despite the extensive clinical trials with rimonabant (and more recently, taranabant) (21–25), few meaningful data have been published to describe the acute effects of the antagonists on subjective appetite ratings. However, there are indications that CB_1 blockade can produce opposite, complementary, effects to the agonists. Blundell and colleagues (26) treated patients with 20 mg/day rimonabant for over 3 months. The study found not only a reduction in energy intake (that was independent of the dietary composition or intrinsic pleasantness of foods), but also a reliable attenuation of food craving and hunger ratings prior to periodic test meals. The size of these motivational effects became more reliable over the course of treatment, leading the authors to conclude that rimonabant enabled patients to gain improved control of their habitual overeating.

ANIMAL STUDIES

Cannabinoid effects in people lay the basis for current hypotheses about the normal role of brain endocannabinoids in appetite processes. But, although even the insights contained within anecdotal reports can inform our model building, we are largely dependent on animal studies for the development of theoretical accounts about ECS involvement in the control of appetite.

Anorectic Effects of CB_1 Antagonists

The first indirect indications of a role for endocannabinoids in feeding came from demonstrations of the anorectic action of rimonabant in animals (27–28), potentially indicating tonic endocannabinoid activity in feeding-related systems. Reliable anorectic actions of a variety of CB_1 antagonists/inverse agonists (e. g., AM281, AM251, O-3259 and O-3257, surinabant, taranabant) have since been reported, following systemic or central administration in satiated or food-deprived animals, and after acute or chronic treatments [e. g., (28–33)]. Additionally, CB_1 blockade can attenuate the phenotypic hyperphagia in genetic models of obesity (34,35).

An important consideration in the interpretation of antagonist effects relates to their behavioral specificity. There are numerous reports that the antagonists may suppress food intake through the induction of nonspecific malaise, conditioned taste aversion, anxiety, or by stimulation of behaviors that are incompatible with the expression of eating, such as compulsive grooming and scratching (36–40).

Hyperphagic Effects of CB_1 Agonists

Systemic or central THC administration can potently stimulate feeding in a variety of animal models (41–43) and this hyperphagia is mediated by CB_1 receptors, being reversed by rimonabant but not the CB_2 selective antagonist SR144258 (44). Of greater significance is the discovery that the hyperphagic actions of exogenous cannabinoids may be replicated with the endocannabinoids anandamide, 2-AG and noladin ether, following systemic or central injection. Again, these actions appear to be CB_1-mediated and can be blocked by very low, sub-anorectic doses of CB_1 antagonists that are devoid of the above noted non-specific behavioral actions (45–49). Importantly, anandamide and 2-AG will promote feeding when administered into brain regions that are closely associated with eating motivation, including various hypothalamic nuclei and the shell of the nucleus accumbens (see below) (3,47–48).

ENDOCANNABINOIDS AND APPETITE: MOTIVATIONAL MECHANISMS AND THE NUCLEUS ACCUMBENS

Reflecting the limited human evidence related to cannabis and THC, hypotheses about how cannabinoids affect eating motivation have largely focused on the heightened food craving, enhanced sensitivity to the sensory properties of food, and apparently preferential effects of CB_1 ligands on preferred, highly palatable foods. Notably, rimonabant's anorectic action was initially reported to be enhanced when animals were fed sweet, palatable foods. As the drug also suppressed sucrose and ethanol drinking, it was proposed that the drug modifies the hedonic value of ingesta via actions on reward pathways (27,28).

Research now supports a role for endocannabinoids in the distinct incentive and reward aspects of appetite, modulating not only the motivation to obtain food and to engage in eating, but also the hedonic evaluation—or palatability—of food that maintains consumption within a meal (50–51). Thus, rats will work harder to obtain palatable ingesta after administration of CB_1 receptor agonists, while antagonist treatments attenuate responding (52–53). Additionally, $CB_1{}^{-/-}$ mice show lower levels of responding for sucrose than wild-type mice (54).

Observational and meal pattern analyses reveal that exogenous and endogenous cannabinoids directly increase the salience of food, independent of need or energetic status. Thus, CB_1 agonists can induce feeding almost as soon as food becomes available. Our animal studies show that, within a finite test interval after cannabinoid treatment, increased food intake primarily results from the advance of meal onset, with only modest increases in meal duration or meal size. Importantly, apart from reduced eating latency, the microstructure of cannabinoid-induced feeding behavior is identical to that of normal, spontaneous eating (1,48,55), indicating that cannabinoids provoke feeding through adjustments to natural feeding processes and hence supporting a normal physiological role of the ECS in appetite control.

Of the various brain loci linked to feeding, the shell subregion of the accumbens (AcbSh) has particularly strong associations with incentive-reward processes (56). The AcbSh contains a relatively high density of CB_1 receptors (57,58) and is particularly sensitive to endocannabinoid-induced feeding. Administration of 2-AG or anandamide into this region induces substantial short-term, antagonist-reversible hyperphagia (48,59). In line with the notion that endocannabinoids mediate the incentive value of food, intra-accumbens 2-AG dramatically advances the onset of feeding. Fasting, which naturally increases food incentive value (and reduces eating latency), significantly increases anandamide and 2-AG levels within the forebrain regions containing the AcbSh (48); effects, which may underlie the enhanced anorectic potency of rimonabant in fasted animals (1,3) and the reduced hyperphagic response to fasting in $CB_1^{-/-}$ animals (60). Emphasizing the importance of accumbens circuitry in endocannabinoid influences on appetite, Soria-Gómez and colleagues found that intra-AcbSh injection of the FAAH inhibitor *N*-arachidonoyl-serotonin increased both accumbens 2-AG levels and stimulated food intake (59).

Endocannabinoid–Dopamine Interactions in Food Wanting

Mesolimbic dopamine (DA) neurons, arising in the ventral tegmental area (VTA) and projecting to the nucleus accumbens, are also central to incentive processes in feeding (61–62), and are key to an organism's orientation toward motivationally significant stimuli and the elicitation of appropriate behavioral responses (63–66). Food stimuli cause DA release in the nucleus accumbens under conditions were food incentive is elevated, such as after fasting, or with the presentation of novel or palatable food. Melis and colleagues (67) have reported that rimonabant reduces the increase in accumbens DA release induced by a novel, highly palatable food. Hyperphagic doses of THC stimulate accumbens DA release (66–68), while THC hyperphagia is attenuated by the D1 antagonist SCH23390 (69). Additionally, SCH23390 and the D2 antagonist reticlopride, respectively, increase anandamide and 2-AG levels in limbic forebrain (70). Complementing those findings, anandamide has been shown to increase extra-cellular DA levels in the AcbSh (70).

Endocannabinoid–Opioid Interactions in Food Liking

In addition to incentive processes, endocannabinoids may also contribute to the pleasure (reward) derived from eating. Such a role is evident in anecdotal reports of cannabis users (10), and animal studies show that CB_1 stimulation or blockade/deletion can, respectively, render food more or less pleasurable. For example, rimonabant was reported to preferentially attenuate the intake of palatable, sweet foods (27–28) and reduce operant responding for sweet food (72); while CB_1 knockout mice do not display the hyperphagia characteristic of the wild-type when fed a palatable, high-fat diet (73).

It should be noted that CB_1 agonist and antagonist effects are not only obtained with highly palatable test foods. For example, antagonist suppression of operant responding is also evident with low palatability foods (72–74), rimonabant is equi-anorectic when tested with foods of differing macronutrient content (75), and agonists will increase intake of the blandest diets (44,45,48). It is probable, therefore, that endocannabinoids modulate appetitive processes per se to provide a general gain in the incentive and reward value of food. Indeed, in taste reactivity tests, THC has been shown to increase the acceptability of even bitter, normally aversive, quinine solutions (76).

The actions of exogenous and endogenous cannabinoids on the microstructure of sucrose drinking match those observed in drug-free animals through a simple increase in the palatability of the test solution (77). Conversely, antagonists alter drinking patterns and hedonic reactions to sweet solutions in a way that is wholly consistent with a reduction in palatability (76,77). Additionally, $CB_1^{-/-}$ mice are less responsive to sweet taste, consistently drinking less sucrose solution than the wild type (54). Key components of the neural mechanisms underlying food palatability lie within the AcbSh and, as already noted, 2-AG administered here produces a profound hyperphagic response (48). Interestingly, in taste reactivity tests, intra-accumbens administration of anandamide specifically increases the number of positive ingestive responses to intra-oral infusions of sweet solutions, indicating that anandamide specifically enhances their hedonic impact, or liking (78). Moreover, accumbens CB_1 receptors are downregulated in rats that chronically overconsume palatable foods (79), presumably in response to increased activation of these receptors by endocannabinoids.

Endocannabinoids may have important functional relationships with the endogenous opioid systems that have an established role mediating food palatability (80–82). Notably, there is ultrastructural evidence that cannabinoid–opioid interactions are mediated by activation of CB_1 and μ-opioid receptors within the same, or synaptically linked, reward-relevant neurons in the AcbSh (83). In rats, THC hyperphagia is blocked by the general opioid receptor antagonist, naloxone (44), and the facilitatory effects of the CB_1 agonist CP55940 on responding for palatable solutions are reversed by both a CB_1 antagonist and naloxone (53). Moreover, low doses of rimonabant and opioid antagonists that are behaviorally inactive when administered separately, combine synergistically to suppress food intake (84,85). In addition, the accumbens shell sites at which anandamide increases the liking of sweet solutions in taste reactivity tests overlap those where morphine administration produces similar behavioral effects (78,86). Moreover, systemic administration of THC has been shown to stimulate β-endorphin release in both the VTA and AcbSh (87), and CB_1 agonist-induced DA release in the accumbens is blocked by intra-VTA infusion of the μ1-selective antagonist, naloxonazine (88).

Typically, the consequences of cannabinoid or opioid manipulations on eating motivational can be easily distinguished. For example, cannabinoids primarily reduce eating latency without affecting meal duration (i.e., actions on appetitive processes) (55); while opioids generally do not alter eating latency but extend meal duration by enhancing palatability (i.e., actions on consummatory processes) (80). However, Solinas and Goldberg (89) found that increased responding for food after both THC or morphine can be blocked by either rimonabant or naloxone, suggesting that activation of endocannabinoid and endogenous opioid systems jointly facilitate the motivational effects of food. Arguably, such co-operativity between cannabinoid and opioid systems could provide a mechanism whereby direct, primary cannabinoid influences on appetitive motivation (wanting) and their secondary facilitation of opioid-mediated consummatory motivation (liking) merge to provide the anticipatory component of the psychological experience of conditioned hunger and food craving.

CONCLUSION

The combined human and animal data outlined here, although still relatively limited, converge to support a model in which the ECS is critical to the processes that underlie the normal controls of appetite and eating motivation. Specifically, it can be proposed that endocannabinoids are intimately associated with the brain mechanisms (particularly those involving the nucleus accumbens) that mediate food craving and the pleasure that is derived from eating. Endocannabinoids, acting in part by modulation of mesolimbic DA systems, may be key to the wanting of food and to the anticipation of eating. Additionally, endocannabinoids appear to interact with opioid peptides to mediate the rewarding effects, or liking, of food. As such, a deeper understanding of endocannabinoid involvement in these processes may provide important intervention targets to manage the compelling overconsumption of palatable, energy-dense foods that is the major contributor to the development and maintenance of obesity.

REFERENCES

1. Kirkham TC, Williams CM. Endogenous cannabinoids and appetite. Nutr Res Rev 2001; 14:65–86.
2. Kirkham TC. Endocannabinoids in the regulation of appetite and body weight. Behav Pharmacol 2005; 16:297–313.
3. Kirkham TC, Williams CM. Endocannabinoids: Neuromodulators of food craving? In: Hetherington M, ed. Food Cravings and Addiction. Surrey, U. K.: Leatherhead Publishing, 2001:85–120.
4. Kirkham TC, Williams CM. Endocannabinoid receptor antagonists. Treat Endocrinol 2004; 3:1–16.
5. Regelson W, Butler J, Schultz J. Delta-9-tetrahydrocannabinol as an effective antidepressant and appetite stimulating agent in advanced cancer patients. In: Braude M, Szara S, eds. The Pharmacology of Marijuana. New York: Raven Press, 1976:763–776.

6. Beal J, Olson R, Laubenstein L, et al. Dronabinol as a treatment for anorexia associated with weight loss in patients with AIDS. J Pain Symptom Manage 1995; 10:89–97.
7. Plasse T, Gorter R, Krasnow S, et al. Recent clinical experience with dronabinol. Pharmacol Biochem Behav 1991; 40:695–700.
8. Struwe M, Kaempfer S, Geiger C, et al. Effect of dronabinol on nutritional status in HIV infection. Ann Pharmacother 1993; 27:827–831.
9. Haines L, Green W. Marijuana: Use patterns. Brit J Addiction 1970; 65:347–362.
10. Tart C. Marijuana intoxication: Common experiences. Nature 1970; 226:701–704.
11. Abel EL. Effects of marijuana on the solution of anagrams, memory and appetite. Nature 1971; 231:260–261.
12. Hollister L. Hunger and appetite after single doses of marijuana, alcohol, and dextroamphetamine. Clin Pharmacol Ther 1971; 12:44–49.
13. Foltin R, Brady J, Fischman M. Behavioral analysis of marijuana effects on food intake in humans. Pharmacol Biochem Behav 1986; 25:577–582.
14. Foltin R, Fischman M, Byrne M. Effects of smoked marijuana on food intake and body weight of humans living in a residential laboratory. Appetite 1988; 11:1–14.
15. Haney M, Rabkin J, Gunderson E, et al. Dronabinol and marijuana in HIV +marijuana smokers: Acute effects on caloric intake and mood. Psychopharmacology (Berl) 2005; 181:170–178.
16. Hart C, Ward A, Haney M, et al. Comparison of smoked marijuana and oral D9-tetrahydrocannbinol in humans. Psychopharmacology (Berl) 2002; 164:407–415.
17. Budney AJ, Hughes JR, Moore BA, et al. Marijuana abstinence effects in marijuana smokers maintained in their home environment. Arch Gen Psychiatry 2001; 58:917–924.
18. Wachtel SR, El Sohly MA, Ross SA, et al. Comparison of the subjective effects of delta(9)-tetrahydrocannabinol and marijuana in humans. Psychopharmacology 2002; 161:331–339.
19. Huestis M, Gorelick D, Heishman S, et al. Blockade of effects of smoked marijuana by the CB1 selective cannabinoid receptor antagonist SR141716. Arch Gen Psychiatry 2001; 58:322–328.
20. Huestis MA, Boyd SJ, Heishman SJ, et al. Single and multiple doses of rimonabant antagonize acute effects of smoked cannabis in male cannabis users. Psychopharmacology (Berl) 2007; 194:505–515.
21. Van Gaal L, Rissanen A, Scheen A, et al. Effects of the cannabinoid-1 receptor blocker rimonabant on weight reduction and cardiovascular risk factors in overweight patients: 1-year experience from the RIO-Europe study. RIO-Europe Study Group. Lancet 2005; 16:1389–1397.
22. Despres JP, Golay A, Sjostrom, L. Rimonabant in Obesity-Lipids Study Group. Effects of rimonabant on metabolic risk factors in over-weight patients with dyslipidemia. N Engl J Med 2005; 353:2121–2134.
23. Pi-Sunyer FX, Aronne LJ, Heshmati HM, et al. RIO-North America Study Group. Effect of rimonabant, a cannabinoid-1 receptor blocker, on weight and cardiometabolic risk factors in overweight or obese patients: RIO-North America: a randomized controlled trial. JAMA 2006; 295:761–775.
24. Scheen AJ, Finer N, Hollander P, et al. RIO-Diabetes Study Group. Efficacy and tolerability of rimonabant in overweight or obese patients with type 2 diabetes: A randomised controlled study. Lancet 2006; 3681:660–672.
25. Addy C, Wright H, Van Laere K, et al. The acyclic CB1R inverse agonist taranabant mediates weight loss by increasing energy expenditure and decreasing caloric intake. Cell Metabolism 2008; 7:68–78.
26. Blundell JE, Jebb SA, Stubbs RJ, et al. Effect of rimonabant on energy intake, motivation to eat and body weight with or without hypocaloric diet: The REBA study. 2006 International Congress on Obesity, Sydney, Australia (poster presentation).
27. Arnone M, Maruani J, Chaperon F, et al. Selective inhibition of sucrose and ethanol intake by SR 141716, an antagonist of central cannabinoid (CB1) receptors. Psychopharmacology 1997; 132:104–106.
28. Simiand J, Keane M, Keane P, et al. SR 141716, a CB1 cannabinoid receptor antagonist, selectively reduces sweet food intake in marmoset. Behav Pharmacol 1998; 9:179–181.
29. Colombo G, Agabio R, Diaz G, et al. Appetite suppression and weight loss after the cannabinoid antagonist SR 141716. Life Sci 1998; 63:PL113–PL117.
30. Werner N, Koch J. Effects of the cannabinoid antagonists AM281 and AM630 on deprivation-induced intake in Lewis rats. Brain Res 2003; 967:290–292.
31. Shearman L, Rosko K, Fleischer R, et al. Antidepressant-like and anorectic effects of the cannabinoid CB1 receptor inverse agonist AM251 in mice. Behav Pharmacol 2003; 14:573–582.
32. Chen R, Huang R, Shen C, et al. Synergistic effects of cannabinoid inverse agonist AM251 and opioid antagonist nalmefene on food intake in mice. Brain Res Brain Res Rev 2004; 999:227–230.
33. Rutkowska M. The effect of AM251, a cannabinoid CB1 receptor antagonist, on food intake in rats. Acta Pol Pharm 2004; 61:401–403.
34. Vickers S, Webster L, Wyatt A, et al. Preferential effects of the cannabinoid CB1 receptor antagonist, SR 141716, on food intake and body weight gain of obese (fa/fa) compared to lean Zucker rats. Psychopharmacology 2003; 167:103–111.
35. Zhou D, Shearman L. Voluntary exercise augments acute effects of CB1-receptor inverse agonist on body weight loss in obese and lean mice. Pharmacol Biochem Behav 2004; 77:117–125.

36. McLaughlin P, Winston K, Limebeer C, et al. The cannabinoid CB1 antagonist AM251 produces food avoidance and behaviour associated with nausea but does not impair feeding efficiency. Psychopharmacology (Berl) 2005; 180:286–93.
37. Navarro M, Hernandez E, Munoz R, et al. Administration of the CB1 cannabinoid receptor antagonist SR141716A induces anxiety-like responses in the rat. Neuroreport 1997; 8:491–496.
38. Darmani N, Janoyan J, Kumar N, et al. Behaviorally active doses of the CB1 receptor antagonist SR 141716A increase brain serotonin and dopamine levels and turnover. Pharmacol Biochem Behav 2003; 75:777–787.
39. Tallett AJ, Blundell JE, Rodgers RJ. Behaviourally selective hypophagic effects of naloxone in non-deprived male rats presented with palatable food. Behav Brain Res 2008; 187:417–427.
40. Tallett AJ, Blundell JE, Rodgers JR. Acute anorectic response to cannabinoid CB1 receptor antagonist/inverse agonist AM 251 in rats: Indirect behavioural mediation. Behav Pharmacol 2007; 18:591–600.
41. Brown J, Kassouny M, Cross J. Kinetic studies of food intake and sucrose solution preference by rats treated with low doses of delta9-tetrahydrocannabinol. Behav Biol 1977; 20:104–110.
42. Anderson-Baker W, McLaughlin C, Baile C. Oral and hypothalamic injections of barbiturates, benzodiazepines and cannabinoids and food intake in rats. Pharmacol Biochem Behav 1979; 11:487–491.
43. Williams CM, Rogers PJ, Kirkham TC. Hyperphagia in pre-fed rats following oral delta9-THC. Physiol Behav 1998; 65:343–346.
44. Williams CM, Kirkham TC. Reversal of delta 9-THC hyperphagia by SR141716 and naloxone but not dexfenfluramine. Pharmacol Biochem Behav 2002; 7:333–340.
45. Williams CM, Kirkham TC. Anandamide induces overeating: Mediation by central cannabinoid (CB1) receptors. Psychopharmacology 1999; 143:315–317.
46. Hao S, Avraham Y, Mechoulam R, et al. Low dose anandamide affects food intake, cognitive function, neurotransmitter and corticosterone levels in diet-restricted mice. Eur J Pharmacol 2000; 392:147–156.
47. Jamshidi N, Taylor D. Anandamide administration into the ventromedial hypothalamus stimulates appetite in rats. Br J Pharmacol 2001; 134:1151–1154.
48. Kirkham TC, Williams CM, Fezza F, et al. Endocannabinoid levels in rat limbic forebrain and hypothalamus in relation to fasting, feeding and satiation: Stimulation of eating by 2-arachidonoyl glycerol. Br J Pharmacol 2002; 136:550–557.
49. Avraham Y, Ben Menachem A, Okun A, et al. Effects of the endocannabinoid noladin ether on body weight, food consumption, locomotor activity, and cognitive index in mice. Brain Res Bull 2005; 65:117–123.
50. Freedland C, Sharpe A, Samson H, et al. Effects of SR141716A on ethanol and sucrose self-administration. Alcohol Clin Exp Res 2001; 25:277–282.
51. Thornton-Jones Z, Vickers S, Clifton P. The cannabinoid CB1 receptor antagonist SR141716A reduces appetitive and consummatory responses for food. Psychopharmacology (Berl) 2005; 179:452–460.
52. Gallate J, McGregor I. The motivation for beer in rats: Effects of ritanserin, naloxone and SR 141716. Psychopharmacology 1999; 142:302–308.
53. Gallate J, Saharov T, Mallet P, et al. Increased motivation for beer in rats following administration of a cannabinoid CB1 receptor agonist. Eur J Pharmacol 1999; 370:233–240.
54. Sanchis-Segura C, Cline B, Marsicano G, et al. Reduced sensitivity to reward in CB1 knockout mice. Psychopharmacology (Berl) 2004; 176:223–232.
55. Williams CM, Kirkham TC. Observational analysis of feeding induced by Delta9-THC and anandamide. Physiol Behav 2002; 76:241–250.
56. Kelley A. Functional specificity of ventral striatal compartments in appetitive behaviors. Ann N Y Acad Sci 1999; 877:71–90.
57. Herkenham M, Lynn A, Johnson M, et al. Characterization and localization of cannabinoid receptors in rat brain: A quantitative in vitro autoradiographic study. J Neurosci 1991; 11:563–583.
58. Breivogel C, Childers S. The functional neuroanatomy of brain cannabinoid receptors. Neurobiol Dis 1998; 5(6 Pt B):417–431.
59. Soria-Gómez E, Matias I, Rueda-Orozco PE, et al. Pharmacological enhancement of the endocannabinoid system in the nucleus accumbens shell stimulates food intake and increases c-Fos expression in the hypothalamus. Br J Pharmacol 2007; 151:1109–1116.
60. Di Marzo V, Goparaju S, Wang L, et al. Leptin-regulated endocannabinoids are involved in maintaining food intake. Nature 2001; 410:822–825.
61. Berridge K. Measuring hedonic impact in animals and infants: Microstructure of affective taste reactivity patterns. Neurosci Biobehav Rev 2000; 24(2):173–198.
62. Berridge K. Motivational concepts in behavioral neuroscience. Physiol Behav 2004; 81:179–209.
63. Van Der Stelt M, Di Marzo V. The endocannabinoid system in the basal ganglia and in the mesolimbic reward system: Implications for neurological and psychiatric disorders. Eur J Pharmacol 2003; 480:133–150.

64. Lupica C, Riegel A. Endocannabinoid release from midbrain dopamine neurons: A potential substrate for cannabinoid receptor antagonist treatment of addiction. Neuropharmacology 2005; 48:1105–1116.
65. Lupica C, Riegel A, Hoffman A. Marijuana and cannabinoid regulation of brain reward circuits. Br J Pharmacol 2004; 143:227–234.
66. Gardner EL. Endocannabinoid signaling system and brain reward: Emphasis on dopamine. Pharmacol Biochem Behav 2005; 81:263–284.
67. Melis T, Succu S, Sanna F, et al. The cannabinoid antagonist SR 141716 A (rimonabant) reduces the increase of extra-cellular dopamine release in the rat nucleus accumbens induced by a novel high palatable food. Neurosci Lett 2007; 419:231–235.
68. Gardner E, Vorel S. Cannabinoid transmission and reward-related events. Neurobiol Disease 1998; 5:502–533.
69. Verty A, McGregor I, Mallet P. The dopamine receptor antagonist SCH 23390 attenuates feeding induced by Delta9-tetrahydrocannabinol. Brain Res 2004; 1020:188–195.
70. Patel S, Hillard CJ. Cannabinoid-induced Fos expression within A10 dopamine neurons. Brain Res 2003; 963:15–25.
71. Solinas M, Justinova Z, Goldberg, et al. Anandamide administration alone and after inhibition of fatty acid hydrolase (FAAH) increases dopamine levels in the nucleus accumbens shell in rats. J Neurochem 2006; 98:408–419.
72. Perio A, Barnouin M, Poncelet M, et al. Activity of SR141716 on post-reinforcemnt pauses in operant responding for sucrose reward in rats. Behav Pharmacol 2001; 12:641–645.
73. Poncelet M, Maruani J, Calassi R, et al. Overeating, alcohol and sucrose consumption decrease in CB1 receptor deleted mice. Neurosci Lett 2003; 343:216–218.
74. Freedland C, Poston J, Porrino L. Effects of SR141716A, a central cannabinoid receptor antagonist, on food-maintained responding. Pharmacol Biochem Behav 2000; 67:265–270.
75. Verty A, McGregor I, Mallet P. Consumption of high carbohydrate, high fat, and normal chow is equally suppressed by a cannabinoid receptor antagonist in non-deprived rats. Neurosci Lett 2004; 354:217–220.
76. Jarrett MM, Scantlebury J, Parker LA. Effect of delta(9)-tetrahydrocannabinol on quinine palatability and AM251 on sucrose and quinine palatability using the taste reactivity test. Physiol Behav 2007; 90:425–430.
77. Higgs S, Williams CM, Kirkham TC. Cannabinoid influences on palatability: Microstructural analysis of sucrose drinking after delta(9)-tetrahydrocannabinol, anandamide, 2-arachidonoyl glycerol and SR141716. Psychopharmacology 2003; 165:370–377.
78. Mahler SV, Smith KS, Berridge KC. Endocannabinoid hedonic hotspot for sensory pleasure: Anandamide in nucleus accumbens shell enhances 'liking' of a sweet reward. Neuropsychopharmacology 2007; 32:2267–2278.
79. Harrold J, Elliott C, King P, et al. Down-regulation of cannabinoid-1 (CB-1) receptors in specific extrahypothalamic regions of rats with dietary obesity: A role for endogenous cannabinoids in driving appetite for palatable food? Brain Res 2002; 952:232–238.
80. Cooper SJ, Kirkham TC. Opioid mechanisms in the control of food consumption and taste preferences. In: Herz A AH, Simon EJ, eds. Handbook of Experimental Pharmacology, vol. 104 (Part II). Berlin: Springer-Verlag; 1993:239–263.
81. Kelley A, Bakshi V, Haber S, et al. Opioid modulation of taste hedonics. Physiol Behav 2002; 76:365–377.
82. Bodnar R. Endogenous opioids and feeding behavior: A 30-year historical perspective. Peptides 2004; 25:697–725.
83. Pickel V, Chan J, Kash T, et al. Compartment-specific localization of cannabinoid (CB1) and mu-opioid receptors in rat nucleus accumbens. Neuroscience 2004; 127:101–112.
84. Kirkham T, Williams C. Synergistic effects of opioid and cannabinoid antagonists on food intake. Psychopharmacology 2001; 153:267–270.
85. Chen R, Huang R, Shen C, et al. Synergistic effects of cannabinoid inverse agonist AM251 and opioid antagonist nalmefene on food intake in mice. Brain Res Brain Res Rev 2004; 999:227–230.
86. Pecina S, Berridge K. Opioid site in nucleus accumbens shell mediates eating and hedonic 'liking' for food: Map based on microinjection Fos plumes. Brain Res Brain Res Rev 2000; 863:71–86.
87. Solinas M, Zangen A, Thiriet N, et al. Beta-endorphin elevations in the ventral tegmental area regulate the discriminative effects of delta-9-tetrahydrocannabinol. Eur J Neurosci 2004; 19:3183–3192.
88. Tanda G, Pontieri F, Di Chiara G. Cannabinoid and heroin activation of mesolimbic dopamine transmission by a common mu1 opioid receptor mechanism. Science 1997; 276:2048–2050.
89. Solinas M, Goldberg S. Motivational effects of cannabinoids and opioids on food reinforcement depend on simultaneous activation of cannabinoid and opioid systems. Neuropsychopharmacology 2005; 30:2035–2045.

18 The EC System and the HPA Axis

Daniela Cota

INSERM U862, Université Bordeaux 2, Bordeaux, France

INTRODUCTION

The term "stress," as it is currently used, was first coined by Hans Selye in 1936; and the term "stressors" (or stressful stimuli) identifies any physical or psychological event that might threaten the homeostatic balance of an organism (1). Exposure to stress triggers a complex, multi-level response involving neuro-vegetative, hormonal, and motor systems whose function is to restore homeostasis in response to the perturbation (2). Activation of the hypothalamic–pituitary–adrenal (HPA) axis represents the major neuroendocrine response to stress.

This neuroendocrine cascade begins in the central nervous system (CNS) with the release of corticotrophin-releasing hormone (CRH) from the paraventricular nucleus (PVN) of the hypothalamus. CRH induces the release of adrenocorticotrophin hormone (ACTH) from the anterior pituitary, which regulates glucocorticoid production from the adrenal gland. Then, the glucocorticoids complete the negative feedback loop necessary for the regulation of CRH and ACTH release (Fig. 1). The hierarchical regulation of the axis also includes extra-hypothalamic brain structures, such as the pre-frontal cortex, the hippocampus, and amygdala, whose function integrates the HPA hormonal response (Fig. 1). Short-term activation of the HPA axis is usually beneficial for the organism. However, if the HPA-axis response is inadequate or excessive, it might lead to metabolic and behavioral alterations, thus predisposing the organism at an increased risk of illness (1). In fact, dysregulation of the HPA axis is often associated with affective disorders, depression, abdominal obesity, and cardiovascular disease (1).

The EC system is known to have an effect on several neuroendocrine axes as well as on the secretion of both prolactin and growth hormone (3). In particular, several pieces of data point to a role for this system in the modulation of the HPA axis. For instance, CB1 receptors are expressed in extra-hypothalamic structures regulating the stress response, as well as in the hypothalamus (particularly in the PVN), anterior pituitary, and adrenal gland [reviewed in (3,4)]. In addition, endocannabinoids have been found in those tissues and organs [reviewed in (3,4)].

Taking into account the role of the EC system in energy balance regulation, and the association between HPA-axis dysfunctions and body weight disorders, it is worth providing a brief overview of the EC system as a modulator of the HPA-axis function.

CANNABINOIDS AND THE HPA AXIS

Studies conducted in marijuana smokers in the 1970s were the first to report that exogenous cannabinoids were able to modulate several neuroendocrine functions. However, while it was generally described as an inhibitory effect on most neuroendocrine actions, cannabinoids actually stimulated the HPA axis (3,5). Indeed, smoking marijuana or administration of Δ^9-THC stimulates ACTH and glucocorticoids secretion in both humans and experimental animals [reviewed in (5)]. However, these effects seem to disappear over time, suggesting that a rapid tolerance develops [reviewed in (5)].

Several studies have supported the notion that exogenous cannabinoids are able to modulate the HPA axis directly at hypothalamic level. Indeed, intracerebroventricular administration of Δ^9-THC induces a strong stimulation of ACTH release, together with CRH depletion in the median eminence (6). Moreover, chronic treatment with the CB1 agonist CP-55,940 increases both CRH and proopiomelanocortin (POMC) mRNAs in the PVN and pituitary, respectively (7). The ability to modulate CRH release is CB1-dependent, since pre-treatment with the CB1 antagonist SR141716A (rimonabant) inhibits the release of ACTH induced by the central administration of Δ^9-THC (8). Actually, cannabinoids were proposed to act on the HPA axis exclusively

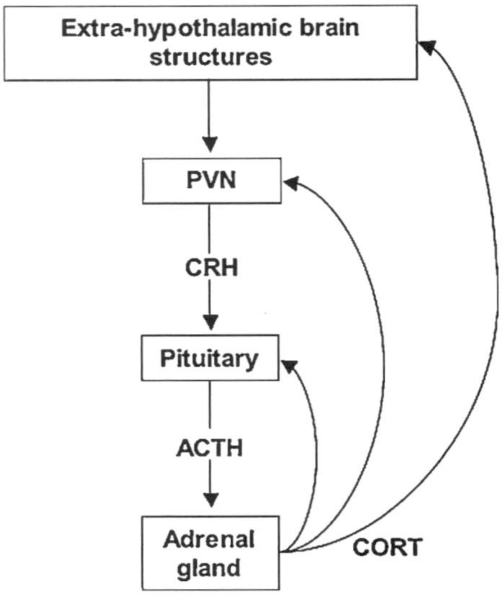

Figure 1 Hierarchical organization of the HPA axis, including feedback inhibition of HPA-axis function by glucocorticoids (CORT). See text for more details.

at hypothalamic level. This hypothesis was supported by initial studies describing the inability of Δ^9-THC to induce ACTH release in hypophysectomized rats [reviewed in (3)]. Moreover, both Δ^9-THC and the CB1 agonist WIN 55,212-2 were found unable to induce ACTH secretion from either isolated pituitary slices or dispersed pituitary cells, suggesting that cannabinoids had no direct effect on the pituitary [reviewed in (3)]. However, as it will be described in the following paragraphs, these findings have been challenged by more recent studies.

It is known that the action of exogenous cannabinoids on the HPA axis is dose-dependent and relies on the activation of CB1. However, the reader should also takes into account that the administration of the CB1 antagonist rimonabant at higher doses than those required for blocking the action of a CB1 agonist, is also able to increase ACTH and corticosterone release [reviewed in (3)]. Thus, an endogenous cannabinoid tone might exist, which is actually inhibiting the release of both hormones (8).

THE EC SYSTEM AND THE HPA AXIS

While initial studies with the endocannabinoid anandamide reported an increase in both ACTH and corticosterone secretion and the induction of *c-Fos* expression in the PVN [reviewed in (3)], subsequent investigations have actually demonstrated that endocannabinoids negatively modulates HPA-axis activity in a context-dependent manner (9). In mice, acute injections of a CB1 agonist, an endocannabinoid transport inhibitor or a fatty acid amide hydrolase (FAAH) inhibitor, all significantly decrease the corticosterone release induced by acute exposure to stress (restraint). Conversely, pre-treatment with the CB1 antagonist rimonabant before restraint robustly potentiates restraint-induced corticosterone release and *c-Fos* expression within the PVN. Finally, while acute exposure to stress is associated with a decrease in hypothalamic 2-AG content, chronic exposure determines and increase in hypothalamic 2-AG (9).

In support of these data, context-dependent effects on ACTH release have been recently described in mice lacking CB1 ($CB1^{-/-}$). After exposure to a more stressful unfamiliar environment, $CB1^{-/-}$ mice have higher ACTH levels than wild-type (WT) mice (10). Actually, normal expression and activation of CB1 is required for the basal modulation of the HPA axis (4). As compared to WT animals, $CB1^{-/-}$ mice show an enhanced circadian drive on the HPA axis, which results in elevated plasma corticosterone levels at the onset of the dark. $CB1^{-/-}$ mice are also characterized by neuro-functional alterations, both at hypothalamic and pituitary levels. In fact, they show increased CRH mRNA expression in the PVN. Moreover, $CB1^{-/-}$-derived pituitary cells have greater responsiveness to CRH- and forskolin-induced ACTH secretion (4). Finally, $CB1^{-/-}$ mice have selective glucocorticoid receptors mRNA down-regulation in the CA1 region of the hippocampus; a possible result of the feedback regulation exerted by increased circulating corticosterone levels (4). Moreover, it is worth mentioning that $CB1^{-/-}$ mice are

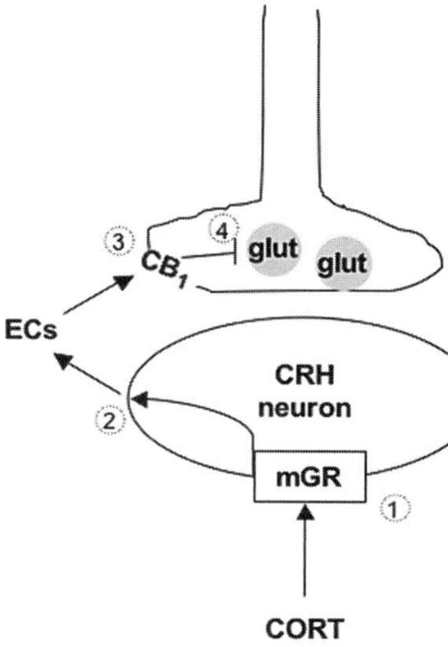

Figure 2 Model of fast-feedback glucocorticoid (CORT) signaling in PVN neuroendocrine neurons (i.e., CRH neurons). 1, glucocorticoids bind to membrane glucocorticoid receptors (mGR) localized on neuroendocrine cells in the PVN; 2, activation of mGR initiates an intracellular cascade leading to synthesis and retrograde release of endocannabinoids (ECs); 3, ECs bind to presynaptic CB1 receptors; 4, activation of CB_1 receptors leads to suppression of glutamate release from glutamate synapses onto the CRH neuron. See also (11,13).

resistant to the actions of anxiolytic drugs and have anxiogenic-like and depressive-like responses under different behavioral paradigms [reviewed in (3)].

The findings aforementioned clearly point to the ability of the EC system to modulate the HPA axis at extra-hypothalamic, hypothalamic, and pituitary levels; however, how does the EC system actually affect the HPA-axis function? A series of studies from Jeffrey Tasker's laboratory has elegantly elucidated the role of endocannabinoids in mediating the negative fast-feedback actions of glucocorticoids on CRH-containing neurons in the PVN. In particular, glucocorticoids, after binding to membrane glucocorticoid receptors localized on neuroendocrine cells in the PVN, induce synthesis and release of endocannabinoids, which in turn inhibit presynaptic excitatory transmission via CB1 (11) (Fig. 2). Thus, these findings might provide a possible mechanism for the rapid feedback inhibition of the HPA axis by glucocorticoids (11). Interestingly, leptin, which has been found to lower hypothalamic endocannabinoids levels (12), counteracts the glucocorticoid-induced endocannabinoid-release in the PVN (13). The mutually exclusive action of glucocorticoids and leptin on endocannabinoid secretion is particularly compelling; also bearing in mind that both glucocorticoids and endocannabinoids increase food consumption, while leptin does the opposite.

CONCLUSIONS

In summary, differently from what initially suggested by pharmacological studies using exogenous cannabinoids, recent data have highlighted a role for the EC system as a negative modulator of the HPA axis. These latest findings also suggest that alterations of the endocannabinoid tone might be associated with the development of stress-related diseases. In this regard, it is worth mentioning that a low number of obese subjects treated with the weight-reducing CB1 antagonist rimonabant suspended the treatment due to the occurrence of anxiety and mood disorders (14–17). Thus, particular care should be used in administering CB1 antagonists to obese patients that show anxiety or other mood disorders.

REFERENCES

1. de Kloet ER, Joels M, Holsboer F. Stress and the brain: From adaptation to disease. Nat Rev Neurosci 2005; 6(6):463–475.
2. Herman JP, Figueiredo H, Mueller NK, et al. Central mechanisms of stress integration: Hierarchical circuitry controlling hypothalamo–pituitary–adrenocortical responsiveness. Front Neuroendocrinol 2003; 24(3):151–180.
3. Pagotto U, Marsicano G, Cota D, et al. The emerging role of the endocannabinoid system in endocrine regulation and energy balance. Endocr Rev 2006; 27(1):73–100.

4. Cota D, Steiner MA, Marsicano G, et al. Requirement of cannabinoid receptor type 1 for the basal modulation of hypothalamic–pituitary–adrenal axis function. Endocrinology 2007; 148(4):1574–1581.
5. Murphy LL, Munoz RM, Adrian BA, et al. Function of cannabinoid receptors in the neuroendocrine regulation of hormone secretion. Neurobiol Dis 1998; 5(6 Pt B):432–446.
6. Weidenfeld J, Feldman S, Mechoulam R. Effect of the brain constituent anandamide, a cannabinoid receptor agonist, on the hypothalamo–pituitary–adrenal axis in the rat. Neuroendocrinology 1994; 59(2):110–112.
7. Corchero J, Fuentes JA, Manzanares J. Chronic treatment with CP-55,940 regulates corticotropin releasing factor and proopiomelanocortin gene expression in the hypothalamus and pituitary gland of the rat. Life Sci 1999; 64(11):905–911.
8. Manzanares J, Corchero J, Fuentes JA. Opioid and cannabinoid receptor-mediated regulation of the increase in adrenocorticotropin hormone and corticosterone plasma concentrations induced by central administration of delta(9)-tetrahydrocannabinol in rats. Brain Res 1999; 839(1):173–179.
9. Patel S, Roelke CT, Rademacher DJ, et al. Endocannabinoid signaling negatively modulates stress-induced activation of the hypothalamic–pituitary–adrenal axis. Endocrinology 2004; 145(12):5431–5438.
10. Haller J, Varga B, Ledent C, et al. Context-dependent effects of CB1 cannabinoid gene disruption on anxiety-like and social behaviour in mice. Eur J Neurosci 2004; 19(7):1906–1912.
11. Di S, Malcher-Lopes R, Halmos KC, et al. Nongenomic glucocorticoid inhibition via endocannabinoid release in the hypothalamus: A fast feedback mechanism. J Neurosci 2003; 23(12):4850–4857.
12. Di Marzo V, Goparaju SK, Wang L, et al. Leptin-regulated endocannabinoids are involved in maintaining food intake. Nature 2001; 410(6830):822–825.
13. Malcher-Lopes R, Di S, Marcheselli VS, et al. Opposing crosstalk between leptin and glucocorticoids rapidly modulates synaptic excitation via endocannabinoid release. J Neurosci 2006; 26(24):6643–6650.
14. Scheen AJ, Finer N, Hollander P, et al. Efficacy and tolerability of rimonabant in overweight or obese patients with type 2 diabetes: A randomised controlled study. Lancet 2006; 368(9548):1660–1672.
15. Van Gaal LF, Rissanen AM, Scheen AJ, et al. Effects of the cannabinoid-1 receptor blocker rimonabant on weight reduction and cardiovascular risk factors in overweight patients: 1-year experience from the RIO-Europe study. Lancet 2005; 365(9468):1389–1397.
16. Despres JP, Golay A, Sjostrom L. Effects of rimonabant on metabolic risk factors in overweight patients with dyslipidemia. N Engl J Med 2005; 353(20):2121–2134.
17. Pi-Sunyer FX, Aronne LJ, Heshmati HM, et al. Effect of rimonabant, a cannabinoid-1 receptor blocker, on weight and cardiometabolic risk factors in overweight or obese patients: RIO-North America: a randomized controlled trial. JAMA 2006; 295(7):761–775.

19 The EC System and Gut–Brain Interactions Relevant to Satiety

Richard Jones and David G. Thompson
Division of Gastroenterology, Hope Hospital, University of Manchester, Manchester, U.K.

Galina Burdyga and Graham J. Dockray
School of Biomedical Sciences, University of Liverpool, Liverpool, U.K.

INTRODUCTION

Interactions between the gut and the brain are well recognized to play important roles in the control of energy intake (1). In particular, hormones released from the gut signal information to the CNS regarding the ingestion of nutrient and these signals in turn influence food intake (2). Some effects of the gut hormones may be mediated by direct action on CNS neurons, for example, in the hypothalamus. Many effects, however, are mediated by afferent fibers in the vagal nerve (1). The same afferent neurons may also function as mechanoreceptors. Cholecystokinin (CCK) was the first of the gut hormones to be shown to influence food intake (3), and its action via vagal neurons, which also function as gastric mechanoreceptors, is now well defined (4). Subsequently, a variety of other peptide hormones from the gut were shown to inhibit nutrient ingestion, including peptide YY (PYY) and glucagon-like peptide (GLP)-1 (5). In recent years, gut peptide hormones that stimulate food intake have also been identified, for example, ghrelin. It is now clear that there are complex interactions at the level of vagal afferent neurons between anorexic and orexigenic hormones such as CCK and ghrelin (6,7). Interestingly, this signaling system has been shown to involve not just peptide hormones and their receptors but also the endocannabinoid (EC) system (8,9). Moreover, the role of the latter in controlling feeding behavior appears to be independent of EC signaling within the CNS. The present chapter provides an overview of recent progress in elucidating gut–brain signaling mechanisms with special relevance to the role of the EC system.

THE VAGUS NERVE AND GUT–BRAIN SIGNALING

The vagus nerve trunk carries both afferent and efferent fibers. The cell bodies of the former are located in the nodose ganglion: their central projections terminate in the *nucleus tractus solitarius* (NTS) in the brainstem, and peripheral projections are made to virtually all regions of the gastrointestinal tract with the exception of the distal colon. Afferent fibers predominate, but parasympathetic efferent fibers play important roles in controlling postprandial gastric and pancreatic secretion, and motility (in particular gastric emptying); they are regulated by vago-vagal reflexes through which delivery of nutrient to the gut triggers the appropriate secretory and motor responses. The peripheral projections of vagal afferent neurons are the primary target of a wide variety of signaling molecules including gut hormones, classical neurotransmitters, cytokines, fatty acids, and endocannabinoids (1). It should be noted that many of these molecules may act at multiple levels on the gut–brain axis. The endocannabinoids are a case in point, since there is evidence for actions within the gastrointestinal tract on intrinsic enteric neurons (10), on vagal afferent neurons (see below), within the dorsal motor complex of the vagus including the NTS (11), as well as at higher CNS sites.

CCK: PRIMARY DETERMINATION OF VAGAL AFFERENT SIGNALING

The release of CCK from the upper small intestine occurs in response to ingestion of lipid or protein. CCK stimulates gallbladder contraction, pancreatic enzyme secretion, inhibition of gastric emptying, and inhibition of food intake. It therefore acts to balance delivery of nutrient to the small intestine with the capacity to digest fat and protein (1). The actions of CCK on pancreas, gastric emptying, and food intake all depend on intact vagal afferent neurons, and electrophysiological evidence, together with immunohistochemistry and in situ hybridization, indicates that CCK acts at CCK1 receptors expressed by neurons of the nodose ganglion which are then transported to peripheral nerve terminals (12). There appear to be potentiating interactions between CCK and leptin in stimulating the discharge of vagal afferent neurons (13). Conversely, orexigenic factors like ghrelin inhibit the action of CCK in stimulating vagal afferent nerve discharge (6). In addition, and importantly, CCK is now recognized to regulate the expression of genes encoding some other receptors and peptide transmitters in vagal afferent neurons, including the CB_1 receptor (8,14). Thus, CCK can be viewed as a primary regulator not just of vagal afferent discharge after a meal, but also of the capacity of vagal afferent neurons to respond to other neurohumoral agents including endocannabinoids.

ENDOCANNABINOIDS AND VAGAL AFFERENT SIGNALING

Intestinal Endocannabinoids

It has been recognized for some time that CB_1 receptors are expressed extensively by enteric neurons and there is evidence for CB_1 regulation of gastrointestinal motility and secretion (10). Until recently, little was known of the control of endocannabinoid production in the gut. However, Gomez et al. have reported that in rats, the abundance of anandamide increases 7-fold in the small intestine in response to a 24-hour period of fasting (9). This appears to be a selective increase since there were no changes in brain or stomach. Refeeding of fasted rats was associated with a return of anandamide concentrations to normal. The relevance of peripheral changes in anandamide for control of food intake was shown by the demonstration that on intraperitoneal administration it stimulated food intake, as did the CB_1 receptor agonist WIN 55212–2, in partially satiated rats (9). In fasted rats, in which the EC system was assumed to be already activated, peripheral anandamide had no effect. However, peripheral administration of the CB_1 receptor antagonist rimonabant decreased food intake in both partially satiated and fasted animals, while a CB_2 receptor antagonist had no effect. Interestingly, the effects of peripheral anandamide on food intake were inhibited by vagotomy and by perivagal capsaicin indicating a dependency on vagal afferent neurons (9). Thus, in addition to the evidence indicating a role within the CNS for regulation of feeding behavior by EC, it appears that there are also peripheral mechanisms involving endocannabinoids that are brought into play during energy withdrawal.

CB_1 Receptor Expression in Vagal Afferent Neurons

Expression of CB_1 receptors by vagal afferent neurons has been described in rat, ferret, and humans (8,15). In rats fed ad libitum, CB_1 receptor expression is found in neurons in the proximal parts of the nodose ganglion that are thought to project predominately to the airways. Expression of CB_1 in neurons of the mid- and distal parts of the ganglion that project to sub-diaphragmatic structures is barely detectable in these animals (8). However, CB_1 receptor expression in these neurons is dramatically upregulated between 8 and 12 hours of fasting (Fig. 1). There is also relatively rapid downregulation after refeeding so that expression of the protein is virtually undetectable 5 hours after refeeding a fasted rat. Downregulation of CB_1 receptors in fasted rats is produced by intraperitoneal administration of CCK, and since the downregulation that occurs with refeeding is blocked by administration of the CCK1 receptor antagonist, lorglumide, it would appear that endogenous CCK regulates CB_1 receptor expression (8). Taken together, the available data therefore indicate that there is the potential for peripheral EC regulation of food intake mediated by vagal afferent neurons, during fasting and in the period of 1–2 hours following refeeding of fasted rats.

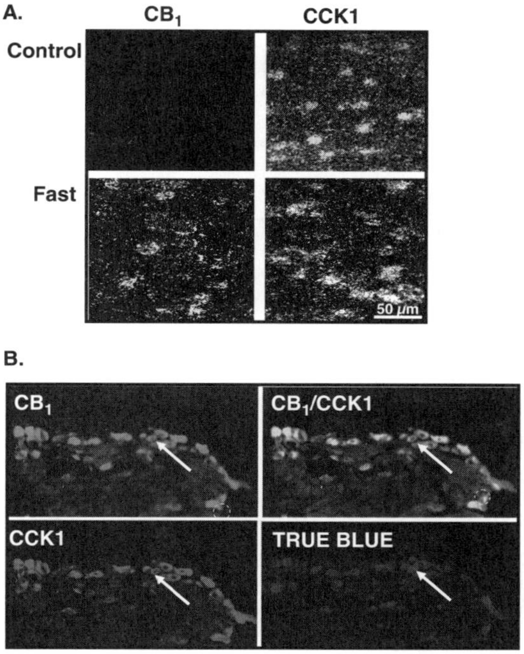

Figure 1 Expression of CB_1 receptors in rat nodose ganglion. **(A)** In situ hybridization indicates expression of CB_1 in fasted rats, but not fed ad libitum, while CCK1 receptors are expressed similarly. **(B)** Immunohistochemistry indicates that CB_1 and CCK1 receptors are expressed by the same neurons, and that these project to the stomach as indicated by retrograde tracing of TRUE BLUE (they also project to the duodenum, not shown).

Integrative Functions of Vagal Afferent Neurons

The vagal afferent neurons that express CB_1 and CCK1 receptors also express ghrelin (GHS-1), orexin (Ox-R1), leptin (Ob-R), and MCH-1 receptors (8,14,16–18). Two patterns of expression are readily distinguishable. On present evidence, CCK1, Ob-R, Ox-R1 and GHS-1 receptors are all expressed constitutively and do not change with feeding. In contrast, expression of both CB_1 and MCH-1 receptors is increased during energy withdrawal when plasma CCK concentrations are low, and depressed by refeeding in response to increasing plasma concentrations of CCK (Fig. 2). In addition, vagal afferent neurons exhibit CCK-dependent, reciprocal expression of two neuropeptide transmitters. Thus, cocaine and amphetamine regulated transcript (CART), which is associated with inhibition of food intake, is expressed in response to CCK (7); in contrast, the expression of MCH, which stimulates food intake, is inhibited by CCK (18). Recent studies on the relevant cellular mechanisms indicate that CCK acts via protein kinase C and the transcription factor CREB to control CART and MCH (7). These observations point, therefore, to a simple form of memory that exists at the level of vagus nerve: withdrawal of food for periods of about 12-hour long is associated with a neurochemical phenotype that includes CB_1 receptor expression allowing responses to orexigenic stimuli such as anandamide from the intestine, and associated with production of an orexigenic peptide transmitter. Conversely, in animals fed ad libitum, this system is suppressed, and instead there is induction of an anorexic peptide transmitter. Interestingly, administration of ghrelin inhibited the downregulation of CB_1 receptor expression with refeeding, although it did not stimulate expression in rats fed ad libitum (14). Thus, the potential for peripheral EC stimulation of appetite during fasting may subsequently be modulated during the refeeding period depending on interactions between CCK and ghrelin. Moreover, there is also evidence that EC stimulation maintains plasma ghrelin concentrations (19), indicating ghrelin–EC interactions at several levels.

CONCLUSIONS

An increasing body of evidence suggests a role for the gastrointestinal EC system in the stimulation of appetite via gut–brain signaling pathways. Food withdrawal induces both the synthesis in the gut of anandamide, and the expression of CB_1 receptors by vagal afferent neurons. Induction of both receptor and ligand, therefore, appears to provide a mechanism to stimulate

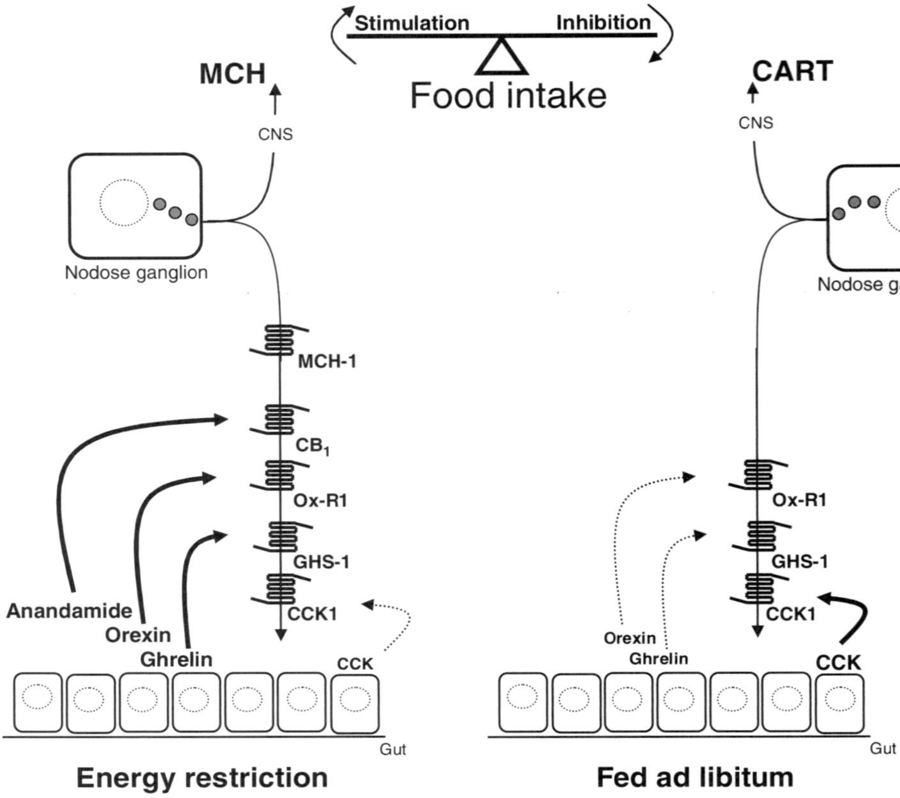

Figure 2 Schematic representation of the neurochemical phenotype of vagal afferent pathways relevant to control of food intake, in rats after energy restriction compared with fed ad libitum. Vagal afferent fibers innervate all relevant regions of the gut apart from the distal colon; for simplicity the different regions are not indicated here. In addition to the pathways shown, there is also evidence that gastric distension, leptin, PYY, and GLP-1 signaling may inhibit food intake by vagal pathways. See text for further details and references.

appropriate increases in food intake after energy restriction. The available data have largely been obtained in animal studies; human experiments are now required to determine whether similar mechanisms exist in man and provide opportunities for therapeutic interventions in feeding-related disorders.

REFERENCES

1. Dockray GJ. The brain–gut axis. In: Yamada T, ed. Textbook of Gastroenterology. New York: Raven Press, 2006:77–92.
2. Dockray GJ. Gut endocrine secretions and their relevance to satiety. Curr Opin Pharmacol 2004; 4(6):557–560.
3. Gibbs J, Young RC, Smith GP. Cholecystokinin elicits satiety in rats with open gastric fistulas. Nature 1973; 245(5424):323–325.
4. Smith GP, Jerome C, Cushin BJ, et al. Abdominal vagotomy blocks the satiety effect of cholecystokinin in the rat. Science 1981; 213(4511):1036–1037.
5. Murphy KG, Bloom SR. Gut hormones in the control of appetite. Exp Physiol 2004; 89(5):507–516.
6. Date Y, Toshinai K, Koda S, et al. Peripheral interaction of ghrelin with cholecystokinin on feeding regulation. Endocrinology 2005; 146(8):3518–3525.
7. de Lartigue G, Dimaline R, Varro A, et al. Cocaine- and amphetamine-regulated transcript: Stimulation of expression in rat vagal afferent neurons by cholecystokinin and suppression by ghrelin. J Neurosci 2007; 27(11):2876–2882.
8. Burdyga G, Lal S, Varro A, et al. Expression of cannabinoid CB1 receptors by vagal afferent neurons is inhibited by cholecystokinin. J Neurosci 2004; 24(11):2708–2715.

9. Gomez R, Navarro M, Ferrer B, et al. A peripheral mechanism for CB1 cannabinoid receptor-dependent modulation of feeding. J Neurosci 2002; 22(21):9612–9617.
10. Pertwee RG. Cannabinoids and the gastrointestinal tract. Gut 2001; 48(6):859–867.
11. Van Sickle MD, Oland LD, Ho W, et al. Cannabinoids inhibit emesis through CB1 receptors in the brainstem of the ferret. Gastroenterology 2001; 121(4):767–774.
12. Moran TH, Kinzig KP. Gastrointestinal satiety signals II. Cholecystokinin. Am J Physiol Gastrointest Liver Physiol 2004; 286(2):G183–G188.
13. Barrachina MD, Martinez V, Wang L, et al. Synergistic interaction between leptin and cholecystokinin to reduce short-term food intake in lean mice. Proc Natl Acad Sci USA 1997; 94(19):10455–10460.
14. Burdyga G, Varro A, Dimaline R, et al. Ghrelin receptors in rat and human nodose ganglia: Putative role in regulating CB-1 and MCH receptor abundance. Am J Physiol Gastrointest Liver Physiol 2006; 290(6):G1289-G1297.
15. Partosoedarso ER, Abrahams TP, Scullion RT, et al. Cannabinoid1 receptor in the dorsal vagal complex modulates lower oesophageal sphincter relaxation in ferrets. J Physiol 2003; 550(Pt 1):149–158.
16. Burdyga G, Spiller D, Morris R, et al. Expression of the leptin receptor in rat and human nodose ganglion neurones. Neuroscience 2002; 109(2):339–347.
17. Burdyga G, Lal S, Spiller D, et al. Localization of orexin-1 receptors to vagal afferent neurons in the rat and humans. Gastroenterology 2003; 124(1):129–139.
18. Burdyga G, Varro A, Dimaline R, et al. Feeding-dependent depression of melanin-concentrating hormone and melanin-concentrating hormone receptor-1 expression in vagal afferent neurones. Neuroscience 2006; 137(4):1405–1415.
19. Cani PD, Montoya ML, Neyrinck AM, et al. Potential modulation of plasma ghrelin and glucagon-like peptide-1 by anorexigenic cannabinoid compounds, SR141716A (rimonabant) and oleoylethanolamide. Br J Nutr 2004; 92(5):757–761.

20 The Endogenous Cannabinoid System in the Gastrointestinal Tract

Angelo A. Izzo

Endocannabinoid Research Group, Department of Experimental Pharmacology, University of Naples Federico II, Naples, Italy

INTRODUCTION

Preparations of *Cannabis sativa* have been known for centuries to stimulate appetite, inhibit emesis, and improve a variety of other gastrointestinal disorders including gastrointestinal pain, flatulence, gastroenteritis, Crohn's disease, diarrhoea, and diabetic gastroparesis (1–5). The main psychotropic constituent of *Cannabis sativa* is Δ^9-tetrahydrocannabinol, which activates CB_1 receptors (present in central and peripheral nerves, including the enteric nervous system) and CB_2 receptors (expressed mainly in immune cells) (6,7). A general feature of CB_1 activation is the reduction in the release of a variety of neurotransmitters, including acetylcholine from enteric nerves. Endogenous ligands for the cannabinoid receptors have been identified; the best knowns are anandamide and 2-arachidonylglycerol (2-AG) (8). Endocannabinoids are biosynthesized "on demand" and released from cells immediately after their production. Endocannabinoid levels in the gut appear to be elevated as an adaptive reaction to re-establish normal homeostasis when this is acutely and pathologically perturbed. For example, noxious stimuli (9–12), food deprivation (13), or clinically diagnosed gut diseases [e.g., inflammatory bowel disease (IBD), colorectal cancer, diverticulitis, and celiac disease] (14–17) produced measurable increases in intestinal endocannabinoid (mainly anandamide) levels.

Anandamide and 2-AG are removed from extracellular compartments by a carrier-mediated re-uptake process, and once within the cell, both endocannabinoids are hydrolyzed by the enzyme fatty acid amide hydrolase (FAAH) (8). There is no direct evidence for the existence of this putative membrane transporter in the gut as yet; although functional studies suggest that this process might be involved in some experimental pathophysiological states (e.g., ileus, diarrhoea, and IBD) (9,11,17). FAAH mRNA and activity have been detected in different regions of the rodent intestinal tract (18) and FAAH inhibition results in anticancer (12), antiinflammatory (16,19) and constipant effects (18).

In addition to the two cannabinoid receptors, anandamide can also activate the transient receptor potential vanilloid subtype 1 (TRPV1), the molecular target for the pungent plant compound capsaicin (20). Activation of TRPV1 receptors by anandamide results in enteritis in rat in vivo (10) and enhanced acetylcholine release from myenteric guinea pig nerves (21).

Cannabinoid receptors, their endogenous ligands (endocannabinoids), and the proteins involved in endocannabinoid synthesis and inactivation are collectively referred as to the endogenous cannabinoid system. This article will review data on the role of the endogenous cannabinoid system in physiology and pathophysiology of the gastrointestinal tract.

GASTROPROTECTION

Cannabinoids (via CB_1 activation) have been shown to exert protective effects in two models of experimental ulcer (e.g., stress- and aspirin-induced gastric damage) (22–24). The gastric antiulcer action of cannabinoids could be due, at least in part, to their antisecretory effect (25,26). Indeed, experimental data have clearly indicated that activation of CB_1 receptors, located on vagal efferent pathways to the gastric mucosa, decreases the acid secretion induced by cholinergically mediated secretagogues, such as 2-deoxy-D-glucose and pentagastrin, but not by histamine, which activates H_2 receptors on parietal cells. The gastric antiacid action of cannabinoids is relevant in the light of the observation that these compounds (via CB_1 activation) also inhibit transient lower esophageal sphincter relaxation (TLESR) in dogs and ferrets (27,28). Reduction in both acid secretion and TLESR could be beneficial for patients with gastroesophageal reflux disease.

INTESTINAL MOTILITY

Cannabinoids have been shown to reduce gastric and intestinal motility in randomized clinical trials (29,30). Experimental evidence suggests that cannabinoid agonists act on prejunctional CB_1 receptors to reduce excitatory enteric transmission (mainly cholinergic transmission) in different regions of the gastrointestinal tract (1–4), including the human intestine (17,31). Animal studies in vivo have shown that endocannabinoids (via CB_1 activation) constitute a physiological "brake" for the gut, both in the small and in the large intestine (32–34). This was mainly based on the findings of (a) high amount of endocannabinoids in intestinal tissues; (b) strategic location of CB_1 receptors on neurons of the myenteric plexus (a neuronal network important in the control of intestinal motility); (c) inhibitory actions of cannabinoid agonists, including the endocannabinoid anandamide, on intestinal motility; (d) prokinetic effect of the CB_1 receptor antagonist rimonabant, and (e) inhibitory action on motility of inhibitors of anandamide inactivation (32,33).

Depending upon the experimental model, activation of both CB_1 and CB_2 receptors can limit the increase in intestinal motility induced by an inflammatory stimulus. In the croton oil model of intestinal hypermotility associated to ileitis, the potency of cannabinoid agonists in reducing motility (via CB_1 activation) is greatly increased compared to control mice (32). By contrast, in the model of intestinal hypermotility induced by an endotoxic inflammatory agent, the CB_1-mediated reduction of gastrointestinal transit was absent and was replaced by CB_2-mediated inhibition of stimulated transit (35).

Finally, Mascolo and colleagues (11) provided the evidence for the involvement of the enteric endocannabinoid system in the induction of experimental paralytic ileus induced by peritoneal irritation. Reduced gastrointestinal motility associated with intraperitoneal acetic acid in mice was restored by the CB_1 receptor antagonist rimonabant, while it was exaggerated by the cellular re-uptake inhibitor VDM11. Ileus was characterized by increased intestinal levels of anandamide (but not 2-AG) and by an increase in the number and density of CB_1 receptors on cholinergic and substance P–containing neurones (11).

INTESTINAL SECRETION

Studies monitoring electrolyte movement in muscle-stripped sheets of tissues mounted in using chambers revealed that activation of CB_1 receptors located on submucosal neurones and extrinsic primary afferents in the submucosa, reduces ion transport in the isolated intestine (36,37). In vivo, experimental data suggest that anandamide inhibits, via CB_1 activation, secretion in mice treated with cholera toxin (9). In mice, oral cholera toxin increases the intestinal levels of anandamide and cannabinoid CB_1 mRNA expression. The overstimulation of endocannabinoid signaling with an antisecretory role was strengthened by the following pharmacological experiments: (i) the CB_1 antagonist rimonabant further increased cholera toxin–induced fluid accumulation, (ii) the anandamide re-uptake inhibitor VDM11 reduced fluid accumulation, and (iii) the cannabinoid agonist CP55940 or the selective CB_1 agonist ACEA inhibited secretion in a CB_1 antagonist–sensitive manner (9).

INTESTINAL INFLAMMATION

Many patients with IBD anecdotally reported that they experience relief from smoking marijuana. Moreover, experimental inflammation enhances cannabinoid signaling, as revealed by the increased expression of cannabinoid receptors and/or increased intestinal levels of endocannabinoids (38). The endocannabinoid anandamide is increased in intestinal tissues from patients with ulcerative colitis (16), diverticular disease (17), and from celiac patients (15). Experimental evidence suggests that both CB_1 and CB_2 receptors can exert protective effects against gut inflammation. In the experimental model of colitis induced by oil of mustard,

Kimball and colleagues found that both ACEA (a CB_1 receptor agonist) and JWH-133 (a CB_2 receptor agonist) reduced colon weight gain, colon shrinkage, colon inflammatory damage score, and diarrhoea (39). Massa and colleagues (19) reported that genetic ablation of CB_1 receptors rendered mice more sensitive to colitis, induced by intracolonic dinitrobenzene sulphonic acid (DNBS); in addition, the cannabinoid agonist HU-210 inhibited, while the CB_1 receptor antagonist rimonabant exacerbated intestinal inflammation. There is also evidence that the increase of anandamide levels could represent an endogenous mechanism and a pharmacological strategy to limit colon inflammation. Indeed, (a) FAAH-deficient mice, which are expected to have higher levels of anandamide, showed significant protection against intestinal inflammation due to DNBS administration (19) and (b) inhibitors of anandamide re-uptake or enzymatic hydrolysis strongly reduce DNBS-induced colonic inflammation (16).

In vitro studies have highlighted the importance of both CB_1 and CB_2 receptors in modulating inflammatory processes. Cannabinoids have been shown to promote epithelial wound healing in a CB_1-sensitive manner in the human colon (40). In the same study, the importance of CB_2 receptors was emphasized by the presence of CB_2 receptors in the epithelium of colonic tissue characteristic of irritable bowel syndrome (IBS) (40). In a different study, Ihenetu and colleagues found that CB_2 receptor activation by cannabinoids exerted an inhibitory effect on the expression of TNF-α–induced interleukin-8 release in human colonic epithelial cells, which are recognized to exert a major influence in the maintenance of intestinal immune homeostasis (41).

VISCERAL SENSATION

Heightened visceral sensation is commonly accepted as an explanation for the symptoms of pain and discomfort of IBD and, importantly, IBS (42). Recent findings have provided evidence that cannabinoid receptors activation inhibits visceral afferent nerve activity in rodents. Sanson and colleagues (43) showed that both CB_1 and CB_2 receptor agonists reduced the degree of visceral sensitivity (abdominal response to colorectal distension) under basal conditions and that this effect was more evident if the abdominal hypersensitivity was induced by an inflammatory stimulus (43). In a different study, Hillsley and colleagues evoked a visceral afferent response by the administration of the algesic agent bradykinin (44). It was found that the CB_2 receptor agonist AM1241 inhibited the bradykinin response of murine mesenteric afferent nerves. The effect of AM1241 on the bradykinin response was blocked by the selective CB_2 receptor antagonist AM630 and, most importantly, no effect of AM1241 was observed in CB_2-deficient mice. In line with these observations, a relevant study (45) has recently shown that probiotics, which play a role in the clinical management of IBS (46), may induce the expression of CB_2 receptors on intestinal epithelial cells that locally contribute to the restoration of the normal perception of visceral pain in rodents.

COLON CANCER

Cannabinoids have been licensed for clinical use as palliative treatment of chemotherapy, but increasing evidence shows direct antiproliferative actions of cannabinoid agonists on several tumor cells in vitro and in animal models (47). The formation of aberrant crypt foci (ACF; precancerous lesions) in the mouse colon has been shown to be associated to increased levels of 2-AG. The FAAH inhibitor *N*-arachidonoylserotonin increased colon endocannabinoid levels and reduced ACF formation, the latter effect being mimicked by the cannabinoid receptor agonist HU-210 (12). In vitro, a number of cannabinoid agonists, including the endocannabinoids anandamide and 2-AG preferentially inhibited cell proliferation of CaCo-2 cells, which express CB_1 receptor, compared to DLD-1 cells (which express both CB_1 and CB_2 receptors, with CB_1 receptor less expressed than CaCo-2 cells). Such data suggest that CB_1 receptors are more important than CB_2 receptors in reducing the proliferation of colorectal carcinoma cells (14). In line with these results, in a study performed on SW480 colon carcinoma cells, Joseph and colleagues (48) reported that CB_1 activation by anandamide inhibited tumor-cell migration, which is of paramount importance in metastasis development. In a different study, it has been proposed that anandamide inhibits cell death in colorectal carcinoma cells by targeting cells that are high expressors of cyclooxygenase-2 (49).

INTESTINAL ANANDAMIDE IN THE CONTROL OF ENERGY INTAKE

Many gut molecules (mainly peptides) have been shown to influence energy intake. The most well studied in this regard are cholecystokinin (CCK), pancreatic polypeptide, peptide YY, glucagons-like peptide-1, oxyntomodulin, and ghrelin (50). These messengers diffuse through interstitial fluids to activate nearby nerve fibers and/or enter the bloodstream to function as hormones (51). With the exception of ghrelin, these hormones act to increase satiety and decrease food intake (50,51). Experimental evidence suggests that the intestinal endocannabinoid system might be involved in the control of appetite and this action be modulated by peripheral peptides (e.g., CCK) which are known to have a role in feeding.

The endogenous cannabinoid system in the gut undergoes adaptive changes in response to diet. Food deprivation produced a 7-fold increase in anandamide content in the small intestine but not in the brain or stomach (13). This effect was associated to increased expression of vagal CB_1 receptors (52). Refeeding normalized intestinal anandamide levels and CB_1 expression. Moreover, capsaicin deafferentation abolished the hyperphagic action of a cannabinoid agonist (13). These findings suggest that CB_1 receptors, located on capsaicin-sensitive sensory neurons, may be involved in cannabinoids-induced modulation of appetite and that anandamide acts as a "hunger signal". Interestingly, the intestinal levels of the anorexic compound oleoylethanolamide (OEA; a natural analogue of anandamide which does not activate cannabinoid receptors) may change in response to nutrient status (53–56)—they are lower in food-deprived than free-feeding rodents, and return to baseline values upon refeeding. Overall, it appears that intestinal levels of anandamide and OEA are inversely correlated to feeding. Food deprivation increases intestinal levels of anandamide (an orexic fatty-acid ethanolamide), while it decreases the levels of OEA (an anorexic fatty-acid ethanolamide); conversely, food ingestion decreases intestinal levels of anandamide while it increases the levels of OEA. Thus, it is possible that the two acylethanolamides act in a coordinated manner to control feeding through their opposing actions on food intake (13,53).

CCK is an anorexigenic peptide produced in gall bladder, pancreas, and stomach, and concentrated in the small intestine (50,51). Like CB_1 activation (2), CCK receptor agonism inhibits gastric emptying and primarily increases central signaling of satiety through vagal afferent signals to the brain resulting in short-term inhibition of food intake (50,51). It is, therefore, noteworthy that gastric and intestinal vagal afferents that express CCK receptors also express CB_1 receptors. Moreover, food intake produced a rapid loss of CB_1 receptor expression, an effect blocked by a CCK-1 receptor antagonist and mimicked by administration of CCK to fasted rats. Because CCK is a satiety factor that acts via the vagus nerve and CB_1 agonists stimulate food intake, the data suggest a new mechanism modulating the effect on food intake of satiety signals from the gastrointestinal tract (52).

CONCLUSIONS

Cannabinoids exert different important physiological and pathophysiological functions in the gut, which include inhibition of gastrointestinal motility, gastric acid and intestinal secretion, inflammation, cell proliferation, and visceral pain. Most of these actions are mediated by CB_1 receptors, although the CB_2 receptor may have a role in pathophysiological states such as gut inflammation. Potential therapeutic applications of cannabinoid drugs include the treatment of gastrointestinal reflux disease, IBD, IBS, and colon cancer. In relation to the possible role of intestinal endocannabinoids in the control of energy balance, there is evidence that anandamide in the gut may act as a "hunger signal", an action which could be counterbalanced by intestinal oleoylethanolamide, which exerts opposite effect on food intake.

REFERENCES

1. Duncan M, Davison JS, Sharkey KA. Endocannabinoids and their receptors in the enteric nervous system. Aliment Pharmacol Ther 2005; 22:667–683.
2. Coutts AA, Izzo AA. The gastrointestinal pharmacology of cannabinoids. An update. Curr Opin Pharmacol 2004; 4:572–579.

3. Hornby PJ, Prouty SM. Involvement of cannabinoid receptors in gut motility and visceral perception. Br J Pharmacol 2004; 141:1335–1345.
4. Massa F, Storr M, Lutz B. The endocannabinoid system in the physiology and pathophysiology of the gastrointestinal tract. J Mol Med 2005; 83:944–954.
5. Izzo AA, Capasso F. Marijuana for cholera therapy. Trends Pharmacol Sci 2006; 27:7–8.
6. Pacher P, Batkai S, Kunos G. The endocannabinoid system as an emerging target of pharmacotherapy. Pharmacol Rev 2006; 58:389–462.
7. Pertwee RG. The pharmacology of cannabinoid receptors and their ligands: An overview. Int J Obes 2006; 30(Suppl. 1):S13–S18.
8. Di Marzo V, Petrosino S. Endocannabinoids and the regulation of their levels in health and disease. Curr Opin Lipidol 2007; 18:129–140.
9. Izzo AA, Capasso F, Costagliola A, et al. An endogenous cannabinoid tone attenuates cholera toxin-induced fluid accumulation in mice. Gastroenterology 2003; 125:765–774.
10. McVey DC, Schmid PC, Schmid HH, et al. Endocannabinoids induce ileitis in rats via the capsaicin receptor (VR1). J Pharmacol Exp Ther 2003; 304:713–722.
11. Mascolo N, Izzo AA, Ligresti A, et al. The endocannabinoid system and the molecular basis of paralytic ileus in mice. FASEB J 2002; 16:1973–1975.
12. Izzo AA, Aviello G, Petrosino S, et al. Increased endocannabinoid levels reduce the development of precancerous lesions in the mouse colon. J Mol Med 2008; 86:89–98.
13. Gomez R, Navarro M, Ferrer B, et al. A peripheral mechanism for CB1 cannabinoid receptor-dependent modulation of feeding. J Neurosci 2002; 22:9612–9617.
14. Ligresti A, Bisogno T, Matias I, et al. Possible endocannabinoid control of colorectal cancer growth. Gastroenterology 2003; 125:677–687.
15. D'Argenio G, Petrosino S, Gianfrani C, et al. Overactivity of the intestinal endocannabinoid system in celiac disease and in methotrexate-treated rats. J Mol Med 2007; 85:523–530.
16. D'Argenio G, Valenti M, Scaglione G, et al. Up-regulation of anandamide levels as an endogenous mechanism and a pharmacological strategy to limit colon inflammation. FASEB J 2006; 20:568–570.
17. Guagnini F, Valenti M, Mukenge S, et al. Neural contractions in colonic strips from patients with diverticulosis: Role of endocannabinoids and substance. P Gut 2006; 55:946–953.
18. Capasso R, Matias I, Lutz B, et al. Fatty acid amide hydrolase controls mouse intestinal motility in vivo. Gastroenterology 2005; 129:941–951.
19. Massa F, Marsicano G, Hermann H, et al. The endogenous cannabinoid system protects against colonic inflammation. J Clin Invest 2004; 113:1202–1209.
20. Holzer P. TRPV1 and the gut: From a tasty receptor for a painful vanilloid to a key player in hyperalgesia. Eur J Pharmacol 2004; 500:231–241.
21. Mang CF, Erbelding D, Kilbinger H. Differential effects of anandamide on acetylcholine release in the guinea-pig ileum mediated via vanilloid and non-CB1 cannabinoid receptors. Br J Pharmacol 2001; 134:161–167.
22. Germano MP, D'Angelo V, Mondello MR, et al. Cannabinoid CB1-mediated inhibition of stress-induced gastric ulcers in rats. Naunyn Schmiedebergs Arch Pharmacol 2001; 363:241–244.
23. Dembinski A, Warzecha Z, Ceranowicz P, et al. Cannabinoids in acute gastric damage and pancreatitis. J Physiol Pharmacol 2006; 57:137–154.
24. Rutkowska M, Fereniec-Goltbiewska L. ACEA (arachidonyl-2-chloroethylamide), the selective cannabinoid CB1 receptor agonist, protects against aspirin-induced gastric ulceration. Pharmazie 2006; 61:341–342.
25. Adami M, Frati P, Bertini S, et al. Gastric antisecretory role and immunohistochemical localization of cannabinoid receptors in the rat stomach. Br J Pharmacol 2002; 135:1598–1606.
26. Coruzzi G, Adami M, Guaita E, et al. Effects of cannabinoid receptor agonists on rat gastric acid secretion: Discrepancy between in vitro and in vivo data. Dig Dis Sci 2006; 51:310–317.
27. Partosoedarso ER, Abrahams TP, Scullion RT, et al. Cannabinoid-1 receptor in the dorsal vagal complex modulates lower oesophageal sphincter relaxation in ferrets. J Physiol 2003; 550(Pt 1):149–158.
28. Lehmann A, Blackshaw LA, Branden L, et al. Cannabinoid receptor agonism inhibits transient lower esophageal sphincter relaxations and reflux in dogs. Gastroenterology 2002; 123:1129–1134.
29. Esfandyari T, Camilleri M, Busciglio I, et al. Effects of a cannabinoid receptor agonist on colonic motor and sensory functions in humans: A randomized, placebo-controlled study. Am J Physiol Gastrointest Liver Physiol 2007; 293, G137–G145.
30. Esfandyari T, Camilleri M, Ferber I, et al. Effect of a cannabinoid agonist on gastrointestinal transit and postprandial satiation in healthy human subjects: A randomized, placebo-controlled study. Neurogastroenterol Motil 2006; 18:831–838.
31. Hinds NM, Ullrich K, Smid SD. Cannabinoid 1 (CB1) receptors coupled to cholinergic motorneurones inhibit neurogenic circular muscle contractility in the human colon. Br J Pharmacol 2006; 148:191–199.
32. Izzo AA, Fezza F, Capasso R, et al. Cannabinoid CB_1-receptor mediated regulation of gastrointestinal motility in mice in a chronic model of intestinal inflammation. Br J Pharmacol 2001; 134:563–570.

33. Pinto L, Izzo AA, Cascio MG, et al. Endocannabinoids as physiological regulators of colonic propulsion in mice. Gastroenterology 2002; 123:227–234.
34. Carai MA, Colombo G, Gessa GL, et al. Investigation on the relationship between cannabinoid CB1 and opioid receptors in gastrointestinal motility in mice. Br J Pharmacol 2006; 148:1043–1050.
35. Mathison R, Ho W, Pittman QJ, et al. Effects of cannabinoid receptor-2 activation on accelerated gastrointestinal transit in lipopolysaccharide-treated rats. Br J Pharmacol 2004; 142:1247–1254.
36. Tyler K, Hillard CJ, Greenwood-Van Meerveld B. Inhibition of small intestinal secretion by cannabinoids is CB_1 receptor-mediated in rats. Eur J Pharmacol 2000; 409:207–211.
37. MacNaughton WK, Van Sickle MD, Keenan CM, et al. Distribution and function of the cannabinoid-1 receptor in the modulation of ion transport in the guinea pig ileum: Relationship to capsaicin-sensitive nerves. Am J Physiol Gastrointest Liver Physiol 2004; 286:G863–G871.
38. Di Marzo V, Izzo AA. Endocannabinoid overactivity and intestinal inflammation. Gut 2006; 55:1373–1376.
39. Kimball ES, Schneider CR, Wallace NH, et al. Agonists of cannabinoid receptor 1 and 2 inhibit experimental colitis induced by oil of mustard and by dextran sulfate sodium. Am J Physiol Gastrointest Liver Physiol 2006; 291:G364–G371.
40. Wright K, Rooney N, Feeney M, et al. Differential expression of cannabinoid receptors in the human colon: Cannabinoids promote epithelial wound healing. Gastroenterology 2005; 129:437–453.
41. Ihenetu K, Molleman A, Parsons ME, et al. Inhibition of interleukin-8 release in the human colonic epithelial cell line HT-29 by cannabinoids. Eur J Pharmacol 2003; 458:207–215.
42. Sharkey KA. Visceral sensation and colitis: Inflammation and hypersensitivity do not always go hand in hand. Neurogastroenterol Motil 2006; 18:87–90.
43. Sanson M, Bueno L, Fioramonti J. Involvement of cannabinoid receptors in inflammatory hypersensitivity to colonic distension in rats. Neurogastroenterol Motil 2006; 18:949–956.
44. Hillsley K, McCaul C, Aerssens J, et al. Activation of the cannabinoids 2 (CB2) receptor inhibits murine mesenteric afferent nerve activity. Neurogastroenterol Motil, May 21; [Epub ahead of print].
45. Rousseaux C, Thuru X, Gelot A, et al. Lactobacillus acidophilus modulates intestinal pain and induces opioid and cannabinoid receptors. Nat Med 2007; 13:35–37.
46. Camilleri M. Is there a role for probiotics in irritable bowel syndrome? Dig Liver Dis 2006; 38(Suppl. 2):S266–S269.
47. Bifulco M, Laezza C, Pisanti S, et al. Cannabinoids and cancer: Pros and cons of an antitumour strategy. Br J Pharmacol 2006; 148:123–135.
48. Joseph J, Niggemann B, Zaenker KS, et al. Anandamide is an endogenous inhibitor for the migration of tumor cells and T lymphocytes. Cancer Immunol Immunother 2004; 53:723–728.
49. Patsos HA, Hicks DJ, Dobson RR, et al. The endogenous cannabinoid, anandamide, induces cell death in colorectal carcinoma cells: A possible role for cyclooxygenase 2. Gut 2005; 54:1741–1750.
50. Chaudhri O, Small C, Bloom S. Gastrointestinal hormones regulating appetite. Philos Trans R Soc Lond B Biol Sci. 2006; 361:1187–1209.
51. Cummings DE, Overduin J. Gastrointestinal regulation of food intake. J Clin Invest 2007; 117:13–23.
52. Burdyga G, Lal S, Varro A, et al. Expression of cannabinoid CB1 receptors by vagal afferent neurons is inhibited by cholecystokinin. J Neurosci 2004; 24:2708–2715.
53. Lo Verme J, Gaetani S, Fu J, et al. Regulation of food intake by oleoylethanolamide. Cell Mol Life Sci 2005; 62:708–716.
54. Rodriguez de Fonseca F, Navarro M, Gomez R, et al. An anorexic lipid mediator regulated by feeding. Nature 2001; 414:209–212.
55. Fu J, Gaetani S, Oveisi F, et al. Oleylethanolamide regulates feeding and body weight through activation of the nuclear receptor PPAR-a. Nature 2003; 425:90–93.
56. Fu J, Astarita G, Gaetani S, et al. Food intake regulates oleoylethanolamide formation and degradation in the proximal small intestine. J Biol Chem 2007; 282:1518–1528.

21 The EC System in the Adipose Tissue and Endocrine Pancreas

Isabel Matias

U862 Centre de Recherche INSERM François Magendie, Université de Bordeaux 2, Bordeaux, France

INTRODUCTION

Over past centuries, cannabis and its major psychoactive component Δ^9-tetrahydocannabinol (Δ^9-THC) have been extensively used for recreational use, and one of its widely effects was the onset of a ravenous appetite and eating behavior (1). Moreover, the discovery of the EC system and the cloning of the cannabinoid receptors, which are activated by the Δ^9-THC, suggested that the EC system might have a key role in the regulation of food intake. Data from CB_1 knockout mice and from pharmacological blockage of the CB_1 receptor by the well-known specific antagonist rimonabant reinforced definitively the concept that CB_1 receptor has a key role in the regulation of food intake (2). A recently expressed view, however, changed the scenario of the mode of action of the EC system not limited to neuronal target and shed light on the peripheral model of action of the EC system. Accordingly, endocannabinoids and CB_1 receptors are present in peripheral cells and tissues controlling energy homeostasis, including the gut (3), the liver and hepatocytes (4), the white adipose tissue (5) and the adipocytes (6–10), the skeletal muscle (11), and the pancreas (9,12–14).

There is increasing evidence for overactivity of the EC system during conditions of unbalanced energy homeostasis (e.g., obesity and hyperglycemia), and for its causative role in these disorders, and in particular in organs such as the adipose tissue and the pancreas (15,16). However, it is still not clear whether the EC system hyperactivity is a consequence or a cause of obesity even if a selective CB_1 receptor rimonabant is already commercially available to normalize the overactive EC system in obese pathological states (17–20). At this point it might be interesting to better understand how the EC system participates in the regulation of the metabolic and endocrine processes, in particular in the adipose tissue and pancreas.

ROLE OF THE EC SYSTEM IN THE ADIPOSE TISSUE (SEE FIG. 1)

Role of the EC System in Lipogenesis and in Adipogenesis

Several studies, carried out either on adipose tissue or on isolated adipocytes, demonstrated the presence of the EC system and seem to favor the idea that the endocannabinoid system is involved in fatty acid homeostasis in this tissue and that the activation of CB_1 receptors increases de novo lipogenesis. Cota and coworkers suggested, for the first time, a role for the EC system at the peripheral level, and in particular in adipocytes and adipose tissue, demonstrating the presence of the CB_1 receptors (7). In fact, they showed that $CB_1{}^{-/-}$ mice exhibits lower body weight due to a reduction of fat mass during a period of 12 weeks after birth accompanied by an increase in lean mass. Since CB_1 receptor knockout and wild-type mice show similar circadian variations in body temperature and locomotor activity, and only a trend toward higher energy expenditure (which corresponds to the energy combustion and fat and carbohydrates oxidation), the fat mass reduction observed in CB_1 receptor knockout mice must be directly connected to the absence of CB_1 receptors and to their role in fat mass accumulation and in fatty acid synthesis (7). The importance of the CB_1 receptor in fat mass regulation had already been pointed out by studies carried out with the use of the antagonist rimonabant in a diet-induced obesity mouse model. While its inhibitory effect on food-intake was only transient, the CB_1 antagonist induced a persistent fall in energy intake and a reduction in fat content after 5-weeks treatment of diet-induced obese (DIO) mice in comparison to the vehicle-treated mice (21). Moreover, the blockade of the CB_1 receptor in a 40-days regimen with rimonabant in the same animal model also reduced body weight persistently in a dose-dependent way, and this effect was

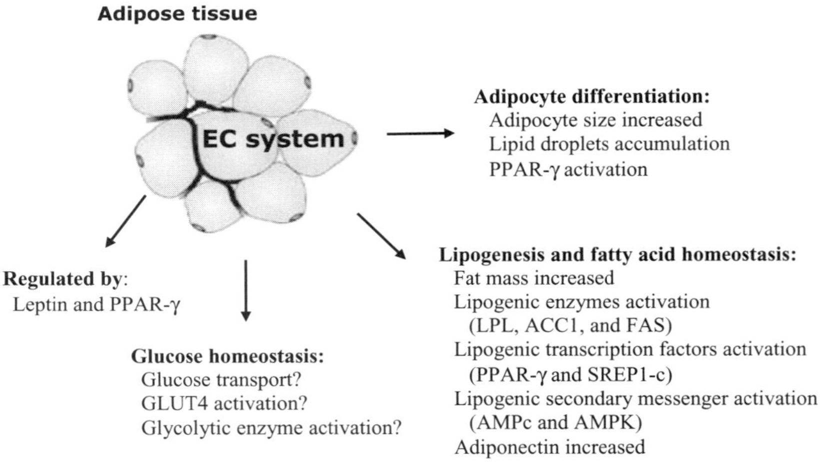

Figure 1 Role of the EC system in the adipose tissue.

accompanied by a decrease of white adipose tissue in epidydimal, perirenal, and lumbar tissues (5). Cota and coworkers also demonstrated that CB_1 was found in the epidydimal fat pads from $CB_1{}^{+/+}$ but not from $CB_1{}^{-/-}$.

The effect of the EC system on lipogenesis is also substantiated by the finding of CB_1 receptors in a primary epidydimal-derived adipocyte cell line 3T3F442 A. In these cells, stimulation of CB_1 by the agonist WIN-55212 leads to activation of the lipoprotein lipase, an enzyme involved in the hydrolysis of the triglycerides for adipocyte adsorption and fat storage, whereas its blockade by rimonabant causes inhibition (7). Bensaid and coworkers have also advanced a hypothesis that could possibly explain the effect of rimonabant on peripheral lipogenesis. In fact, in addition to a direct EC system–dependent effect on lipogenesis, the EC system could also affect lipid metabolism through the release of adipokines. They showed that the expression of one of the major adipocyte-derived hormones, which is playing a crucial role, among other things, in reducing the expression of enzymes involved in lipogenesis, adiponectin (Acrp30) could be enhanced by the CB_1 antagonist rimonabant (6). Blockage of CB_1 receptors by its antagonist rimonabant leads to an increase of adiponectin expression in the adipose tissue of obese zucker (fa/fa) rats, which is more pronounced in lean rats. Rimonabant also induced adiponectin overexpression in the mouse adipocyte cell line, but not on adipocytes from CB_1 receptor knockout mice (6). In agreement with these results, Matias and coworkers (9), using the same adipocyte cell line, demonstrated that the activation of CB_1 receptors by the agonist HU-210 inhibits adiponectin expression in mature/hypertrophic adipocytes. Moreover, HU-210 stimulates the appearance of an early marker of differentiation such as peroxisome proliferator-activated receptor-γ (PPAR-γ) and the accumulation of lipid droplets in the same conditions as assessed by Oil Red O-staining. An almost 2-fold stimulation of PPAR-γ expression was observed in both partially differentiated and mature adipocytes. All these effects were attenuated or reversed by rimonabant, pointing to the direct role of CB_1 receptors in increasing lipid accumulation in adipocytes (9). Considering that stimulation of CB_1 receptors, which has led to inhibition of adenylyl cyclase and of cAMP formation, an intracellular event coupled to lipolysis and inhibition of lipogenesis in adipocytes, one can then hypothesize that the CB_1 receptor–induced lipogenesis or inhibition of lipolysis might be due to inhibition of cAMP formation. The authors studied the effect of the compound on forskolin-induced cAMP formation in mature 3T3F442 A adipocytes and found that HU-210 dose-dependently inhibited cAMP formation in a way that was significantly attenuated by rimonabant but not by a CB_2 receptor antagonist (9). Furthermore, it is well established that cAMP inhibition stimulates lipogenesis by inhibiting the AMP-activated protein kinase (AMPK), which is considered a cellular fuel gauge and plays a key role in the regulation of energy metabolism. Interestingly, it has been demonstrated that Δ^9-THC decreases the AMPK activity in both visceral and subcutaneous adipose tissue and also decreases, in particular in the visceral fat, AMPK phosphorylation on threonine 172 in the similar manner as the orexigenic hormone ghrelin does (22). These data, together with the observation that Δ^9-THC inhibits AMPK and, therefore stimulates fatty acid synthesis in the adipose tissue (22), suggest that the EC system has several potential mechanisms to increase fatty acid storage into white adipocytes and, hence, the mass of adipose tissue. Since CB_1 receptors are expressed in adipose tissue and that rimonabant stimulates adiponectin synthesis (6), which in turn stimulates AMPK activity, these results are in agreement with the inhibition of AMPK activity by a CB_1 agonist like Δ^9-THC. AMPK stimulates catabolism and inhibits fatty acid synthesis by inhibiting ACC and decreasing malonyl-CoA availability (23). It is then important to note that, in fat pads, the activation of CB_1 receptors also stimulates the expression of the important transcription factor SREBP-1 c and its targets, the ACC1 and FAS lipogenic enzymes, suggesting that CB_1 receptors might increase lipid levels by increasing directly fatty acid synthesis (4). In the whole white adipose tissue of DIO mice, using DNA chip technology, it has been demonstrated that rimonabant increases the expression of lipolytic enzymes, such as CAT, CPT2, and crotonase, and of enzymes involved in the TCA cycle, such as fumarase, aconitase, and oxoglutarate dehydrogenase (24). Lipolysis regulators such as the β_3 adrenergic and growth hormone receptors were also upregulated. Since fatty acids can be endogenously synthesized from amino acids in order to increase energy expenditure, Jbilo and coworkers also looked at the expression of three enzymes involved in amino acid degradation and showed that rimonabant in DIO mice increased the expression of the cysteine dioxygenase responsible for the oxidative degradation of the cysteine, and of the methylcrotonoyl-CoA carboxylase and methylmalonyl CoA mutase responsible for valine, leucine, and isoleucine degradation (24). Also in the brown adipose tissue, rimonabant increased the genes involved in energy storage and expenditure and in the regulation of mitochondrial functions (24). In particular in mouse brown adipocytes, it has been recently demonstrated that CB_1 inhibits the thermogenic uncoupling protein-1 (UCP-1), which is a marker of terminal brown fat differentiation and a hallmark of the thermogenic recruitment process (25). Treatment with the CB_1 agonist WIN55212–2 decreases the expression of UCP-1 in a dose-dependent way. Moreover, the CB_1-mediated inhibition was maximal between 2 and 4 hours of stimulation and was paralleled by similar decreases in UCP-1 mRNA levels (25). Blockage of such effects by rimonabant, although interesting in rodents, could be of limited interest since the role of brown adipose tissue is still a matter of debate in humans. However, the authors conclude that CB_1 signaling activation in mice reduces thermogenesis (25) and that rimonabant increased it (26).

Interestingly, in the process of adipocyte differentiation, the endocannabinoid anandamide, whole levels of which we found to peak immediately before adipocyte maturation (9), was also found to stimulate PPAR-γ in a non CB_1-dependent way (27). In fact, the authors observed that anandamide enhances the differentiation of the mouse preadipocyte 3T3L1 by increasing lipid accumulation and adiponectin, lipoprotein lipase and PPAR-γ expression in a way reverted by a PPAR-γ antagonist but not by the CB_1 antagonist rimonabant (27). Recently, Yan and coworkers suggested that not only in the same adipocyte cell line but also in visceral and subcutaneous tissue, CB_1 receptors expression is instead regulated by PPAR-δ, which has received less attention than the other PPARs but appears to be a powerful regulator of lipolysis (28). In white but not in brown adipose tissue, both the high-fat-diet–induced adipocyte fattening and the exercise-induced adipocyte size reduction were accompanied by changes in PPAR-δ levels opposite to those of CB_1 receptors. Accordingly, when 3T3L1 adipocytes were submitted to selective silencing of PPAR-δ mRNA, a significant increase in both CB_1 receptor expression and adipocyte differentiation was observed, whereas adenovirus-mediated overexpression of PPAR-δ significantly reduced both CB_1 expression and adipocyte differentiation. Since PPAR-δ activate genes for fatty acid catabolism and oxidation and then lipolysis, and CB_1 receptor stimulates lipogenesis; it is not surprising to see that PPAR-δ downregulates CB_1 receptor expression (28). These findings reinforce the concept that endocannabinoids actively and directly participate in adipogenesis and fat accumulation.

Role of the EC System in Glycolysis in the Adipose Tissue

Recent findings also suggest that in the adipose tissue, the EC system seems to be involved not only in fatty acid but also in glucose homeostasis and that CB_1 receptors blockage increases glycolysis. In mouse 3T3F442 A adipocytes, rimonabant inhibits cell proliferation in a concentration-dependent manner and stimulates the expression of GAPDH, an enzyme involved in both lipid and glucose metabolism, both at the level of the RNA and the protein (29). Furthermore, also in whole white adipose tissue of DIO mice, rimonabant was shown to increase GAPDH and other glycolytic enzymes such as the glycogen phosphorylase and synthase, the phosphofructokinase, the glyceraldehyde-3-phosphate dehydrogenase, the phosphoglycerate mutase, and the β-enolase (24). Blockage of CB_1 receptors by rimonabant also induced an upregulation of the insulin-responsive glucose transporter, GLUT4, which suggests a facilitated glucose transport and consequently, increased glycolysis and lipogenesis. Recently, in contrast to this finding, Gasperi and coworkers have demonstrated that anandamide stimulates insulin-induced glucose uptake in the adipocyte cell line 3T3L1, and that this effect is antagonized by rimonabant (30). Recently, Pagano and coworkers also observed that CB_1 stimulation increases glucose uptake and translocation of GLUT4 in plasma membrane, mediated by increased $[Ca^{2+}]_i$ and PI3-kinase in human adipocytes, suggesting that endocannabinoids and insulin share a common intracellular signaling pathway (31). In conclusion, blockade of CB_1 receptors might increase glucose uptake and metabolism in the white adipose tissue cells depending on their energy status and insulin sensitivity and resulting in an increased energy loss, which might, at least in part, contribute to the observed 18% to 27% weight loss in DIO mice (21,24).

Regulation of the EC System in the Adipose Tissue

Furthermore, in the 3T3F442 A mouse adipocyte cell line, the levels of endocannabinoids appeared to be regulated by leptin and PPAR-γ according the differentiation status of the adipocytes (9). As previously reported in rodent hypothalamus (32), both anandamide and 2-AG levels in mature adipocytes were decreased after either both acute or prolonged stimulation with leptin. In partially differentiated but not in mature adipocytes, the selective agonist of PPAR-γ ciglitazone decreased 2-AG, but not anandamide levels. The data obtained in 3T3F442 A suggest that the EC system is upregulated immediately before adipocyte differentiation, concurring to induce differentiation and lipogenesis. Consequentially, at the early stage of differentiation, 2-AG might be downregulated by PPAR-γ and then, at late stage of differentiation, both endocannabinoids and PPAR-γ might then be "turned off" by leptin, which is produced by mature adipocytes (9). In agreement with our studies, Pagano and coworkers recently reported an upregulation of PPAR-γ expression induced by WIN55212 only in early differentiated human adipocytes (31). Interestingly, differentiation of human adipocytes with the PPAR-γ agonist rosiglitazone was shown to downregulate CB_1 expression and upregulate FAAH expression (31). All these data suggest a feedback mechanism between PPAR-γ and endocannabinoids at early stage of differentiation, while leptin would then inhibit both endocannabinoids levels and PPAR-γ expression (9,31) at late stage of differentiation.

Deregulation of the EC System in the Adipose Tissue

In the adipose tissue, several authors have recently shown a dysregulation of EC system. Bensaid and coworkers found for the first time an upregulation of the CB_1 receptor expression in adipocyte tissue of zucker (fa/fa) obese rats as compared to lean rats, and at the same time, in differentiated 3T3F442 A mouse adipocyte cell line compared to that of the undifferentiated adipocyte cell line (6). Data from Matias and coworkers demonstrated that not only CB_1 but also CB_2 receptors were expressed only in differentiating 3T3F442 A adipocytes and remained expressed in mature cells, although CB_1 levels significantly decreased in hypertrophic versus partially differentiated preadipocytes (9). Furthermore, they demonstrated that 2-AG levels become hyperregulated in hypertrophic adipocytes (day 12). Accordingly, the differentiation was accompanied by a dramatic increase in the expression of the 2-AG biosynthesizing enzyme, DAGL-α, whereas the 2-AG degrading enzyme, MAGL, was unchanged. In DIO mice, the epididymal fat levels of 2-AG were 2.5-fold higher in DIO versus normoweight mice in agreement with an upregulation of the EC system in the adipocyte 3T3F442 A cell line (9). Moreover, Di Marzo's group recently demonstrated by immunochemistry that both cannabinoid receptors and all the endocannabinoid enzymatic machinery is present in both mice subcutaneous and visceral adipose tissue (33). Importantly, however, no differences in the expression of endocannabinoids metabolic enzymes and endocannabinoids normalized or total levels were found in the visceral fat of mice fed with a high-fat diet (HFD) as compared to standard diet (STD). Instead, in the subcutaneous fat the high fat regimen, starting 8 weeks from its beginning, resulted in an increased expression of endocannabinoids metabolic enzymes and normalized or total levels of AEA and 2-AG that were lower than the corresponding ones in STD mice. The above data on endocannabinoid levels in the adipose tissues do not entirely agree with the previous finding of increased levels of 2-AG in DIO mice (9). Methodologically, different sampling of the visceral and subcutaneous adipose tissue, and high-fat diet differences might account for not only the differences on endocannabinoids levels observed, but also on the expression of CB_1 receptors. Higher or lower CB_1 or CB_2 expression in subcutaneous and visceral adipose tissue of high-fat-diet–fed mice as compared to standard diet fed mice was not observed (9). On the other hand, Yan et al. (28) showed that in rats fed a high-fat diet, the expression of CB_1 in the adipose tissue is increased.

ROLE OF THE EC SYSTEM IN THE ENDOCRINE PANCREAS (SEE FIG. 2)

Role of the EC System in Insulin Release and Glucose Tolerance

Recent findings suggest that endocannabinoids are also involved in the control of metabolism by regulating insulin levels as well as glucose uptake and utilization by tissues, with subsequent impact on glucose tolerance (9,12–14). The role of the EC system has been first investigated in the RIN-m5 F β-cells, a model of rat insulinoma that is a widely used model of pancreatic islet β-cells because of the quantity of insulin they release and also the response they show to this hormone (9). Using quantitative real-time PCR, the author recently demonstrated the presence of both CB_1 and CB_2 in the RIN-m5 F cells of the endocannabinoid biosynthetic enzymes such as the DAGL-α and the NAPE-PLD, and of the degradating enzymes such as MAGL and FAAH (9,34). The author observed that stimulation of cannabinoid receptors by HU-210 enhanced insulin release, as assessed by a specific ELISA. This effect was reversed by rimonabant but not by a cannabinoid CB_2 receptor antagonist and was likely due to elevation of intracellular Ca^{2+} by HU-210, which occurred within a similar range of concentrations (9). Interestingly, since insulin secretion is determined by the $[Ca^{2+}]_i$ transients, De Petrocellis and coworkers recently investigated the functional activity of CB_1 and CB_2 receptors (34). We demonstrated that, like bombesin receptors, but with lower potency, CB_1 and CB_2 receptor activation is coupled to Ca^{2+} mobilization from intracellular stores, possibly from endoplasmic reticulum. This process is sensitive to a specific inhibitor of phosphoinositide selective phospholipase C (PI-PLC), U73122, but not to its inactive analog, U73343, nor to pertussis toxin, adenylyl cyclase stimulation or extracellular Ca^{2+}. This might suggest that CB_1 and CB_2 receptors are coupled to elevation of $[Ca^{2+}]_i$ via G-proteins of the Gq/11 type, activation of the PI-PLC cascade and also $[Ca^{2+}]_i$ mobilization via IP_3 receptors (34).

In mouse Langerhans' islets, Juan-Pico and coworkers showed that stimulation of CB_2 receptors reduces insulin release via inhibition of calcium transients, whereas CB_1 receptors, which were absent from mouse β-cells, exert the same effect to a much lesser extent (12). However, the authors later reported that systemic CB_1, but not CB_2, receptor stimulation in rats causes glucose intolerance in vivo (13). These results from the same group can be interpreted

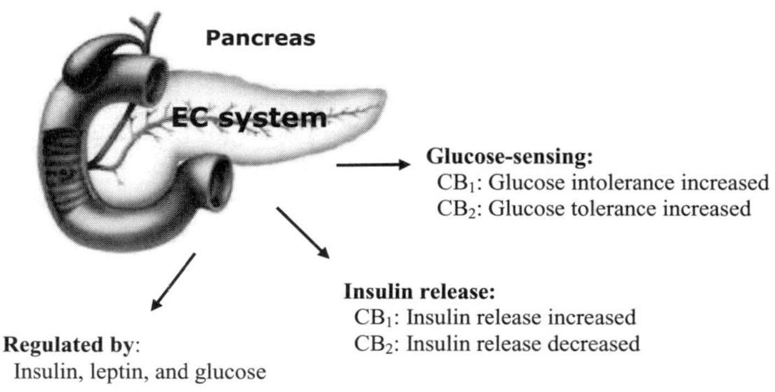

Figure 2 Role of the EC system in the endocrine pancreas.

only by assuming that activation of CB_1 receptor agonists reduce glucose tolerance through an indirect mechanism (i.e., not by targeting β-cells and reducing insulin release directly, but rather by affecting other factors that regulate insulin release, or by inhibiting glucose uptake by tissues in other ways). Alternatively, it is possible that a small population of β-cells do express these receptors under certain conditions. Indeed, the finding of high levels of CB_1 receptors in insulinoma cells (9) might suggest that the expression of these receptors in β-cells might also depend on their differentiation and/or metabolic state. Species differences are also possible, and it has to be underlined that no study in human pancreas has been reported to date. In fact, immunohistochemical data from Di Marzo's group indicate that, in pancreatic islets from lean mice and rats, both CB_1 receptors and endocannabinoid-producing enzymes are mostly located on glucagon-producing α-cells (33).

Furthermore, Bermudez-Silva and coworkers recently established the presence of both CB_1 and CB_2 receptors in rat pancreatic β- and non–β-cells from isolated Langherhans islets and demonstrated that CB_2 receptors improved glucose tolerance (14). Since it has been demonstrated that CB_1 stimulation increases insulin release (9) and that CB_2 stimulation decrease insulin release (12), they suggested that CB_1 and CB_2 have opposite role in glucose homeostasis suggesting a coordinated action of both receptors in the regulation of glycaemia (14). Accordingly, higher glucose levels have been found after CB_1 stimulation while they return to normal levels after CB_2 stimulation. Furthermore, the authors demonstrated that the activation of both CB_1 and CB_2 receptors did not affect glucose levels showing that these receptors inhibited their individual contribution (14). Further detailed studies on the occurrence and function of cannabinoid receptors in cells and tissues producing, regulating, and responding to insulin need to be performed especially in humans.

Regulation of the EC System in Pancreatic Islet β-cells

Furthermore, in RIN-m5 F pancreatic islet β-cells, the levels of endocannabinoids appeared to be under the regulation of glucose and insulin according to the glucose concentration of the cell medium (9). Matias and coworkers reported that a pulse of a "very high" concentration of glucose significantly elevates the levels of both anandamide and 2-AG in these cells. However, we also observed that, contrary to "low" glucose conditions, where insulin reduces the "very high" glucose-induced elevation of endocannabinoid levels and has no effect per se, in β-cells kept for 24 hours in "high" glucose endocannabinoid levels are not depressed any longer by insulin, which instead elevates both AEA and 2-AG levels also in the absence of the "very high" glucose pulse. Additionally, under both conditions, leptin only decreased 2-AG, but not anandamide, levels and that too only after prolonged stimulation (9).

Deregulation of the EC System in the Pancreas

An overactive EC system has also been detected in isolated pancreatic β-cells and in the pancreas in hyperglycaemic and obese states by Matias and coworkers (9). Accordingly, in RIN-m5 F rat insulinoma β-pancreatic cells, in which a high glucose "pulse" elevates both AEA and 2-AG levels, insulin keeps this effect under negative control when the cells are maintained in a relatively low concentration of glucose. However, under conditions mimicking hyperglycemia, insulin no longer inhibits glucose-induced endocannabinoid levels and, instead, it stimulates them per se. In agreement with these findings in isolated cells, enhanced levels of both AEA and 2-AG were observed in the pancreas of hyperglycaemic DIO mice as compared to mice fed a normal diet (9). Recently, they found in the pancreas of mice fed with a HFD, a strong expression of NAPE-PLD and DAGL-α inside the islets, whereas these biosynthetic enzymes are normally expressed in α-cells in the pancreas of mice fed with a STD, suggesting an overexpression of these enzymes in the β-cells of HFD mice (33). On the other hand, the expression of FAAH in these cells decreased starting at 8 weeks from the beginning of the HFD. Following prolonged HFD and development of overt obesity, pancreatic endocannabinoids levels return to normal despite the fact that deregulation of biosynthetic and degradative enzyme persist (33). This overactivity of the EC system in the pancreas is likely to have a strong impact on insulin levels (see below), and hence on glucose utilization and metabolism. Furthermore, it may affect adipo-insular interactions, thus contributing to further hyperinsulinemia and hypoadiponectinemia.

DEREGULATION OF THE EC SYSTEM AND CONSEQUENCE OF SUCH DEREGULATION IN HUMAN

Recently, human subcutaneous or visceral adipocytes and adipose tissue have been found to express CB_1 and CB_2 receptors, suggesting a role for the EC system in the pathophysiology of obesity and hyperglycemia not only in experimental models but also in humans (8,10,31,35). In fact, in overweight/obese patients with mild hyperglycaemia, almost 2-fold higher levels of 2-AG were found in visceral adipose tissue as compared to normoweight controls (9). Importantly, in these patients, visceral fat, known to be the most important determinant in fat mass regulation and obesity-associated disorders, contained significantly higher levels of 2-AG than subcutaneous fat, thus emphasizing the potential implication of the EC system in the link between the metabolic syndrome and visceral adiposity. Engeli and coworkers also found a reduction in CB_1 and FAAH expression in the visceral adipose tissue of obese women. They also observed in obese women a strong correlation between FAAH in the adipose tissue and elevated plasmatic endocannabinoid levels (5). Regarding the expression of CB_1 receptors, discrepancy results have been observed in obese according to, probably, methodological differences. Conversely, a decrease of CB_1 receptor expression in the visceral fat of obese versus normoweight women, and a negative correlation between CB_1 mRNA levels and the amounts of visceral fat in obese patients was reported by another group (5,36), whereas two other studies showed no changes in CB_1 expression (9,37). Nevertheless, a study carried out in human subcutaneous gluteal fat and visceral adipose tissue from normoweight and obese patients, indicates that deregulation of the EC system in adipose tissue is depot-specific, since a decrease in the expression of CB_1 receptors and of the FAAH have been observed in the subcutaneous gluteal fat, whereas an opposite change of these genes was observed in visceral adipose tissue from obese patients (31). These above data are in agreement with the recent data from Di Marzo's group indicating that the expression of endocannabinoids metabolic enzymes and normalized or total levels of endocannabinoids were lower in the subcutaneous fat of HFD mice compared to STD mice (33). Methodologically, different sampling of the subcutaneous adipose tissue which contains two layers of adipose tissue with different biochemical and functional properties, and species differences (see below) might account for not only the different endocannabinoids levels, but also on the expression of CB_1 receptors or endocannabinoids metabolic enzymes. Nevertheless, all these data still suggest that a different distribution between visceral and subcutaneous fat in individuals with the same body mass index (BMI) and overall adiposity might have a dramatic impact on the levels of endocannabinoids in this organ. In fact, it can be predicted that, in both mice and humans, a higher percent of visceral versus subcutaneous fat will result in higher peripheral endocannabinoids levels, thus possibly accounting for the strong association between high-circulating 2-AG levels and intra-abdominal adiposity observed in obese patients with the same BMI (36,39).

Even if endocannabinoids are not normally released from tissues into the bloodstream to act as hormone, plasmatic elevated endocannabinoids levels have been found in obese and diabetic humans suggesting that the deregulation of the EC system, observed in the adipose tissue or in the pancreas or in the other peripheral tissues, might spills over into the blood. In fact, in the blood of women that became obese because of binge eating or menopausa, the levels of anandamide or both endocannabinoids, are also significantly higher than in age-matched nonobese controls (5,38), whereas in the blood of obese, particularly if male, patients, the levels of 2-AG, but not anandamide, correlate with intra-abdominal adiposity and with all the cardiometabolic risks associated with ectopic visceral fat (36,39). Also in the blood of nonobese type 2 diabetes patients, levels of both anandamide and 2-AG are permanently elevated compared to those of age- and gender-matched controls (9).

CONCLUSIONS

This chapter summarized the last evidences pointing to the important role played by the EC system in the control of glucose and fatty acid metabolism at the level of the adipose tissue and pancreas. CB_1 receptor activation has been showed to increase blood glucose levels via different pathways, including the inhibition of insulin release and of glucose utilization by peripheral tissue and brain cells, even if the exact mechanism still needs to be substantiated by future studies. Furthermore, CB_1 receptor activation facilitates the growth of fat deposits rather than burning fat as a fuel for cells. Under normal activation conditions, CB_1 receptor activation is certainly beneficial to ensure the optimal energy homeostasis necessary to compensate for the loss of energy occurring following stressful conditions. As a malignant factor instead, circulating and fat tissue endocannabinoid levels are increased in overweight and especially abdominally adipose patients, thus giving rise to a vicious circle (16). As anticipated above, blockade of CB_1 receptors with specific antagonists seems to be a fruitful and relatively safe pharmacological strategy to reduce body weight in obese humans also. Rimonabant, the first CB_1 receptor antagonist/inverse agonist to be approved for therapeutic use in Europe, might be followed in the future by CB_1 receptor antagonists developed by other companies and now in phase I and II clinical trials. Like rimonabant, these compounds might not only reduce food-intake and body weight in obese patients, but also significantly ameliorate the signs of the metabolic syndrome in overweight/viscerally obese and/or type 2 diabetes patients by directly targeting a potentially overactive EC system in peripheral cells and organs (17–20). This potential additional value of CB_1 receptor antagonists will have to be exploited to add further momentum to the future basic, preclinical and clinical studies that are necessary, now more than ever, to fully appreciate the role of endocannabinoids in the peripheral control of metabolism.

REFERENCES

1. Kirkham TC, Williams CM. Synergistic effects of opioid and cannabinoid antagonists on food intake. Psychopharmacology (Berl) 2001; 153(2):267–270.
2. Cota D, Marsicano G, Lutz B, et al. Endogenous cannabinoid system as a modulator of food intake. Int J Obes Relat Metab Disord 2003; 27(3):289–301.
3. Coutts AA, Izzo AA. The gastrointestinal pharmacology of cannabinoids: An update. Curr Opin Pharmacol 2004; 4(6):572—579, Review.
4. Osei-Hyiaman D, DePetrillo M, Pacher P, et al. Endocannabinoid activation at hepatic CB1 receptors stimulates fatty acid synthesis and contributes to diet-induced obesity. J Clin Invest 2005; 115(5):1298–1305.
5. Engeli S, Bohnke J, Feldpausch M, et al. Activation of the peripheral endocannabinoid system in human obesity. Diabetes 2005; 54(10):2838–2843.
6. Bensaid M, Gary-Bobo M, Esclangon A, et al. The cannabinoid CB1 receptor antagonist SR141716 increases Acrp30 mRNA expression in adipose tissue of obese fa/fa rats and in cultured adipocyte cells. Mol Pharmacol 2003; 63(4):908–914.
7. Cota D, Marsicano G, Tschop M, et al. The endogenous cannabinoid system affects energy balance via central orexigenic drive and peripheral lipogenesis. J Clin Invest 2003; 112(3):423–431.
8. Roche R, Hoareau L, Bes-Houtmann S, et al. Presence of the cannabinoid receptors, CB1 and CB2, in human omental and subcutaneous adipocytes. Histochem Cell Biol 2006; 126(2):177–187.
9. Matias I, Gonthier MP, Orlando P, et al. Regulation, function, and dysregulation of endocannabinoids in models of adipose and beta-pancreatic cells and in obesity and hyperglycemia. J Clin Endocrinol Metab 2006; 91(8):3171–3180.
10. Gonthier MP, Hoareau L, Festy F, et al. Identification of endocannabinoids and related compounds in human fat cells. Obesity 2007; 15(4):837–845.
11. Pagotto U, Marsicano G, Cota D, et al. The emerging role of the endocannabinoid system in endocrine regulation and energy balance. Endocr Rev 2006; 27(1):73–100.
12. Juan-Pico P, Fuentes E, Bermudez-Silva FJ, et al. Cannabinoid receptors regulate Ca(2+) signals and insulin secretion in pancreatic beta-cell. Cell Calcium 2006; 39(2):155–162.
13. Bermudez-Siva FJ, Serrano A, Diaz-Molina FJ, et al. Activation of cannabinoid CB1 receptors induces glucose intolerance in rats. Eur J Pharmacol 2006; 531(1–3):282–284.
14. Bermudez-Silva FJ, Sanchez-Vera I, Suarez J, et al. Role of cannabinoid CB2 receptors in glucose homeostasis in rats. Eur J Pharmacol 2007; 565(1–3):207–211.
15. Di Marzo V, Matias I. Endocannabinoid control of food intake and energy balance. Nat Neurosci 2005; 8(5):585–589.
16. Matias I, Di Marzo V. Endocannabinoids and the control of energy balance. Trends Endocrinol Metab 2007; 18(1):27–37.
17. Van Gaal LF, Rissanen AM, Scheen AJ, et al. Effects of the cannabinoid-1 receptor blocker rimonabant on weight reduction and cardiovascular risk factors in overweight patients: 1-year experience from the RIO-Europe study. Lancet 2005; 365(9468):1389–1397.
18. Despres JP, Golay A, Sjostrom L, et al. Effects of rimonabant on metabolic risk factors in overweight patients with dyslipidemia. N Engl J Med 2005; 353(20):2121–2134.

19. Pi-Sunyer FX, Aronne LJ, Heshmati HM, et al. Effect of rimonabant, a cannabinoid-1 receptor blocker, on weight and cardiometabolic risk factors in overweight or obese patients: RIO-North America: A randomized controlled trial. JAMA 2006; 295(7):761–775.
20. Scheen AJ, Finer N, Hollander P, et al. Efficacy and tolerability of rimonabant in overweight or obese patients with type 2 diabetes: A randomised controlled study. Lancet 2006; 368(9548):1660–1672.
21. Ravinet Trillou C, Arnone M, Delgorge C, et al. Anti-obesity effect of SR141716, a CB1 receptor antagonist, in diet-induced obese mice. Am J Physiol Regul Integr Comp Physiol 2003; 284(2):R345–R353.
22. Kola B, Hubina E, Tucci SA, et al. Cannabinoids and ghrelin have both central and peripheral metabolic and cardiac effects via AMP-activated protein kinase. J Biol Chem 2005; 280(26):25196–25201.
23. Hardie DG, Hawley SA, Scott JW. Activated protein kinase—Development of the energy sensor concept. J Physiol 2006; 574(Pt 1):7–15.
24. Jbilo O, Ravinet-Trillou C, Arnone M, et al. The CB1 receptor antagonist rimonabant reverses the diet-induced obesity phenotype through the regulation of lipolysis and energy balance. FASEB J 2005; 19(11):1567–1569.
25. Perwitz N, Fasshauer M, Klein J. Cannabinoid receptor signaling directly inhibits thermogenesis and alters expression of adiponectin and visfatin. Horm Metab Res 2006; 38(5):356–358.
26. Liu YL, Connoley IP, Wilson CA, et al. Effects of the cannabinoid CB1 receptor antagonist SR141716 on oxygen consumption and soleus muscle glucose uptake in Lep(ob)/Lep(ob) mice. Int J Obes (Lond) 2005; 29:183–187.
27. Bouaboula M, Hilairet S, Marchand J, et al. Anandamide induced PPARgamma transcriptional activation and 3T3-L1 preadipocyte differentiation. Eur J Pharmacol 2005; 517(3):174–181.
28. Yan ZC, Liu DY, Zhang LL, et al. Exercise reduces adipose tissue via cannabinoid receptor type 1 which is regulated by peroxisome proliferator-activated receptor-delta. Biochem Biophys Res Commun 2007; 354(2):427–433.
29. Gary-Bobo M, Elachouri G, Scatton B, et al. The cannabinoid CB1 receptor antagonist rimonabant (SR141716) inhibits cell proliferation and increases markers of adipocyte maturation in cultured mouse 3T3 F442 A preadipocytes. Mol Pharmacol 2006; 69(2):471–478.
30. Gasperi V, Fezza F, Pasquariello N, et al. Endocannabinoids in adipocytes during differentiation and their role in glucose uptake. Cell Mol Life Sci 2007; 64(2):219–229.
31. Pagano C, Pilon C, Calcagno A, et al. The endogenous cannabinoid system stimulates glucose uptake in human fat cells via PI3-kinase and calcium-dependent mechanisms. J Clin Endocrinol Metab 2007:doi:10.1210/jc.2007–0768.
32. Di Marzo V, Goparaju SK, Wang L, et al. Leptin-regulated endocannabinoids are involved in maintaining food intake. Nature 2001; 410(6830):822–825.
33. Starowicz K, Cristino L, Matias I, et al. Endocannabinoid dysregulation in the pancreas and the adipose tissue of mice fed a high fat diet. Obesity 2008; 16(3):553–565.
34. De Petrocellis L, Marini P, Matias I, et al. Mechanisms for the coupling of cannabinoid receptors to intracellular calcium mobilization in rat insulinoma beta-cells. Exp Cell Res 2007; 313(14):2993–3004.
35. Spoto B, Fezza F, Parlongo G, et al. Human adipose tissue binds and metabolizes the endocannabinoids anandamide and 2-arachidonoylglycerol. Biochimie 2006; 88(12):189–197.
36. Bluher M, Engeli S, Kloting N, et al. Dysregulation of the peripheral and adipose tissue endocannabinoid system in human abdominal obesity. Diabetes 2006; 55(11):3053–3060.
37. Lofgren P, Sjolin E, Wahlen K, et al. Human adipose tissue cannabinoid receptor 1 gene expression is not related to fat cell function or adiponectin level. J Clin Endocrinol Metab 2007; 92(4):1555–1559.
38. Monteleone P, Matias I, Martiadis V, et al. Blood levels of the endocannabinoid anandamide are increased in anorexia nervosa and in binge-eating disorder, but not in bulimia nervosa. Neuropsychopharmacology 2005; 30(6):1216–1221.
39. Cote M, Matias I, Lemieux I, et al. Circulating endocannabinoid levels, abdominal adiposity and related cardiometabolic risk factors in obese men. Int J Obes (Lond) 2007; 31(4):692–699.

22 The EC System in the Immune System and the Inflammatory Response

Tracy A. Sherwood and Thomas W. Klein

Department of Molecular Medicine, School of Basic Biomedical Sciences, College of Medicine, University of South Florida, Tampa, Florida, U.S.A.

INTRODUCTION

The first cannabinoid receptor (CB_1) was cloned from rat brain in the early 1990s representing the beginning of the molecular description of the cannabinoid system in this tissue (1). This finding was followed by the isolation and molecular characterization of anandamide (*N*-arachidonoylethanolamine, AEA) (2), an endogenous cannabinoid receptor ligand or endocannabinoid (EC), and also by a report that immune cells expressed a second type of cannabinoid receptor, CB_2 (3). The discovery of CB_2 suggested that the endocannabinoid system (ECS) was functioning in tissues besides brain and further support of this came from studies showing that immune cells produced receptor ligands (4–8) and metabolizing enzymes (5,6,9,10). The demonstration of the molecular components of an immune ECS supported decades of previous work showing that natural cannabinoids, such as THC, modulated immune function in humans and animals (11) and indeed it is now evident that ECs also modulate immune function (11–13). The discovery of the immune endocannabinoid system (IECS) raises two important questions: What is the function of the IECS in regulating normal immune activity? Secondly, can the regulation of the IECS during disease provide new approaches to the management of inflammation? In the following, we will provide a short overview of results establishing that immune cells contain an IECS and also provide evidence supporting a role of the IECS in immune activation and the potential therapeutic benefit of IECS manipulation in the management of inflammation.

THE IMMUNE ENDOCANNABINOID SYSTEM (IECS)

It is now established that cannabinoid receptors (CB_1 and CB_2), their endogenous ligands, and the enzymes responsible for endocannabinoid biosynthesis and degradation are produced and active in immune cells (14,15), thus comprising the IECS. The first studies identifying the components of the ECS, such as ECs and their metabolizing enzymes, were primarily done with cells of the CNS, which provided strategies that were applied to investigate EC synthesis and metabolism in immune cells. ECs are lipid mediators generated on demand by various cells, including activated immune cells (14,15) and neurons (16,17). The most studied and well-characterized ECs are AEA, discovered in porcine brain (18), and 2-AG (2-arachidonylglycerol), first isolated from canine intestines (19). These natural compounds are arachidonic acid derivatives metabolized by cleavage of membrane fatty acids (20,21). From experiments performed in brain, AEA synthesis starts with the combination of arachidonoyl phospholipid and phosphatidylethanolamine by the action of an *N*-acyltransferase (NAT), in the presence of Ca^{2+}, followed by the subsequent hydrolysis of *N*-arachidonoyl-phosphatidylethanolamine (NArPE) catalyzed by phospholipase D (PLD) to yield AEA and phosphatidic acid (12,21,22). 2-AG biosynthesis occurs in response to a rise in intracellular Ca^{2+} and is formed by the hydrolysis of 1,2-diacylglycerol (DAG) by DAG lipase (DAGL) (12,21–23). Degradation of AEA is by fatty acid amide hydrolase (FAAH) (24), while 2-AG hydrolysis is by monoacylglycerol lipase (MAGL) (23–25). There are two well-defined cannabinoid receptors, CB_1 and CB_2 (26), and endocannabinoids bind to CB_1 and CB_2, with 2-AG having affinity for both receptors, whereas AEA having greater affinity for CB_1 (27). Noladin ether and virohdamine have also been describe as endocannabinoids but have not been reported to be produced by immune cells and therefore will not be discussed further.

The initial studies to identify components of the IECS were carried out using mouse J774 macrophages and rat RBL-2 H3 basophils (4,5). These studies showed for the first time that immune cells contained a NAPE-like metabolite that was hydrolyzed by PLD to release AEA, and further demonstrated that ionomycin stimulation caused both cell lines to produced AEA (5) and J774 cells to produced 2-AG (6). To further establish that immune cells have a functional IECS, RBL-2 H3 basophils and J774 macrophages were shown to inactivate AEA (5) and 2-AG (6,9) by re-uptake mechanisms involving either an as-yet-uncharacterized membrane transporter for AEA or by diffusion for 2-AG. This re-uptake was immediately followed by AEA hydrolysis mediated by FAAH (5) and recently in other macrophage systems by NAAA (*N*-acylethanolamine-hydrolyzing acid amidase) (10). 2-AG hydrolysis was mediated minimally by FAAH (9) but more extensively by MGL (6).

Evaluation of endocannabinoid production during immune stimulation has been studied in various models. RBL-2 H3 cells stimulated to release histamine also released AEA at minimal levels (5); on the other hand, immune activation of J774 cells with LPS caused a 2.5-fold increase of 2-AG levels (6) and RAW264.7 macrophages activated with LPS and PAF increased synthesis of AEA (28). However, in another study using RAW246.7 cells, although 2-AG was in greater abundance at basal activity, following stimulation with LPS the level of AEA not 2-AG increased. The increase in AEA was shown to occur independent of PAF stimulation which was shown to induce 2-AG production (29). This supported another study using mouse P388D1 macrophages showing that PAF stimulates the release of 2-AG and not AEA. These studies demonstrate that macrophages can synthesize both AEA and 2-AG with the latter in higher abundance at basal cell activity; however, the upregulation of the endocannabinoids may differ following stimulation with AEA increased by LPS and 2-AG by PAF. More recent studies analyzed the presence of the IECS in brain microglia. It was determined that the rat microglial cell line, RTMGL1, produces 2-AG as well as AEA, with the latter in smaller quantities (30). Microglia cells also produce endocannabinoid hydrolyzing enzymes. For example, BV-2 cells, as well as primary microglia cells, were analyzed for FAAH activity as well as for the presence of MGL. Using a mixture of enzyme inhibitors, it was determined that FAAH hydrolyzed 2-AG as did a "novel MGL" that was not expressed in neurons but had 2-AG hydrolysis activity in microglia (31). Tham et al. (32) using rat microglia cell cultures showed similar results with these cells, showing both FAAH and MGL activity.

Studies with dendritic cells (DC) also showed evidence of an IECS. Human DCs derived from PBMCs were shown to produce AEA and 2-AG at basal activity with the level of 2-AG higher (as in macrophages) than AEA (33). Stimulating the cells with LPS increased 2-AG but not AEA which was different from the response reported above in macrophages wherein LPS increased AEA. From this, it is possible that the upregulation of ECs differs depending on the type of immune cell and that the mobilization of AEA may play a more critical role in macrophage function, while 2-AG mobilization is of greater importance in DC function. In addition to EC production, DCs were shown through RT-PCR and Western blot analysis to express FAAH, CB_1, and CB_2 (33).

Human peripheral blood mononuclear cells (PBMCs) also appear to have a complete IECS. Maccarrone et al. (8) established by PCR and Western blot analysis that PBMCs expressed FAAH, CB_1, and CB_2. FAAH activity and protein were decreased in these cells following LPS stimulation and this was associated with an increase in immune cell AEA level. The PBMCs were also able to take up AEA independent of LPS stimulation and bind AEA through CB_1 receptors. Similar results were obtained in a recent study on Huntington's disease (HD) in which PBMCs were shown to express FAAH, CB_1, and CB_2, synthesize AEA via NAPE-PLD, inactivate AEA by uptake at the AEA transporter (AMT), and hydrolysis by FAAH (34). Interestingly, the HD patients had decreased FAAH activity and increased AEA levels in PBMC.

Human T lymphocytes, purified from PBMCs, also contain endogenous levels of AEA and 2-AG as well as express FAAH activity (35–38). As with data reported above for macrophages and DC, the level of 2-AG in T cells was greater than that of AEA, however, both ECs were decreased by progesterone treatment in culture for 24 hours (36). T cells also expressed FAAH activity and both transcription and translation of the FAAH gene were increased by progesterone treatment suggesting that the hormone is able to regulate the IECS in lymphocytes.

ENDOCANNABINOID MODULATION OF IMMUNE FUNCTION

The immune system is complex and highly regulated and has evolved to combat infection and disease. Regulation involves increasing immunity to mount an effective attack against infections as well as halt immunity after the invading microbes have been cleared. If left unregulated, diseases such as autoimmune, chronic inflammatory, and septic shock can occur. Therefore, immune regulation is vital in maintaining homeostasis and involves regulatory substances, such as cytokines, hormones, and now the endocannabinoids, which lead primarily to immunosuppression. Initial studies (Table 1) on immunomodulation by ECs reported suppression by AEA and 2-AG of mitogen-induced lymphocyte proliferation (39,40). Part of the suppression was due to a reduction in IL-2 secretion since both AEA (41) and 2-AG (42) suppressed IL-2 secretion in activated mouse splenocytes. Natural cannabinoids such as THC have also been reported to suppress human and animal lymphocyte functions (11,26).

There is limited evidence so far that the mechanism of suppression by ECs is mediated through cannabinoid receptors. For example, the suppression of IL-2 by AEA was not due to these receptors but due to EC metabolism by COX-2 and the products of this activating PPAR-γ. Similarly, 2-AG suppression of IFNγ by splenocytes was reported to occur through a decrease in NF-AT activity independent of CB_1 and CB_2 action, instead it depends on a mechanism involving the inhibition of intracellular Ca^{2+} release (43). The suppression of IL-12 production was also shown to be CB_1/CB_2 independent. Using various IL-12p40 gene reporter constructs in RAW264.7 macrophages and specific CB_1/CB_2 antagonists, it was demonstrated that AEA reduced IL-12p40 promoter activity through a GA-12 repressor site and this effect was not attenuated by CB_1/CB_2 antagonist treatment. Replacing AEA with Prostamide E2 (Prostaglandin E2 ethanolamide), a metabolite of AEA hydrolysis by COX-2, exerted the same effects on IL-12p40 as AEA (44). In another model system, 2-AG and THC suppressed IL-12p40 production in stimulated bone marrow–derived dendritic cells (BMDC) from mice and although the mechanism of 2-AG suppression was not examined, the THC effect was shown to be partly mediated by CB_1 and CB_2 mechanisms (45). Cannabinoid receptors were also shown to be involved in AEA-induced apoptosis in mouse BMDCs by receptor antagonist studies (46). From these limited studies, it appears that EC immune suppression might involve both cannabinoid

Table 1 Endocannabinoid Modulation of Immune Function

Immune cell	EC	Function	Reference
Lymphocytes	AEA, 2-AG	Decrease proliferation	(39)
Splenocytes	AEA, 2-AG	Decrease IL-2	(41)
	2-AG	IFN-γ and NF-AT activity,	(42)
		Decrease TNF-α	(43)
		Induces migration	(51)
			(53)
RAW 264.7 macrophages	AEA	Decrease IL-12p40	(44)
Dendritic cells	2-AG	Decrease IL-12p40	(45)
		Induces migration	(55)
	AEA	Induces apoptosis	(46)
J774 macrophages	AEA, 2-AG	Decrease IL-6	(49)
PBMC	AEA	Decrease IL-6, TNF-α, IL-4 and IFN-γ	(50)
Microglial cells	AEA, 2-AG	Decrease TNF-α	(52)
B lymphocytes	2-AG	Induces migration	(56)
			(54)
Eosinophils			(57)
Natural Killer cells			(58)
HL-60 macrophage-like	2-AG	Increase IL-8, MCP-1	(60)
		Induces migration	(59)
T lymphocytes	2-AG	Inhibits CXCL-12-induced chemotaxis	(62)
	AEA	Inhibits SDF-1-induced chemotaxis	(63)
Mast cells	2-AG	Reduce histamine release	(67)
		Increase NO and PGE2 release	

receptor and nonreceptor mechanisms. However, this is not surprising because ECs are lipid mediators which are, as a group, reported to be highly reactive; also, it is possible that EC receptors in addition to CB_1 and CB_2 are expressed in immune and other tissues (47,48).

The production of pro-inflammatory cytokines in addition to IL-12 and IFNγ has also been shown to be modulated by ECs. For example, in LPS-stimulated J774 macrophages, AEA and 2-AG suppressed the release of IL-6; however, neither of the ECs had an effect on PGE2 (49). Similarly, AEA was shown to cause a decrease in IL-6 production by LPS-activated human PBMCs and to decrease TNF-α, IL-4, and IFNγ production at higher concentrations (0.3–3 μM) (50). TNF-α was also shown to be suppressed by 2-AG in mouse splenocytes and serum samples (51); furthermore, AEA and 2-AG were shown to inhibit TNF-α production in LPS-activated rat microglial cells (52). From these studies, it is possible that ECs generated during immune cell activation may suppress pro-inflammatory cytokines leading to a dampening of the ongoing immune response. In this regard, it should also be noted that THC and other natural cannabinoids have been shown to suppress cell-mediated, adaptive immunity by suppressing the function of Th1 cells while increasing Th2 activity (11) and that ECs show activity in various anti-inflammatory models (see below).

The effect of ECs on leukocyte migration and chemotaxis has been extensively studied and they have been shown to not only directly stimulate immune cell migration but also to induce cells to produce chemokines that mediate the immune chemotactic response. Numerous reports have demonstrated that 2-AG, but not AEA, induced leukocyte migration via CB_2 receptor in models with mouse splenocytes (53), naïve B lymphocytes (54), and DCs in vitro and in vivo (55). 2-AG was also reported to induce migration in human Raji B cells (56), eosinophilic leukemia Eol-1 cells and peripheral blood eosinophils (57), natural killer cell lines and peripheral blood natural killers cells (58), PBMCs, and macrophage-like HL-60 cells (59). In addition to acting as a chemoattractant, 2-AG was also shown to enhance the production in HL-60 cells, of the chemokines, IL-8 (CXCL8) and MCP-1 (CCL2) (60), through activation of p42/44 MAP kinase cascade (61). Not all immune cells appear to be attracted by ECs. For example, 2-AG was reported to inhibit CXCL12-induced chemotaxis of human, resting and activated, T lymphocytes (62) and AEA was also shown to inhibit CXCL12-induced chemotaxis (63). The migration and influx of cells into a site of infection or injury is a fundamental first step in the inflammatory response. The results to date suggest that ECs produced locally might promote the influx of a variety of immune cells into the area of inflammation and, therefore, drugs that inhibit the EC effect might be of value in suppressing swelling and inflammation. It is also intriguing, but the meaning unclear, that other neuroimmune agents, such as opioids, are chemotactic for immune cells and can even cross-desensitize the function of chemokine receptors (64).

ENDOCANNABINOID EFFECTS IN MODELS OF INFLAMMATION

EC effects on mast cells and several models of skin hypersensitivity have been reported (Table 2). These hypersensitivities result from different mechanisms ranging from TPA-induced inflammation related to the acute production and release of leukotrienes (65), allergic dermal hypersensitivity due to IgE-mediated degranulation of mast cells, and contact hypersensitivity due to T cell activation with cell-mediated immunity. Initial studies in this area were centered on EC effects on mast cell cultures using rat peritoneal mast cells and RBL-2 H3 cells and showed that cannabinoids inhibited degranulation, but AEA antagonized this effect via the CB_2 receptor. AEA alone had no effect on serotonin release (66). In other studies, 2-AG was shown to reduce histamine release by activated guinea pig mast cells as well as increase NO and PGE2 release (67). The anti-inflammatory effects of EC were also studied in in vivo dermal rodent models. Using TPA (12-*O*-tetradecanoylphorbol-13-acetate) as an inflammatory stimulus, which when applied to the ear induces acute swelling, it was observed that the tissue level of 2-AG was increased by TPA application and the application of 2-AG alone to the skin induced ear swelling (68,69). Application of the CB_2 antagonist, SR144528, and not a CB_1 antagonist, blocked TPA- and 2-AG-induced ear swelling as well as the production of leukotriene B_4 and infiltration of neutrophils. Application of THC (68) and WIN55212–2 (69) also reduced ear swelling. What is interesting in these experiments is that 2-AG acted as an agonist whereas THC and WIN55212–2 acted as antagonists, suggesting that they may interfere with leukotriene metabolism. In a model involving passive cutaneous anaphylaxis by sensitizing mice with anti-dinitrophenol

Table 2 Endocannabinoid Effects on Models of Inflammation

Model	ECS component	Effect on inflammation	Reference
TPA-induced inflammation	2-AG	Levels increased in tissue, Induced ear swelling,	(68)
	CB_2 antagonist SR144528	Applied to skin blocks TPA and 2-AG induced ear swelling and increases leukotriene B_4 and neutrophil infiltration	
	CB_1/CB_2 agonist THC, WIN55212–2	Applied to skin reduced TPA and 2-AG induced ear swelling.	(68,69)
Passive cutaneous anaphylaxis; Sensitize; anti-dinitrophenol IgE Challenge; dinitrofluorobenzene	CB_2 KO mice CB_2 antagonist	Failed to elicit ear swelling, Attenuated inflammation	(70)
Contact hypersensitivity; 2,4-dinitrofluorobenzene	CB_1/CB_2 DKO mice	Enhanced dermatitis,	(71)
	AEA	Increase levels in DKO and WT mice. Greater in WT than DKO.	
	2-AG	Increase levels in DKO and WT mice. Greater in DKO than WT.	
	CB_1/CB_2 antagonist SR141716 A/144528	Enhanced hypersensitivity response.	
	CB_1	Decrease mRNA expression in WT	
	CB_2	Increase mRNA expression in WT	
	CB_1/CB_2 agonist TCH	Oral or skin application, reduce ear swelling.	
Septic shock	AEA, 2-AG	Increase levels in patients with sepsis. However, AEA$\geq$2-AG.	(76)
	AEA	PMB hemoperfusion treated patients blood levels decrease, not 2-AG.	(77)
Traumatic brain injury	2-AG	Increase levels in brain following injury. Reduced oedema. Decrease TNF-α	(78)
Multiple sclerosis	AEA	Elevated levels in active brain lesions, peripheral lymphocytes, and CSF (2-AG minimally higher)	(81,82) (81)
	NAPE-PLD	Increase activity in lymphocytes	
	FAAH	Decrease levels and activity in lymphocytes	
Experimental autoimmune encephalomyelitis (EAE)	AEA	Increase levels in striatum	(81)
	NAPE-PLD	Increase activity in striatum	
	FAAH	Decrease activity in striatum	
	CB_2	Higher expression on microglia, mediated by IFN-γ	(83)
	2-AG	Levels unchanged in spinal cord. Decreased in IFN-γ stimulated microglia.	 (84)
	DAGL	IFN-γ lowers mRNA expression	
Organotypic hippocampal slice culture (OHSC).	AEA	Levels increased, not associated with neuroprotection. Decreases number of microglia.	(82,85)
NMDA-induced neuronal damage	2-AG	Addition to cultures provides neuroprotection by decreasing number of damaged neurons. Also decreases number of microglia	(85)

IgE and then challenging with dinitrofluorobenzene (DNFB), CB_2 knockout, when compared to wild-type mice, failed to elicit ear swelling and CB_2 selective antagonists attenuated the inflammatory response (70). Possible mechanisms for this effect could involve attenuation of histamine release by tissue mast cells and suppression of cell migration, but this was not tested. CB_2 receptors mediate histamine release is contrary to the above studies with mast cell cultures showing that cannabinoids inhibit histamine release. Finally, a role for ECs and the IECS in contact hypersensitivity was recently demonstrated. CB_1/CB_2 double knockout (DKO) mice showed enhanced contact dermatitis to sensitization with nickel and DNFB compared to wild-type (71). As evidence of endogenous EC involvement in this effect, tissue levels of 2-AG and AEA were increased along with other mediators of inflammation and, in addition, the injection of CB_1 and CB_2 antagonists enhanced the hypersensitivity response. Of therapeutic interest and in support of the above, the application, either orally or topically, of CB_2 agonists attenuated the contact hypersensitivity response (71). These experiments seem to suggest that the IECS and exogenously administered cannabinoid ligands attenuate cell-mediated, Th1 immunity as previously suggested in other studies involving resistance to infection (72) and tumors (73).

Septic shock, due to severe bacterial sepsis, is an often fatal feature of the systemic inflammatory response syndrome. Recently, AEA has been implicated as a mediator in septic shock. Early findings demonstrated that ECs such as AEA and 2-AG are generated in the blood during LPS-induced hypotension (74). Furthermore, the hypotensive response to either LPS (75) or ECs (74) was shown to be attenuated by the CB_1 antagonist, SR141716 A, but other pharmacological features suggested that the receptor might be a homologue of CB_1. Additional support for a role of ECs in the pathogenesis of septic shock comes from a report showing a 4-old rise in AEA and 2-AG in the blood of patients with this condition (76) and in vitro studies with LPS stimulated RAW264.7 macrophages showing that AEA levels were increased greater than 10-old whereas 2-AG levels were unchanged (29,76). In addition to preclinical studies, a recent clinical study has shown a correlation between EC blood levels and the severity of septic shock. Polymyxin B (PMB) hemoperfusion has been shown to be useful in the management of septic disease and it was hypothesized that the efficacy was related to absorbing ECs from blood rather than absorbing endotoxin. Therefore, EC blood levels were compared in survivor and non-survivor groups of patients treated with PMB hemoperfusion. Although the study was small (24 eptic shock patients), AEA but not 2-AG blood levels were significantly lower in the survivor group and the lower EC levels were also associated with a better clinical score (77). Thus, although the study is small, the results are compelling in terms of defining the mechanism surrounding the therapeutic efficacy of PMB hemoperfusion as well as putative role of ECs in vascular tone and septic shock.

CNS inflammation resulting from trauma or disease is characterized by the loss of neurons and accumulation of microglial cells. Activated microglia cells secrete mediators, such as cytokines and ECs, and these cells can either cause further neuronal degeneration or mediate anti-inflammatory changes. Early studies examined the role of ECs in traumatic brain injury. Acute inflammation in the brain appeared to be associated with a rise in brain 2-AG (78) and to be attenuated by endocannabinoids and the non-psychoactive synthetic cannabinoid, HU-211 (78–80). This would suggest that both cannabinoid receptor and non-receptor mechanisms are involved in the mechanism of action. 2-AG given IV to mice after closed-head injury was observed to cause a significant reduction in brain oedema and better clinical improvement; the effects were CB_1-mediated (78) but the mechanism was not defined. Other mechanisms of neuroprotection following treatment with HU-211 are reported to involve antagonism of the NMDA receptor and suppression of TNF-α release in the brain. The mechanism of the latter effect is not known but may involve the antioxidant effect of HU-211 (80). More recent evidence suggests that the ECS is dysregulated in neuroinflammatory disease and perhaps plays a role in immune control and neuronal protection (12). Because of the immunomodulating effects reported for cannabinoids and the evidence for an IECS, investigators evaluated EC metabolism in multiple sclerosis (MS). In cerebrospinal fluid (CSF) of MS patients, significant amounts of AEA were observed, whereas a 2-AG levels were minimally higher (81). In addition, elevated AEA levels were observed in active brain lesions (82) and peripheral lymphocytes of MS patients and was associated with increased NAPE-PLD activity and decreases in FAAH levels and activity. This suggested that anti-CNS immune cells activated during MS show signs of an activated IECS.

To explore IECS involvement further, a mouse model of experimental autoimmune encephalomyelitis (EAE) was employed that exhibits similar characteristics as MS. Comparable to human CSF, 2-AG levels remained the same in the spinal cord of EAE mice (83). Also, as seen with human lymphocytes, agonist binding to CBR was unaltered in the cortex though reduced in the striatum of EAE mice (81). In areas of the brain with marked cell damaged in EAE animals, AEA was slightly increased and 2-AG minimally suppressed, but were not significant when compared to healthy mice (84). However, in the striatum of EAE mice, AEA was significantly enhanced, which correlates with an increase in NAPE-PLD activity and decrease in FAAH activity with neither enzyme activity changed in the cortex. Microglia also showed evidence of an altered IECS in EAE mice, in that they expressed significantly higher CB_2 mRNA than resting microglia. This upregulation of CB_2R may be mediated by IFNγ and/or GM-CSF since these were shown to upregulated CB_2R expression on microglia (83). In addition, decreases in 2-AG and Ca^{2+} levels were observed in microglia cultures activated with IFNγ in the presence of ATP, in which IFNγ selectively lowers DAGL mRNA expression (84).

Finally, to analyze a role of the IECS and microglia in the context of neuroprotection, animal organotypic hippocampal slice cultures (OHSC) were employed. Excitotoxic neuronal damage in OHSCs is induced by NMDA (*N*-methyl-D-aspartate) that in addition causes accumulation of microglia. In OHSCs treated with NMDA, the levels of AEA were increased; however, this increase in EC was not associated with neuronal protection, since the addition of AEA to either mouse or rat NDMA-OHSCs did not reduce degeneration of neurons. However, AEA did cause a reduction in the number of microglia. In contrast, the addition of 2-AG to rat NMDA-OHSC provided neuronal protection by decreasing both the number of microglia and damaged neurons (82–85). It is clear that elements of the IECS are perturbed during neuroinflammation in ways similar to the perturbation observed in other immune and inflammatory models. However, it is not clear at this time if the IECS is associated with pro- or anti-inflammatory mechanisms.

CONCLUSION

Marijuana cannabinoids and synthetic analogs have been extensively shown to suppress immunity and inflammation and now reports are beginning to suggest that ECs also play a similar suppressive role in immunity. This effect of ECs was predicted based on the understanding that, like with opioids, the mechanism of action of the natural cannabinoids must be mediated through an endogenous system of receptors and ligands. It is also not surprising that ECs modulate immune cell function because it has been recognized for decades that other metabolites of arachidonic acid, namely, the prostaglandins and leukotrienes, are generated during immune activation and have well-recognized paracrine effects. It is clear from the literature that understanding the role of the IECS in normal immune tone and during immune activation is just beginning and many challenges lie ahead in defining this new immune regulatory system of receptors and ligands. A full understanding of the content and function of the IECS will establish the molecular mode of action of cannabinoid-based drugs and yield new opportunities in designing therapeutics for chronic inflammatory diseases and other immune-mediated disorders.

REFERENCES

1. Matsuda LA, et al. Structure of cannabinoid receptor and functional expression of the cloned cDNA. Nature 1990; 346:561–564.
2. Devane WA, et al. Isolation and structure of a brain constituent that binds to the cannabinoid receptor. Science 1992; 258:1946–1949.
3. Munro S, Thomas KL, Abu-Shaar M. Molecular characterization of a peripheral receptor for cannabinoids. Nature 1993; 365:61–65.
4. DiMarzo V, et al. Biosynthesis of anandamide and related acylethanolamides in mouse J774 macrophages and N18 neuroblastoma cells. Biochem J 1996; 316:977–984.
5. Bisogno T, et al. Biosynthesis, uptake, and degradation of anandamide and palmitoylethanolamide in leukocytes. J Biol Chem 1997; 272:3315–3323.
6. Di Marzo V, et al. Biosynthesis and inactivation of the endocannabinoid 2-arachidonoylglycerol in circulating and tumoral macrophages. Eur J Biochem 1999; 264:258–267.
7. Matias I, et al. Presence and regulation of the endocannabinoid system in human dendritic cells. Eur J Biochem 2002; 269(15):3771–3778.

8. Maccarrone M, et al. Lipopolysaccharide downregulates fatty acid amide hydrolase expression and increases anandamide levels in human peripheral lymphocytes. Arch Biochem Biophys 2001; 393(2):321–328.
9. Di Marzo V, et al. The novel endogenous cannabinoid 2-arachidonoylglycerol is inactivated by neuronal- and basophil-like cells: Connections with anandamide. Biochem J 1998; 331(Pt 1):15–19.
10. Sun YX, et al. Involvement of *N*-acylethanolamine hydrolyzing acid amidase in the degradation of anandamide and other *N*-acylethanolamines in macrophages. Biochim Biophys Acta 2005; 1736(3):211–220.
11. Klein TW, Cabral GA. Cannabinoid-induced immune suppression and modulation of antigen-presenting cells. J Neuroimmune Pharmacol 2006; 1(1):50–64.
12. Ullrich O, et al. Immune control by endocannabinoids—New mechanisms of neuroprotection? J Neuroimmunol 2007; 184(1–2):127–135.
13. Klein TW. Cannabinoid-based drugs as anti-inflammatory therapeutics. Nat Rev Immunol 2005; 5:400–411.
14. Parolaro D, et al. Endocannabinoids in the immune system and cancer. Prostaglandins Leukot Essent Fatty Acids 2002; 66(2–3):319–332.
15. Maccarrone M, et al. Endocannabinoid degradation, endotoxic shock and inflammation. Curr Drug Targets Inflamm Allergy 2002; 1(1):53–63.
16. Hillard CJ, Biochemistry and pharmacology of the endocannabinoids arachidonylethanolamide and 2-arachidonylglycerol. Prostaglandins Other Lipid Mediat 2000; 61(1–2):3–18.
17. Piomelli D, et al. The endocannabinoid system as a target for therapeutic drugs. Trends Pharmacol Sci 2000; 21(6):218–224.
18. Devane WA, et al. Isolation and structure of a brain constituent that binds to the cannabinoid receptor. Science 1992; 258(5090):1946–1949.
19. Mechoulam R, et al. Identification of an endogenous 2-monoglyceride, present in canine gut, that binds to cannabinoid receptors. Biochem Pharmacol 1995; 50(1):83–90.
20. Sugiura T, et al. Biosynthesis and degradation of anandamide and 2-arachidonoylglycerol and their possible physiological significance. Prostaglandins Leukot Essent Fatty Acids 2002; 66(2–3):173–192.
21. Di Marzo V, Bifulco M, De Petrocellis L. The endocannabinoid system and its therapeutic exploitation. Nat Rev Drug Discov 2004; 3(9):771–784.
22. Sugiura T, et al. Biosynthesis and degradation of anandamide and 2-arachidonoylglycerol and their possible physiological significance. Prostaglandins Leukot Essent Fatty Acids 2002; 66(2–3):173–192.
23. Sugiura T, et al. 2-Arachidonoylglycerol: A possible endogenous cannabinoid receptor ligand in brain. Biochem Biophys Res Commun 1995; 215(1):89–97.
24. Day TA, et al. Role of fatty acid amide hydrolase in the transport of the endogenous cannabinoid anandamide. Mol Pharmacol 2001; 59(6):1369–1375.
25. Dinh TP, et al. Brain monoglyceride lipase participating in endocannabinoid inactivation. Proc Natl Acad Sci USA 2002; 99(16):10819–10824.
26. Klein TW, Newton CA. Therapeutic potential of cannabinoid-based drugs. Adv Exp Med Biol 2007; 601:395–413.
27. McAllister SD, Glass M. CB(1) and CB(2) receptor-mediated signalling: A focus on endocannabinoids. Prostaglandins Leukot Essent Fatty Acids 2002; 66(2–3):161–171.
28. Pestonjamasp VK, Burstein SH. Anandamide synthesis is induced by arachidonate mobilizing agonists in cells of the immune system. Biochim Biophys Acta 1998; 1394:249–260.
29. Liu J, et al. Lipopolysaccharide induces anandamide synthesis in macrophages via CD14/MAPK/phosphoinositide 3-kinase/NF-kappaB independently of platelet-activating factor. J Biol Chem 2003; 278(45):45034–45039.
30. Carrier EJ, et al. Cultured rat microglial cells synthesize the endocannabinoid 2-arachidonylglycerol, which increases proliferation via a CB2 receptor-dependent mechanism. Mol Pharmacol 2004; 65(4):999–1007.
31. Muccioli GG, et al. Identification of a novel endocannabinoid-hydrolyzing enzyme expressed by microglial cells. J Neurosci 2007; 27(11):2883–2889.
32. Tham CS, et al. Inhibition of microglial fatty acid amide hydrolase modulates LPS stimulated release of inflammatory mediators. FEBS Lett 2007; 581(16):2899–2904.
33. Matias I, et al. Presence and regulation of the endocannabinoid system in human dendritic cells. Eur J Biochem 2002; 269(15):3771–3778.
34. Battista N, et al. Severe deficiency of the fatty acid amide hydrolase (FAAH) activity segregates with the Huntington's disease mutation in peripheral lymphocytes. Neurobiol Dis 2007; 1:108–116.
35. Maccarrone M, et al. Progesterone up-regulates anandamide hydrolase in human lymphocytes: Role of cytokines and implications for fertility. J Immunol 2001; 166(12):7183–7189.
36. Maccarrone M, et al. Progesterone activates fatty acid amide hydrolase (FAAH) promoter in human T lymphocytes through the transcription factor Ikaros. Evidence for a synergistic effect of leptin. J Biol Chem 2003; 278(35):32726–32732.

37. Maccarrone M, et al. Leptin activates the anandamide hydrolase promoter in human T lymphocytes through STAT3. J Biol Chem 2003; 278(15):13318–13324.
38. Maccarrone M, et al. Differential regulation of fatty acid amide hydrolase promoter in human immune cells and neuronal cells by leptin and progesterone. Eur J Biochem 2004; 271(23–24):4666–4676.
39. Schwarz H, Blanco FJ, Lotz M. Anandamide, an endogenous cannabinoid receptor agonist inhibits lymphocyte proliferation and induces apoptosis. J Neuroimmunol 1994; 55:107–115.
40. Lee M, Yang KH, Kaminski NE. Effects of putative cannabinoid receptor ligands, anandamide and 2-arachidonyl-glycerol, on immune function in B6C3F1 mouse splenocytes. J Pharm Exp Ther 1995; 275:529–536.
41. Rockwell CE, Kaminski NE. A cyclooxygenase metabolite of anandamide causes inhibition of interleukin-2 secretion in murine splenocytes. J Pharmacol Exp Ther 2004; 311(2):683–690.
42. Ouyang Y, et al. Suppression of interleukin-2 by the putative endogenous cannabinoid 2-arachidonyl-glycerol is mediated through down-regulation of the nuclear factor of activated T cells. Mol Pharmacol 1998; 53(4):676–683.
43. Kaplan BL, et al. 2-Arachidonoyl-glycerol suppresses interferon-gamma production in phorbol ester/ionomycin-activated mouse splenocytes independent of CB1 or CB2. J Leukoc Biol 2005; 77(6):966–974.
44. Correa F, et al. Anandamide inhibits IL-12p40 production by acting on the promoter repressor element GA-12: Possible involvement of the COX-2 metabolite prostamide E(2). Biochem J 2008; 409(3):761–770.
45. Lu T, et al. Role of cannabinoid receptors in delta-9-tetrahydrocannabinol suppression of IL-12p40 in mouse bone marrow-derived dendritic cells infected with Legionella pneumophila. Eur J Pharmacol 2006; 532(1–2):170–177.
46. Do Y, et al. Activation through cannabinoid receptors 1 and 2 on dendritic cells triggers NF-kappaB-dependent apoptosis: Novel role for endogenous and exogenous cannabinoids in immunoregulation. J Immunol 2004; 173(4):2373–2382.
47. Baker D, et al. In silico patent searching reveals a new cannabinoid receptor. Trends Pharmacol Sci 2006; 27(1):1–4.
48. Begg M, et al. Evidence for novel cannabinoid receptors. Pharmacol Ther 2005; 106(2):133–145.
49. Chang YH, Lee ST, Lin WW. Effects of cannabinoids on LPS-stimulated inflammatory mediator release from macrophages: Involvement of eicosanoids. J Cell Biochem 2001; 81(4):715–723.
50. Berdyshev EV, et al. Influence of fatty acid ethanolamides and D^9-tetrahydrocannabinol on cytokine and arachidonate release by mononuclear cells. Eur. J. Pharmacol 1997; 330:231–240.
51. Gallily R, Breuer A, Mechoulam R. 2-Arachidonylglycerol, an endogenous cannabinoid, inhibits tumor necrosis factor-alpha production in murine macrophages, and in mice. Eur J Pharmacol 2000; 406(1):R5–R7.
52. Facchinetti F, et al. Cannabinoids ablate release of TNFalpha in rat microglial cells stimulated with lypopolysaccharide. Glia 2003; 41(2):161–168.
53. Jorda MA, et al. Hematopoietic cells expressing the peripheral cannabinoid receptor migrate in response to the endocannabinoid 2-arachidonoylglycerol. Blood 2002; 99(8):2786–2793.
54. Tanikawa T, Kurohane K, Imai Y. Induction of preferential chemotaxis of unstimulated B-lymphocytes by 2-arachidonoylglycerol in immunized mice. Microbiol Immunol 2007; 51(10):1013–1019.
55. Maestroni GJ. The endogenous cannabinoid 2-arachidonoyl glycerol as in vivo chemoattractant for dendritic cells and adjuvant for Th1 response to a soluble protein. Faseb J 2004; 18(15):1914–1916.
56. Rayman N, et al. Distinct expression profiles of the peripheral cannabinoid receptor in lymphoid tissues depending on receptor activation status. J Immunol 2004; 172(4):2111–2117.
57. Oka S, et al. 2-Arachidonoylglycerol, an endogenous cannabinoid receptor ligand, induces the migration of EoL-1 human eosinophilic leukemia cells and human peripheral blood eosinophils. J Leukoc Biol 2004; 76(5):1002–1009.
58. Kishimoto S, et al. Endogenous cannabinoid receptor ligand induces the migration of human natural killer cells. J Biochem (Tokyo) 2005; 137(2):217–223.
59. Kishimoto S, et al. 2-Arachidonoylglycerol induces the migration of HL-60 cells differentiated into macrophage-like cells and human peripheral blood monocytes through the cannabinoid CB2 receptor-dependent mechanism. J Biol Chem 2003; 278(27):24469–24475.
60. Kishimoto S, et al. 2-Arachidonoylglycerol, an endogenous cannabinoid receptor ligand, induces accelerated production of chemokines in HL-60 cells. J Biochem (Tokyo) 2004; 135(4):517–524.
61. Kobayashi Y, et al. Activation by 2-arachidonoylglycerol, an endogenous cannabinoid receptor ligand, of p42/44 mitogen-activated protein kinase in HL-60 cells. J Biochem (Tokyo) 2001; 129(5):665–669.
62. Coopman K, et al. Temporal variation in CB(2)R levels following T lymphocyte activation: Evidence that cannabinoids modulate CXCL12-induced chemotaxis. Int Immunopharmacol 2007; 7(3):360–371.
63. Joseph J, et al. Anandamide is an endogenous inhibitor for the migration of tumor cells and T lymphocytes. Cancer Immunol Immunother 2004; 53(8):723–728.
64. Rogers TJ, Peterson PK. Opioid G protein-coupled receptors: Signals at the crossroads of inflammation. Trends Immunol 2003; 24(3):116–121.

65. Yamazaki R, et al. Anti-inflammatory effect of YPE-01, a novel diarylheptanoid derivative, on dermal inflammation in mice. Inflamm Res 1998; 47(4):182–186.
66. Facci L, et al. Mast cells express a peripheral cannabinoid receptor with differential sensitivity to anandamide and palmitoylethanolamide. Proc Natl Acad Sci USA 1995; 92:3376–3380.
67. Vannacci A, et al. The endocannabinoid 2-arachidonylglycerol decreases the immunological activation of Guinea pig mast cells: Involvement of nitric oxide and eicosanoids. J Pharmacol Exp Ther 2004; 311(1):256–264.
68. Oka S, et al. Evidence for the involvement of the cannabinoid CB2 receptor and its endogenous ligand 2-arachidonoylglycerol in 12-*O*-tetradecanoylphorbol-13-acetate–induced acute inflammation in mouse ear. J Biol Chem 2005; 280(18):18488–18497.
69. Oka S, et al. Suppression by WIN55212–2, a cannabinoid receptor agonist, of inflammatory reactions in mouse ear: Interference with the actions of an endogenous ligand, 2-arachidonoylglycerol. Eur J Pharmacol 2006; 538(1–3):154–162.
70. Ueda Y, Miyagawa N, Wakitani K. Involvement of cannabinoid CB2 receptors in the IgE-mediated triphasic cutaneous reaction in mice. Life Sci 2007; 80(5):414–419.
71. Karsak M, et al. Attenuation of allergic contact dermatitis through the endocannabinoid system. Science 2007; 316(5830):1494–1497.
72. Klein TW, et al. D^9-Tetrahydrocannabinol treatment suppresses immunity and early IFNγ, IL-12, and IL-12 receptor b2 responses to Legionella pneumophila infection. J Immunol 2000; 164:6461–6466.
73. Zhu LX, et al. D-9-Tetrahydrocannabinol inhibits antitumor immunity by a CB2 receptor-mediated, cytokine-dependent pathway. J Immunol 2000; 165:373–380.
74. Varga K, et al. Platelet- and macrophage-derived endogenous cannabinoids are involved in endotoxin-induced hypotension. FASEB J 1998; 12(11):1035–1044.
75. Wagner JA, et al. Cardiovascular actions of cannabinoids and their generation during shock. J Mol Med 1998; 76(12):824–836.
76. Wang Y, et al. Simultaneous measurement of anandamide and 2-arachidonoylglycerol by polymyxin B-selective adsorption and subsequent high-performance liquid chromatography analysis: Increase in endogenous cannabinoids in the sera of patients with endotoxic shock. Anal Biochem 2001; 294(1):73–82.
77. Kohro S, et al. Anandamide absorption by direct hemoperfusion with polymixin B-immobilized fiber improves the prognosis and organ failure assessment score in patients with sepsis. J Anesth 2006; 20(1):11–16.
78. Panikashvili D, et al. An endogenous cannabinoid (2-AG) is neuroprotective after brain injury. Nature 2001; 413(6855):527–531.
79. Shohami E, et al. Cytokine production in the brain following closed head injury: Dexanabinol (HU-211) is a novel TNF-alpha inhibitor and an effective neuroprotectant. J Neuroimmunol 1997; 72:169–177.
80. Mechoulam R, Panikashvili D, Shohami E. Cannabinoids and brain injury: Therapeutic implications. Trends Mol Med 2002; 8(2):58–61.
81. Centonze D, et al. The endocannabinoid system is dysregulated in multiple sclerosis and in experimental autoimmune encephalomyelitis. Brain 2007; 130(Pt 10):2543–2553.
82. Eljaschewitsch E, et al. The endocannabinoid anandamide protects neurons during CNS inflammation by induction of MKP-1 in microglial cells. Neuron 2006; 49(1):67–79.
83. Maresz K, et al. Modulation of the cannabinoid CB2 receptor in microglial cells in response to inflammatory stimuli. J Neurochem 2005; 95(2):437–445.
84. Witting A, et al. Experimental autoimmune encephalomyelitis disrupts endocannabinoid-mediated neuroprotection. Proc Natl Acad Sci U S A 2006; 103(16):6362–6367.
85. Kreutz S, et al. Cannabinoids and neuronal damage: Differential effects of THC, AEA and 2-AG on activated microglial cells and degenerating neurons in excitotoxically lesioned rat organotypic hippocampal slice cultures. Exp Neurol 2007; 203(1):246–257.

23 The Endocannabinoid System in the Liver

Ariane Mallat and Sophie Lotersztajn

INSERM U 841, Université Paris XII-Val de Marne, AP-HP, Groupe hospitalier Henri Mondor-Albert Chenevier, Service d'Hépatologie et de Gastroentérologie, Creteil, France

THE ENDOCANNABINOID SYSTEM

Despite a longstanding history of recreational and therapeutic use of phytocannabinoids derived from *Cannabis sativa*, characterization of the endogenous cannabinoid system emerged only two decades ago with the identification of an endocannabinoid system comprising at least two specific G protein–coupled receptors (CB_1 and CB_2), their endogenous ligands [endocannabinoids, among which anandamide (AEA) and 2-arachidonoyl glycerol (2-AG) are currently the best characterized] and a machinery dedicated to endocannabinoid synthesis and degradation (1,2). The subsequent development of subtype-selective receptor agonists and antagonists (3), and the availabililty of mice invalidated for CB_1 or CB_2 receptors (CB_1 and CB_2 KO) rapidly paved the way to characterization of varied and ubiquitous properties of cannabinoid receptors (4–6). However, functions of the cannabinoid system in liver pathophysiology came into focus very recently, probably given the low-expression level of CB_1 and CB_2 receptors in normal liver.

THE ENDOCANNABINOID SYSTEM AS A KEY PLAYER IN LIVER FIBROGENESIS

Chronic liver injury is associated to liver fibrogenesis, ultimately leading to cirrhosis (7). The latter is a prominent cause of morbidity and mortality worldwide with about 800,000 death/yr, owing to complications of portal hypertension and liver failure, and to a high incidence of hepatocellular carcinoma. In Western countries, prevailing causes of cirrhosis include prolonged alcohol abuse, chronic hepatitis C , and, increasingly, nonalcoholic fatty liver disease (7). Liver fibrogenesis is driven by an heterogenous population of nonparenchymal cells expressing smooth muscle α-actin that originate from hepatic stellate cells and hepatic myofibroblasts. In response to chronic liver injury, both cell types proliferate and accumulate in injured areas, synthetize fibrogenic cytokines, growth factors, chemokines, fibrosis components, and inhibitors of matrix degradation (7). The frequent inability to eradicate the cause of chronic liver disease warrants the development of liver-specific antifibrotic strategies. However, despite encouraging experimental results, proof of efficacy of potential antifibrogenic molecules in a clinical setting is currently lacking.

We recently showed that CB_1 and CB_2 receptors are marginally expressed in the normal liver and upregulated in the cirrhotic human liver, predominating in hepatic myofibroblasts (8,9), an observation that was subsequently confirmed by others (10,11). These findings led us to investigate the impact of the cannabinoid system during liver fibrogenesis.

Antifibrogenic Role of the CB_2 Receptor

The function of CB_2 receptors was investigated in an established liver fibrosis model induced by chronic carbon tetrachloride intoxication. CB_2 KO mice developed significantly enhanced liver fibrosis compared to wild-type mice, following increase in the density of hepatic myofibroblasts (8). Molecular mechanisms were further investigated in cultures of liver fibrogenic cells. Activation of CB_2 receptors in hepatic myofibroblasts and activated hepatic stellate cells triggered both growth inhibition and apoptosis, by a mechanism involving growth inhibition and oxidative stress, respectively (8). This study, therefore, demonstrated that endogenous activation of CB_2 receptors limits progression of experimental liver fibrosis by reducing liver fibrogenic cell accumulation (8).

CB_1 Receptors Enhance Liver Fibrogenesis

The impact of CB_1 receptors was assessed in three distinct models of fibrosis, carbon tetrachloride or thioacetamide intoxication, and bile duct ligation. Concurrent administration of the CB_1 antagonist rimonabant was associated to a reduction in liver fibrosis (9). Rimonabant-treated mice displayed reduced hepatic expression of the profibrogenic cytokine TGF-ß1, and a decrease in the density of hepatic myofibroblasts, following inhibition of their proliferation. As expected, CB_1 KO mice also showed reduced fibrosis and lesser accumulation of fibrogenic cells in the three models, compared to wild-type counterparts (9). Our results were recently confirmed in an independent study of mice submitted to bile duct ligation and treated with another CB_1 antagonist, AM251 (12). Altogether, these results demonstrate that CB_1 receptors enhance liver fibrogenesis, and that a CB_1 receptor antagonist may prove useful in the prevention of fibrosis progression during chronic liver injury.

Impact of Cannabis Use on Fibrosis Progression in Patients with Chronic Hepatitis C

In order to investigate the relevance of experimental findings in a human setting, we examined the impact of cannabis use on progression of liver fibrosis in a cohort of 270 consecutive patients with chronic hepatitis C of known duration (13). Patients were classified according to cannabis smoking habits over the span of HCV infection as nonsmokers, occasional (<1 joint weekly) or daily users (at least 1 joint daily during the course of the disease). Logistic regression analysis indicated that daily cannabis use was a significant independent factor predicting the severity of liver fibrosis. These results therefore support our experimental findings demonstrating profibrogenic properties of CB_1 receptors.

In summary, CB_1 and CB_2 receptors play a central opposite role during chronic liver injury that associates antifibrogenic properties of CB_2 receptors and profibrogenic effects of CB_1 receptors. These findings identify CB_1 and CB_2 receptors as potential novel target for antifibrogenic therapy during chronic liver diseases, and suggest that combined therapy with selective CB_1 antagonists and/or CB_2 agonists might open a new therapeutic avenue for the treatment of liver fibrosis.

ENDOCANNABINOIDS AND FATTY LIVER DISEASES

Chronic alcohol abuse and the metabolic syndrome (6,000,000 subjects worldwide for each condition) are the two major causes of chronic liver diseases, alcoholic liver disease (ALD), and nonalcoholic fatty liver disease (NAFLD). ALD and NAFLD share common pathophysiological mechanisms. In both cases, pathological features range from simple steatosis (as defined by isolated accumulation of triglycerides in greater than 5% of hepatocytes), a condition generally associated to a benign outcome, to steatohepatitis, a stage associated to inflammation and activation of fibrogenic pathways. In contrast to simple steatosis, steatohepatitis carries a 20% risk of cirrhosis after 10 to 20 years; in addition, the severe form of alcoholic steatohepatitis (severe alcoholic hepatitis) is associated to a spontaneous 60% mortality rate, owing to the complications of liver failure. The role of cannabinoid in energy balance has been the focus of numerous recent studies. Indeed, it has been demonstrated that endogenous activation of CB_1 receptors promotes obesity following hypothalamic stimulation of food intake, activation of lipogenesis in adipocytes, and reduction of energy expenditure in peripheral organs. In addition, two recent studies indicate that the endocannabinoid tone is enhanced in the liver of obese mice, as shown by the increased level of hepatic AEA and the upregulation of CB_1 receptors in perivenous hepatocytes (14). Strikingly, CB_1 antagonism prevented development of steatosis, both in obese *fa/fa* rats treated with the CB_1 antagonist rimonabant (15) and in CB_1 KO mice fed a high-fat diet (14). Direct induction of hepatocyte lipogenesis was also demonstrated. Indeed, activation of upregulated CB_1 was associated to an induction of the transcription factor SREBP-1c and of its target lipogenic genes, ACC-1 and fatty acid synthase. In addition, rimonabant decreased hepatic TNF-αlevels, suggesting that CB_1 receptors may also contribute to the inflammatory phase of steatohepatitis (15). Interestingly, upregulation of the endocannabinoid system and steatogenic properties of CB_1 receptors have also recently been reported in an experimental model of ALD induced by chronic intoxication with alcohol (16). In this study, mice with liver-targeted deletion of the CB_1 gene did not develop steatosis following chronic exposure to alcohol, further demonstrating that steatosis is the consequence of a direct activation of hepatic CB_1 receptors (16). Taken together, these findings indicate that CB_1 antagonists may offer a novel therapeutic strategy for ALD and NAFLD. Whether CB_2 may also participate to the pathogenesis of fatty liver diseases remains to be investigated but strikingly, upregulation of CB_2 receptors has been reported in NAFLD (17).

ENDOCANNABINOIDS AND LIVER ISCHEMIA REPERFUSION INJURY

Ischemia/reperfusion (I/R) injury is a severe complication of several conditions, associating hypoxic organ damage followed by return of blood flow and oxygen delivery to the compromised tissue. Transient episodes of hepatic ischemia occur during organ transplantation, trauma, hypovolemic shock, and selective liver resection, following inflow occlusion or total vascular exclusion. The pathophysiology of liver I/R injury associates ischemia-induced cellular injury, followed by prolonged dysfunction resulting from activation of liver inflammatory pathways.

Recent data have shown that endogenous activation of CB_2 receptors reduces liver injury induced by I/R (18). Indeed, the reperfusion phase was associated with an activation of the endocannabinoid system in the liver, associating an induction of CB_2 receptors and an increased synthesis of AEA and 2-AG. Administration of the selective CB_2 agonist JWH-133 prior to vascular occlusion protected against hepatic I/R injury, by a mechanism involving decreased inflammatory cell infiltration, reduced expression of proinflammatory cytokines, chemokines and adhesion molecules, and decreased lipid peroxydation. Consistent with these data, CB_2 KO mice or animals treated with the CB_2 antagonist SR 144528 displayed enhanced liver injury and inflammation following I/R, compared to control mice (18). Altogether, these data represent a novel demonstration of the anti-finflammatory properties of CB_2 receptors and suggest that CB_2 agonists may offer novel perspectives in the prevention of hepatic I/R injury.

ENDOCANNABINOIDS AND PORTAL HYPERTENSION IN CIRRHOSIS

Portal hypertension primarily occurs in patients with cirrhosis and is characterized by increased portal blood flow and intra-hepatic resistance. This syndrome is responsible for a high rate of morbidity and mortality, owing to severe complications. Increased intra-hepatic resistance is related to architectural distorsion and vasoconstriction of portal venules and sinusoidal capillaries. Enhanced portal blood flow develops as a consequence of overproduction of vasodilatory molecules in the splanchnic bed, responsible for arterial hypertension and reactional enhanced splanchnic inflow. Administration of rimonabant to rats with experimental cirrhosis reversed the increase in mesenteric blood flow and portal pressure (19). These results suggested that cirrhosis is associated to enhanced production of vasodilatory endocannabinoïds. In keeping with this hypothesis, anandamide levels were increased in monocytes and blood from cirrhotic rats and cirrhotic patients, compared to healthy controls (19,20). Moreover, infusion of monocytes from cirrhotic patients or cirrhotic rats to control animals elicited a significant reduction mean arterial blood pressure (21).

Finally, CB_1 receptors were upregulated in endothelial cells isolated from human mesenteric arteries, and AEA elicited a selective vasodilation of mesenteric arterioles in cirrhosis, without affecting vasomotricity of peripheral arteries (22). Overall, these results indicate that an enhanced AEA/CB_1-dependent tone participates to the pathogenesis of portal hypertension via vasodilation of mesenteric arterioles.

OTHER ASPECTS OF ENDOCANNABINOID BIOLOGY DURING LIVER DISEASES

Cirrhotic Cardiomyopathy

Cirrhotic cardiomyopathy is characterized by impaired responsiveness to pharmacological stimulation or stress. A role of endocannabinoids in cirrhotic cardiomyopathy has been suggested, based on the increase in cardiac AEA and CB_1 levels in cirrhotic rats and the finding that the CB_1 receptor antagonist AM251 reverses cirrhotic cardiomyopathy (23,24).

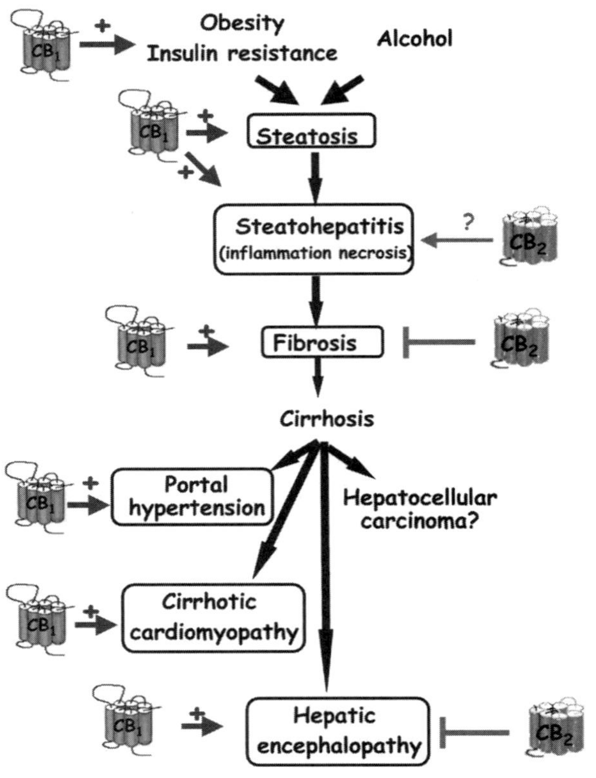

Figure 1 CB receptors as novel targets for the treatment of liver diseases

Hepatic Encephalopathy

Pathogenesis of hepatic encephalopathy, a major complication of acute and chronic liver failure, remains partially understood. Multiple pathways have been incriminated including altered production of neurotransmitters, astrocyte dysfunction, and abnormalities in cerebral perfusion. Recent studies showed that brain levels of CB_2 receptors and of its ligand 2-AG are increased in the model of fulminant liver failure induced by thioacetamide (25,26). In this model, neurological dysfunction was improved by the nonselective CB_1/CB_2 agonist Δ^9-THC (26), the CB_2 agonists HU308 and 2-AG, as well as by the CB_1 antagonist rimonabant (25). The neuroprotective effect of Δ^9-THC occurred despite a similar degree of liver failure, and disappeared in CB_2 KO mice, suggesting that neuroprotection results from a direct effect of THC on brain CB_2 receptors (26). These results identify the endocannabinoid system as a novel protective pathway during hepatic encephalopathy. However, further studies are awaited to fully clarify the respective contribution of CB_1 and CB_2 receptors in this process.

CB-Receptor Independent Effects of Endocannabinoids

CB-receptor independent effects of endocannabinoïds are increasingly described in the liver as in other tissues. Thus, AEA and 2-AG induce apoptosis of fibrogenic cells by CB_1 and CB_2-independent pathways (8,27). Other CB-independent effects of endocannabinoids in the liver include AEA-induced hepatocyte injury in vivo and in cell cultures (27,28), and opposing effects of AEA and 2-AG on cholangiocarcima cell growth (29).

In conclusion, endocannabinoids are increasingly incriminated in a variety of liver diseases and their complications (Fig. 1). Understanding the specific roles of CB_1 and CB_2 receptors opens a potential novel therapeutic approaches for the treatment of nonalcoholic fatty liver diseases, liver fibrosis, ischemia reperfusion, and portal hypertension. The CB_1 agonist rimonabant has recently been approved in Europe for the treatment of overweight and cardiovascular risks and other CB_1 antagonists are already under trial. Additional evaluation of CB_1 antagonists for the treatment of NAFLD or liver-associated fibrosis appears warranted. CB_2 selective modulators are still awaited for clinical development.

ACKNOWLEDGMENTS

This work was supported by the INSERM, the Université Paris-Val-de-Marne, and by grants (to S. L.) of the Agence Nationale de la Recherche, the Fondation de la Recherche Médicale and Sanofi-Aventis.

REFERENCES

1. Mallat A, Lotersztajn S. Endocannabinoids as novel mediators of liver diseases. Endocrinological Investigation 2006; 29(3 Suppl.):58–65.
2. Mallat A, Teixeira-Clerc F, Deveaux V, et al. Cannabinoid receptors as new targets of antifibrosing strategies during chronic liver diseases. Expert Opin Ther Targets 2007; 11(3):403–409.
3. Pertwee RG. Pharmacology of cannabinoid receptor ligands. Curr Med Chem 1999; 6(8):635–664.
4. Ledent C, Valverde O, Cossu G, et al. Unresponsiveness to cannabinoids and reduced addictive effects of opiates in CB1 receptor knockout mice. Science 1999; 283(5400):401–404.
5. Zimmer A, Zimmer AM, Hohmann AG, et al. Increased mortality, hypoactivity, and hypoalgesia in cannabinoid CB1 receptor knockout mice. Proc Natl Acad Sci U S A 1999; 96(10):5780–5785.
6. Buckley NE, McCoy KL, Mezey E, et al. Immunomodulation by cannabinoids is absent in mice deficient for the cannabinoid CB(2) receptor. Eur J Pharmacol 2000; 396(2–3):141–149.
7. Lotersztajn S, Julien B, Teixeira-Clerc F, et al. Hepatic fibrosis: Molecular mechanisms and drug targets. Ann Rev Pharmacol Toxicol 2005; 45:605–628.
8. Julien B, Grenard P, Teixeira-Clerc F, et al. Antifibrogenic role of the cannabinoid receptor CB2 in the liver. Gastroenterology 2005; 128(3):742–755.
9. Teixeira-Clerc F, Julien B, Grenard P, et al. CB1 cannabinoid receptor antagonism: A novel strategy for the treatment of liver fibrosis. Nat Med 2006; 12(6):671–676.
10. Xu X, Liu Y, Huang S, et al. Overexpression of cannabinoid receptors CB1 and CB2 correlates with improved prognosis of patients with hepatocellular carcinoma. Cancer Genet Cytogenet 2006; 171(1):31–38.
11. Biecker E, Sagesser H, Reichen J. Vasodilator mRNA levels are increased in the livers of portal hypertensive NO-synthase 3-deficient mice. Eur J Clin Invest 2004; 34(4):283–289.
12. Yang YY, Lin HC, Huang YT, et al. Effect of chronic CB1 cannabinoid receptor antagonism on livers of rats with biliary cirrhosis. Clin Sci (Lond) 2007; 112(10):533–542.
13. Hezode C, Roudot-Thoraval F, Nguyen S, et al. Daily cannabis smoking as a risk factor for fibrosis progression in chronic hepatitis C. Hepatology 2005; 42(1):63–71.
14. Osei-Hyiaman D, Depetrillo M, Pacher P, et al. Endocannabinoid activation at hepatic CB(1) receptors stimulates fatty acid synthesis and contributes to diet-induced obesity. J Clin Invest 2005; 115(5):1298–1305.
15. Gary-Bobo M, Elachouri G, Gallas JF, et al. Rimonabant reduces obesity-associated hepatic steatosis and features of metabolic syndrome in obese Zucker fa/fa rats. Hepatology 2007; 46(1):122–129.
16. Jeong WI, Osei-Hyiaman D, Park O, et al. Paracrine activation of hepatic CB1 receptors by stellate cell-derived endocannabinoids mediates alcoholic fatty liver. Cell Metab. 2008; 7:227–235.
17. Mendez-Sanchez N, Zamora-Valdes D, Pichardo-Bahena R, et al. Endocannabinoid receptor CB2 in nonalcoholic fatty liver disease. Liver Int 2007; 27(2):215–219.
18. Batkai S, Osei-Hyiaman D, Pan H, et al. Cannabinoid-2 receptor mediates protection against hepatic ischemia/reperfusion injury. FASEB J 2007; 21(8):1788–1800.
19. Batkai S, Jarai Z, Wagner JA, et al. Endocannabinoids acting at vascular CB1 receptors mediate the vasodilated state in advanced liver cirrhosis. Nat Med 2001; 7(7):827–832.
20. Fernandez-Rodriguez CM, Romero J, Petros TJ, et al. Circulating endogenous cannabinoid anandamide and portal, systemic and renal hemodynamics in cirrhosis. Liver Int 2004; 24(5):477–483.
21. Ros J, Claria J, To-Figueras J, et al. Endogenous cannabinoids: A new system involved in the homeostasis of arterial pressure in experimental cirrhosis in the rat. Gastroenterology 2002; 122(1):85–93.
22. Domenicali M, Ros J, Fernandez-Varo G, et al. Increased anandamide induced relaxation in mesenteric arteries of cirrhotic rats: Role of cannabinoid and vanilloid receptors. Gut 2005; 54(4):522–527.
23. Gaskari SA, Liu H, Moezi L, et al. Role of endocannabinoids in the pathogenesis of cirrhotic cardiomyopathy in bile duct-ligated rats. Br J Pharmacol 2005; 146(3):315–323.
24. Batkai S, Mukhopadhyay P, Harvey-White J, et al. Endocannabinoids acting at CB1 receptors mediate the cardiac contractile dysfunction in vivo in cirrhotic rats. Am J Physiol Heart Circ Physiol 2007; 293:H2210–2218.
25. Avraham Y, Israeli E, Gabbay E, et al. Endocannabinoids affect neurological and cognitive function in thioacetamide-induced hepatic encephalopathy in mice. Neurobiol Dis 2005; 12:12.

26. Dagon Y, Avraham Y, Ilan Y, et al. Cannabinoids ameliorate cerebral dysfunction following liver failure via AMP-activated protein kinase. FASEB J 2007; 21:2431–2341.
27. Siegmund SV, Uchinami H, Osawa Y, et al. Anandamide induces necrosis in primary hepatic stellate cells. Hepatology 2005; 41(5):1085–1095.
28. Biswas KK, Sarker KP, Abeyama K, et al. Membrane cholesterol but not putative receptors mediates anandamide-induced hepatocyte apoptosis. Hepatology 2003; 38(5):1167–1177.
29. DeMorrow S, Glaser S, Francis H, et al. Opposing actions of endocannabinoids on cholangiocarcinoma growth: recruitment of Fas and Fas ligand to lipid rafts. J Biol Chem 2007; 282(17):13098–13113.

24 The Endocannabinoid System and Cardiovascular Disease

Pál Pacher

Section on Oxidative Stress Tissue Injury, Laboratory of Physiological Studies, NIAAA, National Institutes of Health, Bethesda, Maryland, U.S.A.

George Kunos

Section on Neuroendocrinology, Laboratory of Physiological Studies, NIAAA, National Institutes of Health, Bethesda, Maryland, U.S.A.

KEY POINTS

- Endocannabinoids (ECs) are endogenous lipid substances which elicit biological effects similar to those of marijuana via activation of G protein–coupled cannabinoid receptors (CB_1 and CB_2, as well as additional, as yet unidentified receptors). The two best characterized ECs are arachidonoyl ethanolamide (anandamide) and 2-arachidonoylglycerol (2-AG).
- Both CB_1 and CB_2 receptors are expressed in the myocardium and the vasculature, and their respective cardiovascular functions are summarized in Fig. 1.
- ECs and their synthetic analogs exert potent hypotension via CB_1 receptor–mediated sympathoinhibitory, negative inotropic, and vasodilatory effects.
- Activation of endothelial CB_2 receptors by endogenous or exogenous ligands limits endothelial inflammatory response, chemotaxis and adhesion of inflammatory cells to the activated endothelium, and consequent release of various proinflammatory mediators (key processes involved in the initiation and progression of reperfusion injury and atherosclerosis). CB_2 receptor activation on immune cells mediates additional anti-inflammatory properties. Selective CB_2 agonists may be useful in the treatment of various forms of reperfusion injury (e.g., myocardial infarction, cardiac transplantation, vascular surgeries and stroke, etc.).
- Activation of the EC system has been implicated in hypotension and/or decreased myocardial contractility associated with hemorrhagic, endotoxic, septic, cardiogenic shock, advanced liver cirrhosis, heart failure secondary to doxorubicin treatment, and as a compensatory mechanism in various forms of hypertension.
- Activation of the EC system contributes to the cardiovascular risk associated with obesity/metabolic syndrome and diabetes (abdominal obesity, plasma lipid alterations, insulin and leptin resistance).

ENDOCANNABINOIDS AND THEIR RECEPTORS

Endocannabinoids are generated by virtually all cell types both in the brain and peripheral tissues and exert a broad range of biological effects similar to those of cannabis (1,2). Anandamide (AEA) and 2-AG are the two most widely studied endocannabinoids that are thought to be autocrine or paracrine mediators acting in close proximity to their site of release. They act on G protein–coupled cannabinoid (CB) receptors, two of which have been identified by cloning: CB_1 and the CB_2 receptors (2). The CB_1 receptor is not only abundantly expressed in the brain, but is also present at lower levels in peripheral tissues including the myocardium, vascular smooth muscle, and endothelium, as well as the liver and adipose tissue (2). The CB_2 receptor is expressed primarily in immune and hematopoietic cells, but has also been identified in various other tissues/cells including the myocardium (3) and coronary endothelial cells (4). Additional cannabinoid receptors may exist based on pharmacological data, but have not yet been identified (5). This chapter provides a brief overview of the emerging role of the EC system in cardiovascular disorders and discusses its therapeutic exploitation. Because of space limitations, recent reviews rather then original studies are cited when possible.

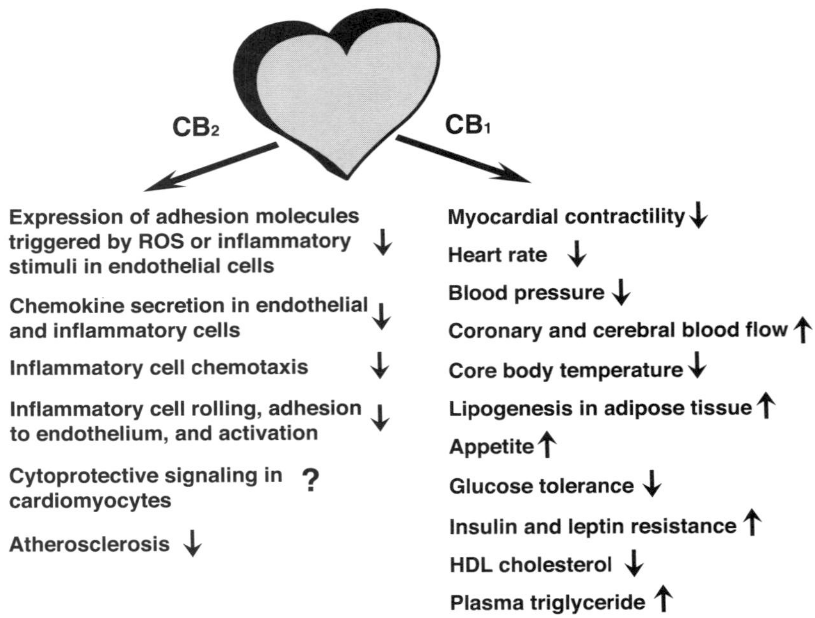

Figure 1 Effects of CB_1 and CB_2 receptor activation relevant to cardiovascular disease.

CARDIOVASCULAR EFFECTS

In addition to their well-known neurobehavioral and immunological actions, cannabinoids exert important cardiovascular effects. In anesthetized rodents, AEA and Δ^9-tetrahydrocannabinol (THC) cause hypotension, bradycardia, and depressed cardiac contractility, which are less pronounced or absent in conscious normotensive animals but are amplified in hypertension (6–8). In humans, chronic use of marijuana may lead to hypotension and bradycardia, while acute exposure generally causes isolated tachycardia. The underlying mechanisms of these in vivo cardiovascular actions are complex and may comprise effects on the vasculature, myocardium, and modulation of autonomic outflow at presynaptic autonomic nerve terminals as well as in the central nervous systems. In the case of ECs, these effects are further complicated by their rapid metabolism, which liberates arachidonic acid that can be further metabolized into vasoactive prostanoids (6,7). CB_1 receptors are present in the myocardium where they decrease contractility. In anesthetized rodents, synthetic cannabinoids and anandamide decrease cardiac contractility and cardiac output via CB_1 receptors, and these effects are potentiated in various forms of hypertension (9). Although the presence of CB_2 receptors has been reported in the myocardium and cardiomyocytes (4,10), their role is elusive. CB_1 receptors appear to be more important than CB_2 receptors in cardiovascular regulation, the latter so far being implicated only in ischemic preconditioning, ischemia-reperfusion (I/R) injury, and atherosclerosis (2,10). ECs and synthetic cannabinoids also elicit vasodilation in vitro in a tissue- and species-dependent manner, which may involve CB_1- and $TRPV_1$-receptor and NO-mediated or NO-independent mechanisms, and also as yet undefined endothelial site(s) of action (5–8). In the cerebral and coronary vasculature, CB_1 receptors and CB_1-mediated vasodilation have been documented (7).

ROLE OF THE ENDOCANNABINOID SYSTEM IN CARDIOVASCULAR DISEASE

The EC system has been implicated in the pathophysiological alterations associated with various forms of circulatory shock (hemorrhagic, endotoxic/septic, and cardiogenic), cirrhotic cardiomyopathy, myocardial infarction, stroke, atherosclerosis, and heart failure (2,5–8).

Myocardial Ischemia Reperfusion and Preconditioning

Overproduction of ECs has been documented in various forms of I/R injury, such as myocardial infarction or whole-body I/R associated with hemorrhagic shock, and it may contribute to the cardiovascular depression associated with these pathologies (2). On the other hand, ECs have been found to protect against myocardial I/R injury and to contribute to the ischemic preconditioning effect of heat stress, endotoxin, or brief periods of ischemia (2,10). Recent studies using selective CB_2 receptor agonists and/or CB_2 receptor knockout mice have provided compelling evidence that CB_2 receptor activation is protective against myocardial, cerebral, and hepatic I/R injuries by decreasing the endothelial cell activation/inflammatory response (expression of adhesion molecules, secretion of chemokines, etc.), and by attenuating leukocyte chemotaxis, rolling and adhesion to endothelium, activation and transendothelial migration, and interrelated oxidative/nitrosative damage (4,11–13). All this indicates that ECs protect against myocardial I/R injury predominantly via CB_2 receptors located both on endothelial and inflammatory cells, and perhaps also on cardiomyocytes, and that targeting CB_2 receptors on coronary artery endothelial cells may also attenuate TNFα- and/or endotoxin-induced vascular inflammatory responses.

Stroke

The first evidence for the neuroprotective effect of cannabinoids came from the stroke research field from studies using synthetic cannabinoids in various in vivo models of cerebral ischemia. These initial studies have suggested the existence of CB_1 receptor–dependent protective mechanisms against cerebral I/R injury in rodents (2). However, several follow-up reports have demonstrated protection afforded by CB_1 receptor antagonists, which does not support the neuroprotective role of endocannabinoids and CB_1 receptor activation (2). Interestingly, CB_2 agonists were found to protect against stroke-induced brain damage by attenuating the transient I/R-induced increase in leukocyte infiltration, rolling and adhesion to vascular endothelial cells, and consequent neuronal activation (13), consistent with results obtained using myocardial (11) and hepatic I/R injury models (12).

Atherosclerosis and Restenosis

Orally administered THC has been shown to inhibit atherosclerosis progression in a mouse model through CB_2 receptor mechanisms and CB_2 receptor-expressing immune cells are present both in human and mouse atherosclerotic plaques (14). In addition, THC treatment of mice reduced the proliferative capacity and interferon-γ production of lymphoid cells, and inhibited macrophage chemotaxis in vitro in a CB_2-dependent manner (14). Proinflammatory cytokines such as TNF-α and bacterial endotoxin(s), which are pro-atherogenic via NF-κB activation in endothelial cells with consequent induction of adhesion molecules and chemokines and the release of factors that promote smooth muscle cell migration and proliferation, play pivotal roles in vascular inflammation associated with atherosclerosis. In human coronary artery endothelial cells, which express CB_1 and CB_2 receptors, TNF-α induced NF-κB and RhoA activation, upregulated ICAM-1 and VCAM-1, increased the expression of monocyte chemoattractant protein, enhanced transendothelial migration of monocytes, and augmented monocyte–endothelial adhesion, and all these responses were markedly attenuated by selective CB_2 agonists. The endotoxin-induced ICAM-1 and VCAM-1 expression in isolated aortas, and the adhesion of monocytes to aortic vascular endothelium were also decreased by CB_2 agonists (4). Thus, targeting CB_2 receptors on endothelial cells may offer a novel approach in the treatment of atherosclerosis and restenosis, which often complicates vascular surgery.

Circulatory Shock and Hypertension

The profound hypotensive response to CB_1 receptor activation suggested a role for ECs in hypotensive states. Indeed, activation of the EC system has been implicated in the hypotension and decreased myocardial contractility associated with hemorrhagic, endotoxic, septic and cardiogenic shock, shock associated with necrotizing pancreatitis (2), as well as advanced liver cirrhosis (15,16) and in doxorubicin-induced heart failure (3). Pathologically overproduced ECs may mediate these effects, and they may be derived from activated macrophages and platelets (2) as well as various parenchymal cells such as cardiomyocytes (3), endothelial cells (12), and hepatocytes (16). Accordingly, treatment with CB_1 antagonists was found to prevent or reverse the hypotension and/or decreased cardiac contractility associated with these conditions.

Numerous early reports demonstrated that chronic use of cannabis in humans, as well as both acute and prolonged administration of THC to experimental animals, can elicit long-lasting decreases in blood pressure and heart rate, which pointed to the potential utility of cannabinoids to treat hypertension, provided that their neurobehavioral and cardiovascular effects could be separated (7). The antihypertensive potential of cannabinoids was further suggested by their greater hypotensive efficacy in hypertensive compared to normotenisve animals (7–9). More recent studies demonstrated that the EC system is tonically activated in various experimental models of hypertension as a homeostatic, hypotensive mechanism. Unexpectedly, this "tone" was found to be due, primarily, to a CB_1 receptor–mediated decrease in cardiac contractility and cardiac output, rather than a decrease vascular resistance (9). Accordingly, pharmacological inhibition of fatty acid amidohydrolase (FAAH), which increases tissue levels of anandamide, was found to reduce blood pressure and cardiac contractility in hypertensive but not in normotensive animals (9). As inhibition of FAAH does not elicit behavioral effects suggestive of addictive properties (17), these findings suggest that the modulation of the EC system in hypertension may be therapeutically exploited.

Metabolic Syndrome

The endocannabinoid system is emerging as a key player in obesity and related metabolic and cardiovascular disorders. In rodent models of obesity, chronic treatment with the CB_1 antagonist rimonabant only transiently reduced food intake, while the associated reduction in body weight was maintained throughout the treatment, indicating direct effects on peripheral fat metabolism (2). Indeed, CB_1 receptors are present on adipocytes and hepatocytes, and their activation can lead to increased lipogenesis in adipose tissue (18) and in the liver (19), whereas CB_1 blockade has the opposite effect, and can also reverse the steatosis associated with obesity (20). CB_1 blockade also improves glucose tolerance and insulin sensitivity in diet-induced or genetically obese animals (21), although the underlying mechanisms are not yet clear.

Recent clinical trials with rimonabant involving obese individuals with the metabolic syndrome, and also with type 2 diabetes, have documented the beneficial effects of chronic CB_1 blockade not only on body weight and waist circumference, but also on plasma triglyceride, HDL-cholesterol levels, and glucose tolerance. In addition, rimonabant decreased markers of inflammation, plasma leptin, and insulin levels, while increasing plasma adiponectin (22–25). A modest reduction of blood pressure was also observed in one study (22). Interestingly, some of these beneficial metabolic effects were weight-loss–independent, confirming the importance of effects mediated through the peripheral EC system. These findings indicate that pharmacological inhibition of CB_1 receptors may represent a promising therapeutic strategy not only to treat obesity/metabolic syndrome, but also to decrease the associated cardiometabolic risk.

CONCLUSIONS

Collectively, the evidence reviewed above suggests that modulation of endocannabinoid system holds enormous therapeutic potential to combat cardiovascular disorders.

REFERENCES

1. Di Marzo V, Bifulco M, De Petrocellis L. The endocannabinoid system and its therapeutic exploitation. Nat Rev Drug Discov 2004; 3:771–784.
2. Pacher P, Batkai S, Kunos G. The endocannabinoid system as an emerging target of pharmacotherapy. Pharmacol Rev 2006; 58:389–462.
3. Mukhopadhyay P, Batkai S, Rajesh M, et al. Pharmacological inhibition of cannabinoid-1 receptor protects against doxorubicin-induced cardiotoxicity. J Am Coll Cardiol 2007; 50:528–536.
4. Rajesh M, Mukhopadhyay P, Batkai S, et al. Cannabinoid-2 receptor stimulation attenuates TNFα-induced human endothelial cell activation, transendothelial migration of monocytes, and monocyte-endothelial adhesion. Am J Physiol Heart Circ Physiol 2007; 293:H2210–H2218.
5. Begg M, Pacher P, Batkai S, et al. Evidence for novel cannabinoid receptors. Pharmacol & Ther 2005; 106:133–145.
6. Randall MD, Harris D, Kendall DA, et al. Cardiovascular effects of cannabinoids. Pharmacol & Ther 2002; 95:191–202.

7. Pacher P, Batkai S, Kunos G. Cardiovascular pharmacology of cannabinoids. Handb Exp Pharmacol 2005; 168:599–625.
8. Mendizabal VE, Adler-Graschinsky E. Cannabinoids as therapeutic agents in cardiovascular disease: A tale of passions and illusions. Br J Pharmacol 2007; 151:427–440.
9. Batkai S, Pacher P, Osei-Hyiaman D, et al. Endocannabinoids acting at cannabinoid-1 receptors regulate cardiovascular function in hypertension. Circulation 2004; 110:1996–2002.
10. Lepicier P, Bibeau-Poirier A, Lagneux C, et al. Signaling pathways involved in the cardioprotective effects of cannabinoids. J Pharmacol Sci 2006; 102:155–166.
11. Di Filippo C, Rossi F, Rossi S, et al. Cannabinoid CB2 receptor activation reduces mouse myocardial ischemia-reperfusion injury: Involvement of cytokine/chemokines and PMN. J Leukocyte Biol 2004; 75:453–459.
12. Batkai S, Osei-Hyiaman D, Pan H, et al. Cannabinoid-2 receptor mediates protection against hepatic ischemia/reperfusion injury. FASEB J 2007; 21:1788–1800.
13. Zhang M, Martin BR, Adler MW, et al. Cannabinoid CB(2) receptor activation decreases cerebral infarction in a mouse focal ischemia/reperfusion model. J Cereb Blood Flow Metab 2007; 27:1387–1396.
14. Steffens S, Veillard NR, Arnaud C, et al. Low dose oral cannabinoid therapy reduces progression of atherosclerosis in mice. Nature 2005; 434:782–786.
15. Lee RF, Glenn TK, Lee SS. Cardiac dysfunction in cirrhosis. Best Pract Clin Gastroenterol 2007; 21:125–140.
16. Batkai S, Mukhopadhyay P, Harvey-White J, et al. Endocannabinoids acting at CB1 receptors mediate the cardiac contractile dysfunction in vivo in cirrhotic rats. Am J Physiol Heart Circ Physiol, June 8, 2007 [Epub ahead of print]
17. Khaturia S, Gaetani S, Fegley D, et al. Modulation of anxiety through blockade of anandamide hydrolysis. Nat Med 2003; 9:76–81.
18. Cota D, Marsicano G, Tschop M, et al. The endogenous cannabinoid system affects energy balance via central orexigenic drive and peripheral lipogenesis. J Clin Invest 2003; 112:423–431.
19. Osei-Hyiaman D, DePetrillo M, Pacher P, et al. Endocannabinoid activation at hepatic CB1 receptors stimulates fatty acid synthesis and contributes to diet-induced obesity. J Clin Invest 2005; 115:1298–1305.
20. Gary-Bobo M, Elachouri G, Gallas JF, et al. Rimonabant reduces obesity-associated hepatic steatosis and features of metabolic syndrome in obese Zucker fa/fa rats. Hepatology 2007; 46:122
21. Poirier B, Bidouard JP, Cadrouvele C, et al. The anti-obesity effect of rimonabant is associated with an improved serum lipid profile. Diab Obes Metab 2005; 7:65–72.
22. Despres JP, Golay A, Sjostrom L. Effects of rimonabant on metabolic risk factors in overweight patients with dyslipidemia. N Engl J Med 2005; 353:2121–2134.
23. Pi-Sunyer FX, Aronne LJ, Heshmati HM, et al. Effect of rimonabant, a cannabinoid-1 receptor blocker, on weight and cardiometabolic risk factors in overweight or obese patients: RIO-North America: A randomized controlled trial. JAMA 2006; 295:761–775.
24. Scheen AJ, Finer N, Hollander P, et al. Efficacy and tolerability of rimonabant in overweight or obese patients with type 2 diabetes: A randomised controlled study. Lancet 2006; 368:1660–1672.
25. Van Gaal LF, Rissanen AM, Scheen AJ, et al. Effects of the cannabinoid-1 receptor blocker rimonabant on weight reduction and cardiovascular risk factors in overweight patients: 1-Year experience from the RIO-Europe study. Lancet 2005; 365:1389–1397.

25 The Endocannabinoid System, Energy Expenditure, and Thermogenesis

Luigi Bellocchio, Cristina Cervino, Valentina Vicennati, Renato Pasquali, and Uberto Pagotto
Endocrinology Unit and Center of Applied Biomedical Research (CRBA), Department of Internal Medicine and Gastroenterology, S. Orsola-Malpighi Hospital, University of Bologna, Bologna, Italy

The endocannabinoid system has emerged as an important modulator of neuronal functions, as demonstrated by the abundance of CB_1 receptor in the brain (1). One of the key functions attributed to the endocannabinoid system in the brain is the control of food intake resulting in a significant orexigenic stimulus. However, more recently, the finding of a peripheral presence of CB_1 receptor in many organs, involved in the regulation of metabolism, has changed the past identification of the endocannabinoid system as a particular neuronal orexigenic promoter, and its role in the regulation of energy balance has started to be completely re-evaluated (2–3).

Only since 2003, it has become evident that the role of the endocannabinoid system in energy expenditure is not only limited to the action at the central nervous system (4). However, the first indirect indication that cannabinoids may affect energy homeostasis, through mechanisms beyond food intake control, came many years ago from a study conducted in marijuana smokers (5). In this study, the marijuana-induced stimulation in caloric intake vanished after a few days, whereas weight gain continued throughout the rest of the observation period, suggesting the presence of an independent effect on peripheral metabolism (5). A similar conclusion, many years later, was reached in rodents, when rimonabant, the first CB_1 antagonist, was tested. In this study, a development of a tolerance to the anorectic effect of rimonabant was noticed after a few days of treatment in rats, whereas the reduction in body weight was maintained throughout the treatment period (6). At that time, the authors were not able to explain the loss in body weight, which was partially independent of food intake reduction; however, they correctly hypothesized a stimulatory action of rimonabant on energy expenditure (6). Later, these intuitions were substantiated by using a rodent model of genetic ablation of CB_1 receptor. The lack of CB_1 receptor in mutant mice was, in fact, shown to cause hypophagia and body-fat reduction (4). However, pair-feeding experiments showed that in young $CB_1^{-/-}$ mice, the lean phenotype was predominantly caused by decreased caloric intake; here metabolic factors appear to be the major cause of the lean phenotype of the adult $CB_1^{-/-}$ mice. On the other hand, energy expenditure evaluated by indirect calorimetry did not show any significant change between the two groups of animals examined (4). Greater differences in terms of body weight regulation were obtained in the same genetically modified animal models when a high-fat diet was administered (7). Although $CB_1^{-/-}$ mice did not show a reduction of energy intake in comparison to the wild type littermates, the genetically transformed animals were resistant to diet-induced obesity (7).

The vast experimental use of CB_1 receptor antagonist has corroborated the hypothesis that a blockade of a peripheral CB_1 receptor may play a relevant role in the final weight loss effect. In fact, prolonged treatment with rimonabant (3 and 10 mg/kg, respectively) was shown to produce only a short-lasting hypophagic effect in DIO mice, followed by the development of tolerance to the anorectic effect of the drug. However, the reduction in body weight and in adipose tissue was continuously observed throughout the period of observation (5 weeks) (8). The data on a development of rapid tolerance to the anorectic action, despite a prolonged effect on body fat loss, was confirmed in other models of obesity (Zucker rats) (9), with longer periods of treatment (10) and even with other CB_1 antagonists such as AM-251 (11). All these experiments in animals were convergent in hypothesizing that an increase in energy expenditure may be a complementary route by which blockade of the endocannabinoid system may affect energy metabolism.

In 2005, searching for nonappetite-related pathways involved in CB_1 receptor antagonist mediating body weight loss, Dernbach et al. noted that on top of the well-known effect on food intake, rimonabant administered for 10 days to DIO rats was able to induce an increase in energy expenditure, while in the pair-feeding group, the lowered food intake led to an expected decrease in the same parameter. The low respiratory quotient observed in the rimonabant-treated group of animals allowed the authors to speculate that a shift to an increase in fat oxidation could have represented one of the possible mechanisms of action of the pharmacological blockade of CB_1 receptor (12). Similar data were obtained by Liu et al. who found that a 7-day treatment with rimonabant induced an increase in basal oxygen consumption as compared to the vehicle in Lep^{ob}/Lep^{ob} mice (13). However, the authors were not able to identify the mechanism by which rimonabant treatment affected energy expenditure. Taking advantage of micro-array analysis and treating DIO mice for a long period with rimonabant, Jbilo et al. were able to screen the changes of a wide panel of genes in adipocytes after treatment (14). They found that the transcriptional patterns of treated obese mice were similar to those obtained in the $CB_1^{-/-}$ mice fed with a high-fat diet, supporting a CB_1 receptor-mediated process. Functional analysis of these gene modulations indicated that the reduction in adipose mass by the drug was due to increased energy expenditure, mainly through futile cycling (calcium and substrate) (14). Other studies by in vivo microdialysis have documented that CB_1 antagonist treatment in rodents may increase noradrenaline outflow in rat anterior hypothalamus, suggesting a possible central stimulation of efferent sympathetic activity (15).

In the same experimental setting mentioned above, Jbilo et al. also demonstrated several expression changes in genes favoring energy dissipation through mitochondrial heat production in brown adipose tissue (14). Several reports have documented a direct role of the endocannabinoid system in modulation of proteins involved in thermogenesis. Shearman et al. was the first to show that a 9-day treatment of DIO mice with the CB_1 receptor antagonist AM251 increases Uncoupling Protein (UCP)-1 and UCP-3 mRNA expression level in brown adipose tissue, suggesting that CB_1 receptor blockade may contribute to increased thermogenesis (16). It has also recently been shown that treatment of differentiated brown adipocytes with a CB_1/CB_2 agonist such as WIN 55212-3 decreased the expression of UCP-1 (17). Brown adipose tissue–mediated thermogenesis importantly contributes to energy expenditure in small animals like rodents. The role of brown adipose tissue is less clear in humans. However, even in humans, it has been speculated that several physiological and pharmacological stimuli may be capable of trans-differentiating white adipocytes into brown ones (18). One can therefore speculate that CB_1 receptor antagonist may increase brown adipocytes, determining an increase in energy expenditure as a final effect. In the same study mentioned above, among the number of genes affected by rimonabant treatment, Jbilo et al. also detected the gene coding for β3-adrenergic receptor, a well-known player in thermogenesis (14). On the other hand, our unpublished data seem to attribute an important stimulation on mithocondriogenesis to the CB_1 receptor blockade, which may represent a further action toward an increase in energy expenditure.

In their study, Jbilo et al. also found that rimonabant gives rise to an increase in gene pattern expression of enzymes of the β-oxidation and tricarbolyxilic acid cycle (14). After the initial description of the presence of CB_1 receptor in rodent mature adipocytes (4,19), a large number of studies have shown that the CB_1 receptor is also present in human mature adipocytes (20–22). The importance of the finding of the CB_1 receptor in the adipocytes is further highlighted by the evidence of the presence of the full biochemical machinery to synthesize and degrade endocannabinoids (20–25). CB_1 receptor blockade has also been demonstrated by several groups to increase adiponectin in white adipose tissue and 3T3-F44 A adipocyte cells (14,17,19,23), although this finding was not reproduced by others (22), whereas WIN55212, a CB_1/CB_2 agonist has been shown to reduce adiponectin mRNA expression (14,17). These data are convergent in showing that cannabinoid modulation by CB_1 antagonist on the endocrine secretive pattern of the adipocytes is compatible with the induction of a negative energy balance. In fact, adiponectin circulating levels have been found to be decreased in visceral obese patients; this protein displays insulin-sensitizing properties and is known to be antiatherosclerotic (26). Moreover, cannabinoids seem to inhibit the AMP-activated protein kinase (AMPK) (27); this inhibition, in addition to an increase in LPL activity (4), leads to an increased lipogenesis and a reduction in fatty acid β-oxidation, probably involving acetyl-CoA carboxilase-1 (ACC-1), the rate-limiting enzyme of fatty acid biosynthesis.

CB_1 receptor has also been recently identified in the rodent liver using a combination of RT-PCR, in situ hybridization, immunoistochemistry, and Western blot (28). In the same study, hepatic CB_1 receptor activation was found to increase de novo lipogenesis as well as the expression of the transcription factor sterol regulatory element binding protein-1 c (SHERBP-1c) and its targets ACC-1 and fatty acid sythase (28). The role of CB_1 receptor in cannabinoid-induced lipogenesis was indicated by the ability of rimonabant to block the increased incorporation of ^3H_2O, induced by HU-210, another CB_1 agonist. Interestingly, this effect was not observed in mice pretreated with rimonabant and in CB_1 knockout mice (28). The hepatic lipogenic pathway may also be directly activated through a cannabinoid-dependent decrease in AMPK phosphorylation and activity, which also occurs in the liver (26).

Finally, a recent study demonstrated CB_1 receptor expression in the soleus muscle, and this expression is increased in obese mice as compared to lean controls (4). In cultured myotubes derived from lean and obese subjects, it was recently shown that anandamide is able to decrease mRNA expression of several enzymes involved in muscle oxidative pathways, such as AMPK-α1 and 2, pyruvate dehydrogenase kinase 4 (PDK-4) and peroxisome proliferator–activated receptor-γ co-activator-1 (PGC-1). Interestingly, these effects could be reversed by CB_1 antagonist treatment, indicating a crucial negative role of the endocannabinoid system on fatty acid and glucose oxidation in skeletal muscle (29). In this scenario, an elegant study showed that, in genetically obese mice, treatment with rimonabant is able to stimulate glucose uptake in soleus muscle (13), and this increase may also explain the improvement in the hyperglycemia observed in DIO mice after pharmacological CB_1 receptor blocking in other experimental settings (10).

Collectively, all these studies seem to point to a role of AMPK as a putative intracellular modulator of endocannabinoid signaling. This kinase acts as a fuel sensor to regulate energy balance at both cellular and whole body levels. The first targets of AMPK to be identified were the acetyl-CoA carboxylase and HMG-CoA reductase, and it was demonstrated that activation of AMPK caused consequent inhibition of fatty acid and cholesterol synthesis in hepatocytes (30). AMPK activation also inhibits muscle glycogen synthesis via phosphorylation of glycogen synthase, and de novo glucose synthesis (gluconeogenesis) in the liver (30). Besides conserving ATP by inhibiting biosynthetic pathways, AMPK activation stimulates catabolic pathways that generate ATP. In skeletal muscle, it stimulates glucose uptake, both via translocation of the glucose transporter GLUT4 to the plasma membrane and, in the longer term, by increasing its expression (31). In other cells, AMPK activation increases the intrinsic activity of the glucose transporter GLUT1 by an unknown mechanism (32). By phosphorylation of the ACC-2 ($-\beta$) isoform of acetyl-CoA carboxylase, AMPK lowers malonyl-CoA, relieving inhibition of uptake of fatty acids into mitochondria via the carnitine carrier system, and thus stimulating fatty acid oxidation (33). In addition to these acute effects on glucose and fatty acid oxidation, AMPK also upregulates mitochondrial biogenesis (34), thus increasing the capacity of tissues for aerobic production of ATP. In this scenario, we can hypothesize, supporting by some recent work, that in AMPK activity, the endocannabinoid system may have an important mediator of its functions. In fact, CB_1 receptor activation by endocannabinoids has been shown to increase AMPK activity in hypothalamus, resulting in a net increase in food intake (26). On the other hand, endocannabinoids are able to decrease AMPK activity in liver, in adipose tissue, and in skeletal muscle (26), resulting in an increase of adiposity and lipogenesis, and an impaired fatty acid and glucose oxidation.

WHAT IS KNOWN IN HUMANS

In the four studies in which overweight and obese subjects completed the 12 or 24 months of treatment with the CB_1 antagonist rimonabant, there was a significant reduction in body weight when compared to placebo (35–38). These studies also showed that the weight loss was accompanied by a decrease in plasma triglycerides, an increase in HDL cholesterol and adiponectin, and an improvement in insulin sensitivity measured by HOMA-IR. When adjusted for weight loss, 50% of the improvements in triglycerides, HDL cholesterol, adiponectin, and insulin sensitivity were not attributable to weight loss (35–38). This suggests that rimonabant has direct effects on fat metabolism. On the other hand, these data have been derived by statistical analysis and no direct evidence has been provided to validate these indirect findings. However, a recent clinical trial in which a new CB_1 antagonist, taranabant, was tested in humans provided new data concerning the effect of CB_1 blockade on energy expenditure. A single-dose administration of 12-mg taranabant caused a small but significant increase in resting energy expenditure and fat oxidation (39). The authors concluded that the modest increases in energy expenditure may exert profound effects on body weight over a period of months. On the other hand, in the same study, Addy et al. were not able to define what proportion of taranabant's effects on resting energy expenditure were mediated centrally via activation of the autonomic nervous system or peripherally by engagement of CB_1 receptor distributed in peripheral organs involved in metabolic functions (39).

A further phase IV clinical trial is supposed to provide solid answers to this kind of question. The ongoing study will investigate the direct effects of rimonabant (i.e., independent of weight loss) in two randomized groups. One group will receive rimonabant for 12 weeks and the other group will have dietary intervention to match the weight loss in the rimonabant group. Energy expenditure (using indirect calorimetry and Actiheart monitors), fatty acid and triglyceride metabolism (using stable isotope techniques), and body fat distribution (by magnetic resonance imaging) will be measured before and after the intervention (40). To determine the possible mechanisms of the changes in metabolism, gene expression of key regulators of fatty acid metabolism in adipose and muscle tissue and circulating levels of adipokines will be measured (40).

CONCLUSIONS

Preclinical studies in rodents have shown that CB_1 receptor is involved in food intake in various brain regions, including hypothalamus, and peripherally in several metabolic functions involving adipose tissue, skeletal muscle, endocrine pancreas, and liver. The net effect of CB_1 activation on metabolism is anabolic. In fact, the activation of CB_1 receptor inhibits adiponectin release and lipolysis in adipose tissue, increases lipogenic gene expression and de novo fatty acid synthesis in liver, and decreases the oxidative pathways in skeletal muscle. On the other hand, the pharmacologic blockade or genetic deletion of CB_1 receptor increases insulin sensitivity, ameliorates serum lipid profile and, more importantly, increases energy expenditure in peripheral tissues, such as liver, adipose tissue, and skeletal muscle, by removing the cannabinoid-dependent inhibition of AMPK activity (Fig.1). Extrapolating from animal studies to the clinic, the reduction of endocannabinoid system activity with the new class of drugs like the CB_1 receptor antagonists

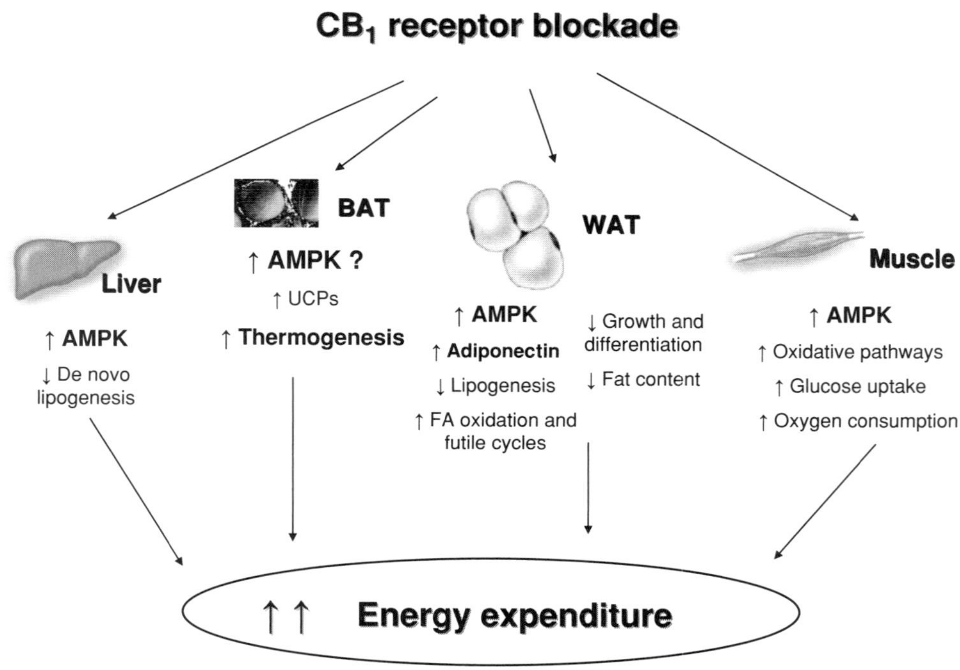

Figure 1 Effects of CB_1 receptor blockade on energy expenditure by acting on peripheral tissues involved in energy metabolism. *Abbreviations*: BAT, brown adipose tissue; WAT, white adipose tissue; AMPK, AMP-activated protein kinase; UCPs, uncoupling proteins; FA, fatty acids.

offers a promising treatment, not only for reduction of body weight and abdominal adiposity but also for increasing energy expenditure and ameliorating metabolic profile.

REFERENCES

1. Herkenham M, Lynn AB, Little MD, et al. Cannabinoid receptor localization in brain. Proc Natl Acad Sci USA 1990; 87:1932–1936.
2. Pagotto U, Marsicano G, Cota D, et al. The emerging role of endocannabinoid system in endocrine regulation and energy balance. Endocrine Rev 2006; 27:73–100.
3. Matias I, Di Marzo V. Endocannabinoids and the control of energy balance. Trends Endocrinol Metab 2007; 18:27–37.
4. Cota D, Marsicano G, Tschoep M, et al. The endogenous cannabinoid system affects energy balance via central orexigenic drive and peripheral lipogenesis. J Clin Invest 2003; 112:423–431.
5. Greenberg I, Kuenlue J, Mendelson JH, et al. Effects of marijuana use on body weight and energy intake in humans. Psycopharmacology (Berlin) 1976; 49:79–84.
6. Colombo G, Agabio R, Diaz G, et al. Appetite suppression and weight loss after the cannabinoid antagonist SR 141716. Life Sci 1998; 63:L113–L117.
7. Ravinet-Trillou C, Delgorge C, Menet C, et al. CB1 cannabinoid receptor knockout in mice leads to leanness, resistance to diet-induced obesity and enhanced leptin sensitivity. Int J Obes Relat Metab Disord 2004; 28:640–648.
8. Ravinet-Trillou C, Arnone M, Delgorge C, et al. Anti-obesity effect of SR141716, a CB1 receptor antagonist, in diet-induced obese mice. Am J Physiol Regul Integr Comp Physiol 2003; 284:R345–R353.
9. Bensaid M, Gary-Bobo M, Esclangon A, et al. The cannabinoid CB1 receptor antagonist SR141716 increases Acrp30 mRNA expression in adipose tissue of obese fa/fa rats and in cultured adipocyte cells. Mol Pharmacol 2003; 63:908–914.
10. Poirier B, Bidouard JP, Cadrouvele C, et al. The anti-obesity effect of rimonabant is associated with an improved serum lipid profile. Diabetes Obes Metab 2005; 7:65–72.
11. Hildebrandt AL, Kelly-Sullivan DM, Black SC. Antiobesity effects of chronic cannabinoid CB1 receptor antagonist treatment in diet-induced obese mice. Eur J Pharmacol 2003; 462:125–132.
12. Dernbach H, Haller J, Kaulisch T, et al. Effects of the CB1 antagonist SR141716 A (Rimonabant) on energy expenditure and respiratory quotient in diet-induced obese rats. Obesity Rev 2005; 6(s1): 172.
13. Liu YL, Connoley IP, Wilson CA, et al. Effects of the cannabinoid CB1 receptor antagonist SR141716 on oxygen consumption and soleus muscle glucose uptake in Lep(ob)/Lep(ob) mice. Int J Obes Relat Metab Disord 2005; 29:183–187.
14. Jbilo O, Ravinet-Trillou C, Arnone M, et al. The CB1 receptor antagonist rimonabant reverse the diet-induced obesity phenotype through regulation of lipolysis and energy balance. FASEB J 2005; 19:1567–1569.
15. Tzavara ET, Perry KW, Rodriguez DE, et al. The cannabinoid CB1 receptor antagonist SR141716 A increases norepinephrine outflow in the rat anterior hypothalamus. Eur J Pharmacol 2001; 426:R3–R4.
16. Shearman LP, Zhou D, Rosko KM, et al. Multiple day CB1R inverse agonist effects on hypothalamic gene expression and energy balance in diet-induced obese mice. Soc Neuroscience San Diego 2003, abstract p 76.4.
17. Perwitz N, Fasshauer M, Klein J. Cannabinoid receptor signalling directly inhibits thermogenesis and alters expression of adiponectin and visfatin. Hom Metab Res 2006; 38:356–358.
18. Klaus C. Adipose tissue as a regulator of energy balance. Curr Drug Targets 2004; 5:241–250.
19. Bensaid M, Gary-Bobo M, Esclangon A, et al. The cannabinoid CB1 receptor antagonist SR141716 increases Acrp30 mRNA expression in adipose tissue of obese *fa/fa* rats and in cultured adipocyte cells. Mol Pharmacol 2003; 63:908–914.
20. Engeli S, Bohnke J, Feldpausch M, et al. Activation of the peripheral endocannabinoid system in human obesity. Diabetes 2005; 54:2838–2843.
21. Roche R, Hoareau L, Bes-Houtmann S, et al. Presence of the cannabinoid receptors, CB1 and CB2, in human omental and subcutaneous adipocytes. Histochem Cell Biol 2007; 4:1–11.
22. Pagano C, Pilon C, Calcagno A, et al. The endogenous cannabinoid system stimulates glucose uptake in human fat cells via phosphatidylinositol 3-kinase and calcium-dependent mechanisms. J Clin Endocrinol Metab 2007; 92:4810–4819.
23. Matias I, Gonthier MP, Orlando P, et al. Regulation, function and dysregulation of endocannabinoids in models of adipose and β-pancreatic cells and in obesity and hyperglicemia. J Clin Endocrin Metab 2006; 91:3171–3180.
24. Gasperi V, Fezza F, Pasquariello N, et al. Endocannabinoids in adipocytes during differentiation and their role in glucose uptake. Cell Mol Life Sci 2007; 64:219–229.

25. Spoto B, Fezza F, Parlogo G, et al. Human adipose tissue binds and metabolizes the endocannabinoids anandamide and 2-arachidonoylglycerol. Biochimie 2006; 88:1889–1897.
26. Kola B, Hubina E, Tucci SA, et al. Cannabinoids and ghrelin have both central and peripheral metabolic and cardiac effects via AMP-activated protein kinase. J Biol Chem 2005; 280:25196–25201.
27. Guerre-Millo M. Adiponectin: An update. Diabetes Metab 2007; 7 December 2007 [Epub ahead of print].
28. Osei-Hyiaman D, DePetrillo M, Pacher P, et al. Endocannabinoids activation at hepatic CB1 receptors stimulates fatty acid synthesis and contributes to diet induced obesity. J Clin Invest 2005; 115:1298–1305.
29. Cavuoto P, McAincha AJ, Hatzinikolas G, et al. Effects of cannabinoid receptors on skeletal muscle oxidative pathways. Mol Cell Endocrin 2007; 267:63–69.
30. Hardie DG, Hawley SA, Scott JW. AMP-activated protein kinase—Development of the energy sensor concept. J Physiol 2006; 574:7–15.
31. Holmes BF, Kurth-Kraczek EJ, Winder WW. Chronic activation of 5′-AMP-activated protein kinase increases GLUT-4, hexokinase, and glycogen in muscle. J Appl Physiol 1999; 87:1990–1995.
32. Barnes K, Ingram JC, Porras OH, et al. Activation of GLUT1 by metabolic and osmotic stress: Potential involvement of AMP-activated protein kinase (AMPK). J Cell Sci 2002; 115:2433–2442.
33. Merrill GM, Kurth E, Hardie DG, et al. AICAR decreases malonyl-CoA and increases fatty acid oxidation in skeletal muscle of the rat. Am J Physiol 1997; 273:E1107–E1112.
34. Winder WW, Holmes BF, Rubink DS, et al. Activation of AMP-activated protein kinase increases mitochondrial enzymes in skeletal muscle. J Appl Physiol 2000; 88:2219–2226.
35. Van Gaal LF, Rissanen AM, Scheen AJ, et al. Effects of the cannabinoid CB1 receptor blocker rimonabant on weight reduction and cardiovascular risk factor in overweight patients: 1 year experience from the RIO-Europe Study. Lancet 2005; 365:1389–1397.
36. Despres JP, Golay A, Sjostrom L, et al. for the RIO-Lipids Study Group. Effects of rimonabant on metabolic risk factors in overweight patients with dyslipidemia. N Engl J Med 2005; 353:2121–2134.
37. Pi-Sunyer FX, Aronne LJ, Heshamati HM, et al. Effects of rimonabant, a cannabinoid-1 receptor blocker. On weight and cardiometabolic risk factors in overweight or obese patients. JAMA 2006; 295:761–775.
38. Scheen AJ, Finer N, Hollander P, et al. Efficacy and tolerability of rimonabant in overweight or obese patients with type 2 diabetes: A randomised controlled study. Lancet 2006; 368:1660–1672.
39. Addy C, Wright H, Van Laere K, et al. The acyclic CB1 r inverse agonist taranabant mediates weight loss by increasing energy expenditure and decreasing caloric intake. Cell Metab 2008;7:68–78.
40. http://clinicaltrialsfeeds.org/clinical-trials/show/NCT00584389 Study ID Number: EC/2006/117/PGMS ClinicalTrials.gov.

26 Effects of Dietary Fatty Acids on Endocannabinoid Signaling in the Brain and Peripheral Organs

Alvin Berger

Metabolon, Inc., Durham, North Carolina, U.S.A.
Department of Nutrition, University of North Carolina, Chapel Hill, North Carolina, U.S.A.

Vincenzo Di Marzo

Endocannabinoid Research Group, Institute of Biomolecular Chemistry, National Research Council, Pozzuoli, Naples, Italy

INTRODUCTION

Two of the most studied long-chain polyunsaturated fatty acids (LC-PUFA) are arachidonic acid (AA) and docosahexaenoic acid (DHA). Both are components of breast milk; whereas the latter is also a component of nervous tissue membranes (1). These fatty acids (particularly AA) have been largely studied for their conversion to classical eicosanoids (prostaglandins, leukotrienes, HETES, lipoxins, resolvins, etc.) and subsequent signaling. As first shown by Berger et al. (2), it is now clear that dietary fatty acids are also precursors to endocannabinoids (eCBs), which bind cannabinoid CB_1 and CB_2 receptors (CB1R and CB2R) (3). It is also noteworthy that the diet is also a minor source of preformed eCBs, as previously reviewed (4–7) (Fig. 1). In this chapter, we review the available data suggesting that the diet, and in particular its fatty acid composition, might influence endocannabinoid levels and, subsequently, affect function in the brain and peripheral organs.

EFFECT OF DIETARY FATTY ACIDS ON BRAIN ENDOCANNABINOID SIGNALING

Effects on Endocannabinoid Levels

In newborn piglets, AA- and DHA feeding in milk formulas, respectively, increased levels of the corresponding NAEs *N*-arachidonoylethanolamine (anandamide, 20:4n6 NAE) and *N*-docosahexaenoyl-ethanolamine (22:6n3 NAE) in specific brain regions (2). Both NAEs are known to bind CB1R, though 22:6n3 NAE is with low affinity (2). In mice, feeding with an AA-rich diet from postnatal day 1 to day 58 similarly increased anandamide in whole brain (2,8), and this was accompanied by changes in corresponding fatty acids in individual phospholipids, and changes to gene expression profile in liver and hippocampus, using lipidomic and microarray approaches, respectively (9–10).

Similar to these observations in mice, increasing dietary DHA did not consistently increase 22:6n3 NAE levels in brain, but did increase the ratio of 22:6n3 NAE/20:4n6 NAE in brain and plasma (11). These authors also reported that fish oil feeding increased 20:5n3 and 22:6n3 2-monoacylglycerols and 22:6n3 NAE in plasma (11). Thus, following dietary fatty acid manipulations, the plasma pool of eCBs and plasma eCB ratios may be predictive of changes occurring in the brain.

In another set of experiments, Watanabe and colleagues (12) fed mice with an n-3 PUFA–deficient diet, which resulted in higher brain 2-AG levels. In a second experiment, these authors found that short-term supplementation of DHA-rich fish oil reduced brain 2-AG level as compared with supplementation with low n-3 PUFA. Concomitantly, a decrease in AA levels and an increase in DHA levels in the major phospholipids occurred in the brains of the mice fed the fish oil diet compared with those fed the low n-3 PUFA diet. These results indicate that n-3 PUFA deficiency elevates, while n-3 PUFA enrichment reduces brain 2-AG levels in mice, suggesting that "physiological and pathological events mediated by 2-AG through cannabinoid

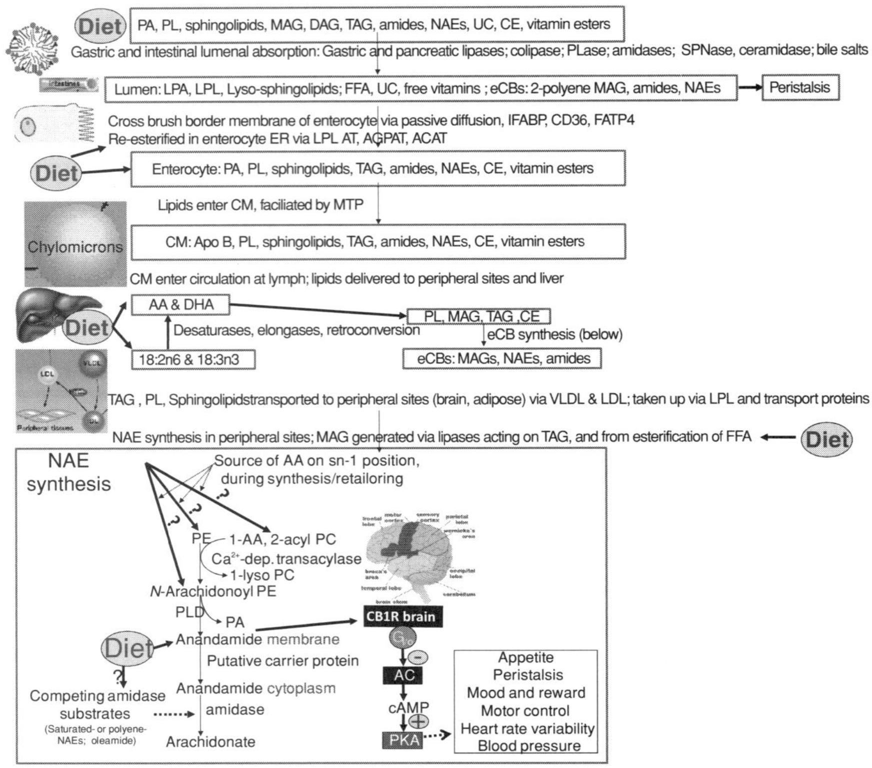

Figure 1 Dietary fatty acid modulation of eCB levels. Diet is a rich source of triacylglycerols (TAG) and to a lesser extent, diacylglycerols (DAG) and monoacylglycerols (MAG), as well as minor amounts of primary amides and NAEs. Following gastric/pancreatic lipases, digestion in stomach and intestinal lumen produces MAGs with polyenes on sn-2 position (e.g., 2-AG and 2-docosahexaenoylmonoacylglycerol), free fatty acids (FFA) derived from the sn-1/-3, unesterified cholesterol (UC) derived from cholesterol esters (CE), lysophosphatidate (LPA) derived from phosphatidate (PA), lysophospholipids (LPL) derived from phospholipids (PL), and fat soluble vitamins. At the lumen, NAEs, 2-AG, and other MAGs bind intestinal CB_1 receptors affecting peristalsis. FFA and MAG enter enterocytes via passive diffusion and are re-esterified inside the endoplasmic reticulum by MAG acyltransferase (MAGAT) and DAGAT reforming TAG. Lysophospholipids (via LPL AT), LPA (via 1-acyl-glycerol-3-phosphate acyltransferase; AGPAT), and cholesterol (via acyl-CoA: cholesterol acyltransferase; ACAT) are re-esterified forming PL, phosphatidate (PA), and cholesterol esters (CE), respectively. Diet affects molecular species of TAG, PL, PA, and CE. Facilitated by microsomal triglyceride transfer protein (MTP), TAG joins CE and apolipoprotein B (ApoB), forming chylomicrons (CM), which enter circulation via lymph, delivering lipids to peripheral sites and liver. At liver, dietary derived essential fatty acids, such as linoleate (LA, 18:2n6), and linolenate (ALA, 18:3n3) compete for the same desaturases elongases, and retroconversion systems, forming free AA and DHA, respectively. This AA and DHA pool from precursors, along with pre-formed dietary-derived AA and DHA, and other dietary- and endogenously derived FA form a FFA pool for generating specific molecular species of PL, TAG, and CE, via retailoring (deacylation, reacylation). At liver and peripheral sites, PL may be precursors in synthesis of eCBs. MAGs with specific acyl chains (generated via TAG- and DAG-lipases) have eCB activity. Primary amides (e.g., oleamide) also have eCB activities and may be influenced by dietary FA. PL, TAG, and CE are packaged into VLDL for delivery via lipoprotein lipase (LPL) to peripheral sites such as adipose and brain. At adipose, dietary FA influence the FA taken up by adipose tissue and the FA released during lipolysis. At brain, FA is delivered via lipoproteins and specific FA transport proteins (FATP) and binding proteins (FABP) to facilitate delivery of LC-PUFA across blood–brain barrier (BBB). Brain also forms AA and DHA from LA and ALA precursors, respectively. Anandamide synthesis in cells and dietary influences are shown in the bottom box. Unique PL pools [e.g., phosphatidylcholine (PC) with AA on sn-1 rather than sn-2] are possible precursors in transacylase reactions leading to *N*-acylphosphatidylethanolamines (NAPEs). *N*-Arachidonylphosphatidylethanolamine represents one NAPE molecular species. Dietary AA could enrich sn-1-arachidonyl 2-polyene acyl PC pool of lipids by affecting direct synthesis or retailoring. Likewise, dietary FA could alter acyl chains of phosphatidylethanolamine (PE), a donor in a transacylase reaction. Dietary lipids could also influence retailoring of *N*-arachidonylphosphatidylethanolamine. Thereafter, *N*-arachidonylphosphatidylethanolamine is converted to anandamide via phospholipase D (PLD). Dietary FA could also influence levels of anandamide by acting as alterative substrates for amidase, which degrades anandamides and other eCBs. NAEs with acyl chains other than AA may serve as competing substrates for amidase, and bind CB_1 receptors (CB1-R). CB1-R–triggered intracellular signaling, for example, downregulation of adenylate cyclase (AC), leads to various physiological sequealae including changes in appetite, peristalsis, mood and reward, motor control, heart rate variability, and blood pressure.

receptor in the CNS could be modified by the manipulation of the dietary n-3 LCPUFA status". It has been established by previous generations of lipid researchers that phospholipid pools, such as PC, PE, and cardiolipin (CL), are more modifiable by dietary fish oil than sphingomyelin (SPN), and other sphingolipids, PS, and PI (13). In understanding how dietary fatty acids affect endocannabinoid levels, particularly in brain regions, it is necessary to examine acyl changes in specific phospholipid molecular species, using modern lipidomic approaches to increase sensitivity (14).

The role of the diet in determining brain levels of eCBs are in agreement with the results showing that food restriction of dams, either during gestation or lactation, or both, causes a decrease in hypothalamic anandamide levels in pups, which persists until weaning, but not in adult rats (15). In fact, pups depend on the diet of the dams for their LC-PUFA, as their ability to synthesize AA and DHA from dietary precursors is limited. Interestingly, the observed dam dietary restriction–induced decrease in hypothalamic anandamide levels of the pups is directly and strongly correlated with their reduced body weight.

A general rule in adult rodent feeding trials with LC-PUFA is that at least 2 weeks are required to reach steady state levels in phospholipid acyl profiles (16) and the same may hold for dietary fatty acid modulation of eCBs. Absolute amounts of dietary fatty acids and total fat content, and competition amongst n3, n6, and n9 fatty acids are also important considerations. In a feeding trial of only 1 week in rats, Artmann et al. (17) fed rats five different dietary fats [palm oil, olive oil (OA), safflower oil (LA), fish oil (FO), and AA] and examined tissue levels of 2-arachidonoylglycerol, anandamide, *N*-oleoylethanolamine (an anorectic compound), *N*-palmitoylethanolamine, *N*-stearoylethanolamine, *N*-linoleoyl-ethanolamine, *N*-eicosapentaenoylethanolamine, and *N*-docosahexaenoylethanolamine. The LA-diet increased *N*-linoleoylethanolamine in the brain, whereas the OA-diet increased brain levels of anandamide and *N*-oleoylethanolamine (but not 2-AG). Importantly, the AA-diet and FO-diet had no effect on NAEs and eCBs in the brain after this 1-week period, but a longer feeding period may yield a different results. Importantly, the study demonstrated that dietary monoenes and dienes can also influence corresponding NAEs in the brain, which has ramifications for populations consuming large amounts of oleic acid (Mediterranean diet) and linoleic acid (American Diet) in the diet.

Dietary AA- and FO-derived fatty acids are not the only LC-PUFA that can be incorporated into eCBs and affect eCB signaling, but numerous naturally occurring fatty acids also comprise the acyl chain of eCBs. As one important example, 5,11,4-eicosatrienoate (sciadonic acid; like AA but lacking the internal double bond essential for classical eicosanoid production and thus an anti-inflammatory fatty acid) can be incorporated into monoacylglycerols forming 2-sciadonoylglycerol, which exhibits cannabimimetic activity in NG108-15 neuroblastoma × glioma hybrid cells (18). Sciadonic acid may also have eCB activity in vivo since it is readily incorporated into phospholipid pools when administered as a minor dietary component (19), and it may have eCB activity in the gymnosperm plant species where it is derived (20).

Effects on Cannabinoid CB_1 Receptor–Mediated Behaviors

One of us (A.B.) investigated changes in behaviors typically affected by CB1R activation of either a control diet (CONT), adequate in 18:2n6 and 18:3n3 fatty acid content, or of diets containing a fungal oil enriched in AA (AA), a fish oil enriched in DHA (DHA), or a combination (AA+DHA) diet containing an even mixture of the AA- and DHA-containing oils. In particular, it was evaluated whether dietary LC-PUFA may affect CB1R-mediated behaviors including catalepsy, hypothermia, antinociception/analgesia, plus maze anxiolysis, and forced swim test antidepression, and whether any observed change in behavior was sensitive to blockade of CB1R with the specific antagonist AM251. Diets contained 90% fat-free AIN93G powdered rodent diet, 0.4% milk fat, 1.2% palm olein, 1.9% sunflower oil, 1.5% soybean oil and 2.1–5.1% medium chain triacylglycerol oil. Part of medium chain triacylglycerol oil in CONT was replaced with 1.1% fungal oil (providing 0.5 dietary wt% AA and 1.0en% AA) in AA diet; 1.9% fish oil (providing 0.5 dietary wt% DHA and 1.0en% DHA) in DHA diet; and 1.1% fungal oil and 1.9% fish oil in AA+DHA diet. These levels of AA and DHA affect neurotransmitter levels and behavior in rats (21), and were not excessively high, 2–3-fold higher than recommended for human babies, with a slower Δ6 desaturase activity than rodents. Male Rj:NMRI mice weighed 10 to 11 g at delivery and 33 to 51 g on experimental day 42. They were housed 10/cage and received purified powdered diets (7.5 g/mouse) from day 1 to day 58, and were thereafter

Table 1 Timing and Design of Behavioral Tests

Group/tests	Feeding	Tetrad test	Plus maze test	Porsolt test	Sacrifice and dissection
Days	D 1–56[a]	D 29–30[b]	D 44–45[b]	D 47[c]	D 57–59[d]
Timing of diet or drug	Ad libitum	P.o. 15 min	P.o. 60 min	P.o. 60 min	–
A	CONT	Vehicle	Vehicle	Vehicle	Brain, liver, carcasses[e]
B	CONT	THC	Clobazam	Imipramine	Carcasses
C	CONT	AM251	AM251	AM251	Brain, liver, carcasses[e]
D	AA	Vehicle	Vehicle	Vehicle	Brain, liver, carcasses[e]
E	DHA	Vehicle	Vehicle	Vehicle	Brain, liver, carcasses[e]
F	AA+DHA	Vehicle	Vehicle	Vehicle	Brain, liver, carcasses[e]
G	AA+DHA	AM251	AM251	AM251	Carcasses

Drug doses across tests were THC-45, AM251-64, clobazam-32, and imipramine-128 mg/kg BW.
[a] Food consumption and body weights were measured daily, and the experiment was divided into two sub-experiments: $n = 5$/group and $n = 70$ in total.
[b] Two sub-experiments were performed on 2 consecutive days.
[c] Two sub-experiments were performed on the same day.
[d] Sacrifice and dissection were performed on 3 consecutive days in total for two subgroups.
[e] Brain was sectioned in 5 mice; whole brain and liver were extracted in the remaining 5 mice/group.

sacrificed in the AM by cervical dislocation over the last 2 experimental days. Food was not removed the night before, and since nocturnal mice eat during the normal dark cycle period employed, mice were likely fasted 0 to 6 hours at sacrifice (12–16 hours being a complete fast). These conditions and dietary levels of AA were previously found to increase by 5.8-fold of the brain levels of anandamide (2). Behavioral testing was performed on 10 mice/group (5/cage). Effective reference substance doses were determined in prestudy trials. The seven experimental groups are designated in Table 1: CONT plus drug vehicle administered p.o. at time of testing (CONT-A); CONT plus specific pharmacologic agents to validate individual behavioral tests (CONT-B); CONT+AM251 to inhibit CB1R-mediated activities (CONT+AM251-C); AA (AA-D); DHA (DHA-E); AA+DHA (AA+DHA-F); and AA+DHA+AM251 (AA+DHA+AM251-G) to inhibit CB1R-mediated activities. For logistical reasons, AA+AM251 and DHA+AM251 were excluded from the experimental design. It was reasoned that AA+DHA group should have a strong (AM251-inhibitable) affect on CB1R-mediated signaling since AA- and DHA-derived NAEs were formed from LC-PUFA precursors in prior work with pigs (2). Behavioral tests were spaced out to avoid and minimize carry over effects of one behavioral test upon another. Tetrad tests were conducted first. There was thereafter 15 days between tetrad and plus maze testing (for anxiolytic activity), and 2 days between plus maze and forced swim testing (for antidepressant activity). As plus maze testing can induce stress for up to 24 hours posttest, the 2 to 3 days between plus maze and forced swim testing should have been sufficient to reduce stress and washout effects of reference drugs used in CONT-B groups (22–25).

Open-Field Rearings, Ambulations and Fecal Droppings, Ring Test Immobility, Hot-Plate Analgesia, and Hypothermia

Relative to CONT-A, other groups (including AA-D, DHA-E, AA+DHA-F, AA+DHA+AM251-G) did not affect rearing, open field ambulations, fecal droppings, ring test immobility, nor hot plate foot-licking latency ($p \geq 0.1$) (Table 2). Relative to CONT-A and DHA-E, body temperature showed a trend ($p \leq 0.1$) to decrease with AA-D and AA+DHA-F (Table 2). In the AA-D group, higher anandamide levels in whole mouse brain were found (2,8), and the reduction in body temperature with AA feeding is consistent with the reduction in body temperature previously observed with gavaged anandamide relative to control mice (4,6). Yehuda and Carasso (26) previously noted that dietary LC-PUFA could modulate agonist-induced hypothermia. In addition to potential signaling through CB1R, LC-PUFA could affect body temperature through other mechanisms. For example, as part of the same experiment reported herein, hippocampal prostaglandin D_2 (PGD_2) synthase (ptgds) transcripts were increased 3–5-fold by AA-D, DHA-E, and AA+DHA-F relative to CONT-A ($p \leq 0.05$; no differences between the noncontrol groups) (8). PGD_2 is a major prostaglandin in rodent and human hippocampus with roles in body temperature regulation and sleep (27–29).

Table 2 Results of "Tetrad" Behavioral Tests

Group	Ambulation #	Rearing #	Fecal drops #	Ring test immobility (%)	Temperature (°C)	Foot-licking latency (sec)
A	95.7	42.1	3.4	10.5	38.28	4.23
B	$18.1^{1\ddagger}$	$1.4^{1\ddagger}$	$0.5^{1\ddagger}$	$58.8^{1\ddagger}$	$35.15^{1\ddagger}$	$8.65^{1\ddagger}$
C	66.9^{2}	23.4^{2}	3.89	9.11	37.98	4.62
D	93.0	32.8	2.6	8.7	38.02^{3}	4.38
E	113.8	35.9	3.2	6.6	38.30^{6}	3.86
F	101.2	36.0	2.4	13.3	$37.87^{5,7}$	4.19
G	92.6	23.7^{9*a}	2.8	11.7	37.72	5.46

Values represent means from $n = 10$. Levels of significance from a two sided, unpaired student's t-test with unequal variance are indicated with superscripted symbols. Superscripted numbers refer to t-test pairwise group comparisons. Not all possible pairwise comparisons were conducted. Group designations A–G are shown in Table 1.
A superscripted number with: no asterisk, $p \leq 0.1$; $^{*}p \leq 0.05$; $^{\dagger}p \leq 0.01$; $^{\ddagger}p \leq 0.001$.
^{a} Comparison is significant after eliminating a single outlier. ^{1}B vs. A; ^{2}C vs. A; ^{3}D vs. A; ^{4}E vs. A; ^{5}F vs. A; ^{6}E vs. D; ^{7}F vs. E; ^{8}G vs. C; ^{9}G vs. F.

Depression

In the Porsolt forced swim test, antidepressants decrease immobility duration (increase duration of mobility) when mice are forced to swim in a situation from which they cannot escape rapidly. CONT-A mice showed a high level of immobility, and the antidepressant imipramine administered 60 minute pretest, decreased immobility duration, validating the test (Table 3). DHA and AA+DHA did not affect immobility. AA-D showed a trend to reduce immobility duration (antidepressant-like activity) relative to CONT-A, from 171.5 to 152.0 seconds ($p \leq 0.1$; time immobile during last 4 minutes of the 6-minute test). This behavioral activity could be eCB-CB1R–mediated as the AA-D diet increased anandamide in whole brain (2,8). There is precedent for LC-PUFA and eCBs affecting immobility/antidepression (30–37). eCB levels and enhancement of eCB signaling produced antidepression in forced swim tests (34–36), supporting our findings. Immobility was reported to be affected in some studies with LC-PUFA deficiencies (37,38), but not others (30). Unlike our findings, supplementation with n3 LC-PUFA in rats induced antidepressant activities in forced swim tests after 30 days (32).

Anxiety

Elevated plus maze tests evaluate anxiolytic and anxiogenic responses. Caveats are that the test requires rigorous standardized conditions; results are strain-specific with differences in sensitivity between rats and mice (39); and the test is influenced by environmental factors (40,41). The test is also influenced by prior experience of mice to the plus maze with test-experienced mice being more anxiogenic than plus maze naïve mice (42). Closed- and open-arm entries were positively correlated (Spearman's rank correlation = 0.40, $p \leq 0.001$). Clobazam slightly increased open-arm entries (CONT-Clobazam-B vs. CONT-A; $p \leq 0.05$) (Table 3). AM251 showed a trend to decrease open-arm entries in CONT-AM251-C versus CONT-A ($p \leq 0.1$) and in

Table 3 Results of Plus Maze and Forced Swim Tests

Group	Plus maze Closed-arms (epm)	Open-arms (epm)	Time open arms (sec)	Forced swim test Time immobiity (sec)
A	3.6	2.3	40.0	171.5
B	6.3^{1}	2.4^{1*}	68.4	$71.5^{1\ddagger}$
C	2.3	0.2^{2}	0.2^{2*}	171.9
D	6.4^{3*}	2.0	21.3	152.0^{3}
E	6.0^{4*}	1.6	21.1	161.7
F	$6.8^{5\dagger}$	1.9	17.8	163.7
G	$4.6^{8,9}$	0.8^{9}	6.4	161.9

Values represent means from $n = 10$. Levels of significance from a two sided, unpaired student's t-test with unequal variance are indicated with superscripted symbols. Superscripted numbers refer to t-test pairwise group comparisons. Not all possible pairwise comparisons were conducted. Epm: entries per minute. Group designations A–G are shown in Table 1.
A superscripted number with: no asterisk, $p \leq 0.1$; $^{*}p \leq 0.05$; $^{\dagger}p \leq 0.01$; $^{\ddagger}p \leq 0.001$. ^{1}B vs. A; ^{2}C vs. A; ^{3}D vs. A; ^{4}E vs. A; ^{5}F vs. A; ^{6}E vs. D; ^{7}F vs. E; ^{8}G vs. C; ^{9}G vs. F.

AA+DHA-AM251-G versus AA+DHA-F ($p \leq 0.1$). AM251 also substantially decreased the amount of time spent in the open arms, most notably for the CONT diet (CONT-AM251-C vs. CONT-A ($p \leq 0.05$). AM251 thus showed potential CB1R-mediated anxiogenic properties as previously reported (42–46). Relative to CONT-A, none of diets (AA-D, DHA-E, and AA+DHA-F) affected entries or time spent in open arms ($p \geq 0.1$). Closed arm entries increased from 3.6 to 6.3 with clobazam (CONT-A vs. −B; $p \leq 0.1$), partially validating the test for evaluating anxiolysis with closed-arm entries. Closed-arm entries increased from 3.6 with CONT-A to 6.0–6.8 with AA-D ($p \leq 0.05$), DHA-E ($p \leq 0.05$), and AA+DHA-F ($p \leq 0.01$) indicating that these LC-PUFA–enriched diets may induce anxiolytic (clobazam-like) effects. Closed-arm entries showed a statistical trend to decrease from 6.8 to 4.6 with AA+DHA+AM251 (AA+DHA+AM251-G vs. AA+DHA-F; $p \leq 0.1$). The p-value for this comparison is slightly reduced to 0.08 after $\log_{10}$ transformation (which minimizes affects of outliers). This reduction is not surprising as AM251 alone can antagonize CB1R, induce anxiogenesis, and decrease closed-arm entries in mice (42), and might suggest that part of the effects of the diets might be due to elevation of eCB levels. Closed-arm entries showed a trend to increase from 2.3 with CONT+AM251-C to 4.6 with AA+DHA+AM251-G ($p \leq 0.1$), indicating that CB_1 inhibition with AM251 could not completely block dietary affects on closed-arm entries. LC-PUFA could affect closed-arm entries via CB1R, receptors related to CB1R (47), and via signaling cascades independent of eCBs. Since the dietary treatments did not affect open-field ambulations and ring-test immobility, it is unlikely that mobility per se is responsible for changes observed in closed-arm entries (48). In the present experiment, levels of 22:6n3 NAE in whole mouse brain were not affected by DHA feeding, but 20:4n6 NAE levels were elevated 5.8-fold following AA feeding (2,8). The diets also increased LC-PUFA in phospholipids pools. AA increased 20:4n6 and 22:4n6, and DHA increased 20:5n3, 22:5n3, and 22:6n3 in whole brain, hippocampal, and hepatic phospholipid pools confirming that the diets were consumed, bioavailable, and incorporated into phospholipids (9). Changes to NAEs (e.g., following DHA feeding) may have been partly masked by examining levels in whole brain rather than individual sections (2). A related point is that there is differential expression of CB1R on distinct neuronal populations within specific brain regions, such as the amygdala and hypothalamus (49). Although these experiments do not provide conclusive evidence, there is the possibility that the anxiolytic effects of AA+DHA (and potentially AA and DHA alone) may involve anandamide–CB1R interactions, based on closed-arm entries. Accordingly, other researchers have found that addition of eCBs or drug-induced manipulation of endogenous eCBs can induce anxiolysis in the plus maze test. In adult rats, i.p. administration of AM404 (an eCB transport inhibitor) increased anandamide in hippocampus, prefrontal cortex, and thalamus, which was associated with increased time spent in open arms (36). This anxiolytic effect was reversed with the CB1R antagonist, rimonabant (SR141716A). Similarly, inhibitors of fatty-acid amide hydrolase (an enzyme that degrades NAEs and related molecules) increased brain anandamide, inducing anxiolytic-, benzodiazepine-like effects in the elevated zero-maze test that could be inhibited by blocking CB1Rs (50). Dietary LC-PUFA are also reported to affect plus maze responses. For example, in a generational study in which mouse dams and offspring received diets rich in either 18:2n6 (a 20:4n6 precursor) or 18:3n3 (a DHA precursor), open- and closed-arm entries were less, and time spent in dark enclosed arms tended to be longer with 18:3n3 feeding (suggesting anxiogenesis), in 6-week offspring (51). With DHA feeding in our experiments, closed-arm entries increased relative to the 18:2n6 control (DHA vs. CONT-A) showing an opposite effect. Deficiency of dietary 18:3n3 did not affect plus maze responses in other reports (30,52). In addition to potential signaling through CB1R, LC-PUFA could affect plus maze responses through other mechanisms. For example, we previously reported that transcripts for 5-hydroxytryptamine receptor 4 (htr4) were increased 6.5-fold by AA-D relative to CONT-A in the hippocampus (8) as part of the same experiment reported herein. 5-Hydroxytryptamine receptor signaling is known to affect plus maze anxiolysis (53–55). It is conceivable that the AA-induced increase in 20:4n6 NAE (2,8,56) could displace ligands from binding 5-hydroxytryptamine receptors (57), contributing to plus maze anxiolysis. DHA feeding in rats were previously reported to increase 5-hydroxytryptamine levels (58), further supporting associations between LC-PUFA feeding and 5-HT signaling. LC-PUFA could also signal through somatostatin receptors (sst), which affect stress responses (59) and potentially results in some of the behavioral tests we evaluated. As part of the same experiment reported herein AA-D, DHA-E, and AA+DHA-F significantly increased sst transcripts 1.8–2.1 fold in hippocampus ($p \leq 0.05$) (8). Sst transcripts were similarly reported to be elevated following DHA feeding in rats (60).

Appetite Control

Although brain eCB levels appear to be strongly modified by diets enriched in LC-PUFA and the brain eCB system is deeply involved in appetite control (see other chapters in this book), no specific study has been carried out to date to investigate whether dietary-induced changes in eCB signaling are paralleled by changes in food-intake. Previous studies showed that perinatal deficiency in dietary n-3 PUFA is accompanied by increased food-intake in rats (61), a finding that would be in agreement with the inhibitory effects of chronic dietary n-3 PUFA on brain eCB (2-arachidonylglycerol) levels (12). On the other hand, studies carried out in human volunteers have so far investigated only the effect of different acute dietary fatty acids on appetite and satiety (62,63).

EFFECTS OF DIETARY FATTY ACIDS ON PERIPHERAL ENDOCANNABINOID SIGNALING AND THEIR POTENTIAL CONSEQUENCES ON ENERGY HOMEOSTASIS

Three studies have investigated so far the effect of high fat diets or dietary fatty acids on peripheral tissues and cells involved in energy homeostasis. Matias et al. (64) showed that incubation of 3T3F442A mouse adipocytes with AA strongly elevates 2-AG levels and amounts of AA esterified in triacylglycerols and on glycerol sn-2 carbon but not sn-1, in phospholipids. The sn-2 position is the most common placement on the glycerol backbone for polyenes, although rare phospholipids enriched with AA on the sn-1 position may serve as precursors for *N*-arachidonoyl-PE in the synthesis of anandamide (3). Incubation with DHA, instead, decreased 2-AG and anandamide levels and the amounts of AA esterified on both sn-2 and sn-1 position of phospholipids, but not on triacylglycerols. The authors suggested that dietary LC-PUFA and/or their biosynthetic precursors might modulate levels of adipocyte phospholipids that act as eCB precursors, and that this, in view of the lipogenic actions of eCBs in adipocytes (65–67), might participate in the beneficial effects of n-3 PUFA and in the worsening effect of dietary n-6 PUFA in abdominal obesity, dyslipidemia, and insulin resistance (see other chapters in this book).

In a 1-week feeding trial examing five different dietary fats [palm oil, olive oil (OA), safflower oil (LA), fish oil (FO), and AA], Artmann et al. (17) reported that (1) the LA-diet increased *N*-linoleoylethanolamine in the jejunum and liver; (2) the OA-diet increased *N*-oleoylethanolamine in the liver, a finding potentially relevant to the anti-lipogenic effects of this compound in hepatocytes (68) and to the beneficial effects of the Mediterranean diet; (3) all five dietary fats decreased *N*-oleoylethanolamine in the jejunum without changing levels of anandamide, thus suggesting that dietary fat may have an orexigenic action (*N*-oleoylethanolamine is a potent anorectic lipid); (4) the AA-diet increased anandamide and 2-arachidonoylglycerol in the jejunum with no effect on the liver, thus suggesting that dietary AA might also cause orexigenic effects (eCBs exert potent orexigenic actions at both the central and small intestine levels; see other chapter in this book); and (5) the FO-diet decreased liver levels of NAEs, except for *N*-eicosapentaenoylethanolamine and *N*-docosahexaenoyl-ethanolamine.

Finally, Matias et al. (66) recently reported new data on the dysregulation of eCB levels in organs with endocrine function (adrenal glands and thyroid), involved in energy expenditure (brown adipose tissue and skeletal muscle), or affected by the consequences of metabolic disorders (heart and kidney), obtained from mice fed for 3, 8, and 14 weeks with two different high-fat diets (HFDs), with different fatty acid compositions and impact on fasting glucose levels. In particular, although the two diets used for experiments exhibited similar n-6/n-3 PUFA precursor ratios and nonsaturated fatty acid amounts, HFD2 was characterized by significantly higher amounts of monounsaturated fatty acids and PUFA than HFD1, and by capability of inducing high fasting glycemia not after 3 weeks but only after 14 weeks of the dietary regimen. The authors observed elevations (in skeletal muscle, heart, and kidney) or reductions (in thyroid) of levels of either anandamide or 2-AG, or both. Depending on the diet, these changes preceded or accompanied development of overt obesity and/or hyperglycemia. In adrenal gland, there was first a reduction and then an elevation of eCBs. In brown fat, a very early elevation of both anandamide and 2-AG normalized levels was observed with one of the diets, whereas delayed decreases appeared to be caused by increased amounts of fat tissue weight induced by HFDs. Although the authors did not observe strong correlations between abundance of a certain family of dietary fatty acids and effects on eCB levels, in those organs where eCBs first decreased and then increased by diet (i.e., adrenal gland), HFD2 (higher in PUFA) produced this effect earlier.

On the other hand, in some organs where an increase of eCBs was observed with diet (i.e., kidney and heart), this effect was often extended to 2-AG only with HFD1. These differences might be due to the higher amounts, in HFD2 versus HFD1, of precursors for n-3 PUFA, which were shown to reduce both anandamide and 2-AG levels in adipocytes (64), and the effect of which might predominate over the stimulatory one (64) of n-6 PUFA.

These studies highlight the possibility that both the type and amount of fatty acids present in the diet and the duration of the diet itself might differentially alter levels of eCBs and NAEs not only in the brain but also in peripheral organs involved in the control of energy homeostasis, contributing to the adverse consequences of prolonged HFD and related metabolic disorders (dyslipidemia, dyslipoproteinemia, insulin resistence, glucose intolerance, and type 2 diabetes). In particular, prolonged exposure to diets rich in n-3 PUFA or their precursors seem to cause a decrease in eCB levels in most of the tissues analyzed, and, in view of the strong contribution of an overactive eCB system in hyperphagia, dyslipidemia, and insulin resistance (see other chapters in this book), this phenomenon might be responsible in part for some of the beneficial metabolic effects of such diets. By contrast, prolonged exposure to diets rich in n-6 PUFA or their precursors might indirectly participate in ectopic fat formation by enhancing levels of lipogenic eCBs in the adipose tissue and liver. Clearly, specific studies are required to fully investigate this possibility, utilizing CB1R blockers or eCB degradation inhibitors to better understand the metabolic consequences of prolonged dietary consumption of LC-PUFA.

CONCLUSIONS

In our quest to better understand how dietary LC-PUFA affect eCB levels and subsequent signaling, there are numerous important dietary variables to consider in designing proper nutritional experiments and to minimize covariates. First, the amount of total fat and importantly, the ratio of different classes (n-9, n-7, n-6, and n-3) of dietary fatty acids (69) ultimately will affect the final phospholipid and eCB acyl profile and must be considered. Second, nonfatty acid components of oils containing fatty acids have their own influences on obesity. For example, plant sterols (70–72), gangliosides (73,74), and sphingolipids (75) can affect fat absorbability and inflammatory and obesity potential of the overall diet. Third, different mammals metabolize dietary fatty acids differently. For example, humans have a slower elongase and desaturase system than rodents and hence in humans, dietary precursors of AA and DHA may be less effective than in rodents for synthesizing AA and DHA end products. Fourth, there are fundamental differences in how different mammals synthesize and store fatty acids. For example, humans synthesize fatty acids in the liver and store them in adipose tissue and liver, whereas rodents synthesize fatty acids in both liver and adipose tissue, and store fatty acids in both locations. Fifth, the intestinal flora of species (itself influenced by diet, maternal nutrition, environment, and drugs) can affect the absorbability of fat and nutrients and influence obesity (76,77). In this regard, mammals should be thought of as mammal–microbe superorganism hybrids (78). Sixth, dietary fatty acids are introduced into the diet mainly as triacyglycerols and converted to 2-monoacylgycerols and free fatty acids by lipases during digestion (79). These 2-monoacylglycerols may then affect the activity of gut CB receptors and, subsequently, peristalsis (80) and absorbability of the lipid components, whereas free fatty acids, monoacylglycerols (81,82), and gangliosides (74,83) in the diet, may have positive effects on the immune system by killing or binding to dietary toxins.

ACKNOWLEDGMENTS

Concerning the newly described behavioral results (A. B.), the authors thank Sylvain Roux, Anne Marie Hay, and Martine Lemaire of Porsolt & Partners Pharmacology (Boulogne-Billiancourt, France) for performing feeding experiments, behavioral testing, and tissue preparations. The Nestlé Research Center (Lausanne, Switzerland) is thanked for their overall support to the project, particularly Oliver Ballèvre and Andrea Pfeifer.

REFERENCES

1. Wainwright PE. Dietary essential fatty acids and brain function: A developmental perspective on mechanisms. Proc Nutr Soc 2002; 61(1):61–69.

2. Berger A, Crozier G, Bisogno T, et al. Anandamide and diet: Inclusion of dietary arachidonate and docosahexaenoate leads to increased brain levels of the corresponding *N*-acylethanolamines in piglets. Proc Natl Acad Sci U S A 2001; 98(11):6402–6406.
3. Di Marzo V, Petrosino S. Endocannabinoids and the regulation of their levels in health and disease. Curr Opin Lipidol 2007; 18(2):129–140.
4. Di Marzo V, Sepe N, De Petrocellis L, et al. Trick or treat from food endocannabinoids? [letter]. Nature 1998; 396(6712):636–637.
5. Crozier Willi G, Berger A, Di Marzo V, et al. Lipids in neural function: Modulation of behavior by oral administration of endocannabinoids found in foods. Nestle Nutr Workshop Ser Clin Perform Programme 2001; (5):169–184, discussion 185–167.
6. Di Marzo V, De Petrocellis L, Bisogno T, et al. Biology of endocannabinoids. In: Onaivi E, ed. The Biology of Marijuana from Gene to Behavior. London: Taylor & Francis, 2002:125–173.
7. Berger A, Crozier-Willi G, Di Marzo V. Anandamides and diet. A new pot of nutritional research is simmering. In: Neeser J-R, German BJ, eds. Bioprocesses and Biotechnology for Functional Foods and Nutraceuticals. New York: Marcel Dekker, 2003:225–261.
8. Berger A, Roberts MA. Dietary effects of arachidonate-rich fungal oil and fish oil on murine hippocampal gene expression. In: Berger A, Roberts MA, eds. Unraveling Lipid Metabolism with Microarrays. New York: Marcel Dekker, 2005:69–100.
9. Berger A, Mutch DM, German BJ, et al. Dietary effects of arachidonate-rich fungal oil and fish oil on murine hepatic and hippocampal gene expression. Lipids Health Dis 2002; 1(1):2.
10. Berger A, Roberts MA, Hoff B. How dietary arachidonic- and docosahexaenoic-acid rich oils differentially affect the murine hepatic transcriptome. Lipids Health Dis 2006; 5:10.
11. Wood JT, Williams JS, Pandarinathan L, et al. Plasma and brain endocannabinoid level correlation studies after increasing DHA dietary intake. FASEB J 2007; 21(6):A1067.
12. Watanabe S, Doshi M, Hamazaki T. n-3 Polyunsaturated fatty acid (PUFA) deficiency elevates and n-3 PUFA enrichment reduces brain 2-arachidonoylglycerol level in mice. Prostaglandins Leukot Essent Fatty Acids 2003; 69(1):51–59.
13. Berger A, Gershwin ME, German JB. Effects of various dietary fats on cardiolipin acyl composition during ontogeny of mice. Lipids 1992; 27:605–612.
14. Williams J, Wood J, Pandarinathan L, et al. Quantitative method for the profiling of the endocannabinoid metabolome by LC-atmospheric pressure chemical ionization-MS. Anal Chem 2007; 79 (15):5582–5593.
15. Matias I, Leonhardt M, Lesage J, et al. Effect of maternal under-nutrition on pup body weight and hypothalamic endocannabinoid levels. Cell Mol Life Sci 2003; 60(2):382–389.
16. Berger A, German JB. Phospholipid fatty acid composition of various mouse tissues after feeding alpha-linolenate (18;3n-3) or eicosatrienoate (20;3n-3). Lipids 1990; 25(8):473–480.
17. Artmann A, Petersen G, Hellgren LI, et al. Influence of dietary fatty acids on endocannabinoid and *N*-acylethanolamine levels in rat brain, liver and small intestine. Biochim Biophys Acta 2008; 1781(4):200–212.
18. Nakane S, Tanaka T, Satouchi K, et al. Occurrence of a novel cannabimimetic molecule 2-sciadonoylglycerol (2-eicosa-5′,11′,14′-trienoylglycerol) in the umbrella pine *Sciadopitys verticillata* seeds. Biol Pharm Bull 2000; 23(6):758–761.
19. Berger A, Monnard I, Baur M, et al. Epidermal anti-inflammatory properties of 5,11,14 20:3: Effects on mouse ear edema, PGE2 levels in cultured keratinocytes, and PPAR activation. Lipids Health Dis 2002; 1:5.
20. Wolff RL. Sources of 5,11,14 20:3 (sciadonic) acid, a structural analog of arachidonic acid. JAOCS 1998; 75(12):1901–1902.
21. Chalon S, Delion-Vancassel S, Belzung C, et al. Dietary fish oil affects monoaminergic neurotransmission and behavior in rats. J Nutr 1998; 128(12):2512–2519.
22. Schulkin J, Gold PW, McEwen BS. Induction of corticotropin-releasing hormone gene expression by glucocorticoids: Implication for understanding the states of fear and anxiety and allostatic load. Psychoneuroendocrinology 1998; 23(3):219–243.
23. Rodgers RJ, Haller J, Holmes A, et al. Corticosterone response to the plus-maze: High correlation with risk assessment in rats and mice. Physiol Behav 1999; 68(1–2):47–53.
24. Netto SM, Silveira R, Coimbra NC, et al. Anxiogenic effect of median raphe nucleus lesion in stressed rats. Prog Neuropsychopharmacol Biol Psychiatry 2002; 26(6):1135–1141.
25. Hill MN, Patel S, Carrier EJ, et al. Downregulation of endocannabinoid signaling in the hippocampus following chronic unpredictable stress. Neuropsychopharmacology 2005; 30(3):508–515.
26. Yehuda S, Carasso RL. Modulation of learning, pain thresholds, and thermoregulation in the rat by preparations of free purified α-linolenic and linoleic acids: Determination of the optimal ω3-to-ω6 ratio. Proc Natl Acad Sci U S A 1993; 90(21):10345–10349.
27. Forstermann U, Heldt R, Hertting G. Studies on the mechanism of central cardiovascular and temperature responses to prostaglandin D2. Prostaglandins Leukot Med 1985; 18(3):301–308.

28. Mong JA, Devidze N, Goodwillie A, et al. Reduction of lipocalin-type prostaglandin D synthase in the preoptic area of female mice mimics estradiol effects on arousal and sex behavior. Proc Natl Acad Sci U S A 2003; 100(25):15206–15211.
29. Chen C, Bazan NG. Lipid signaling: Sleep, synaptic plasticity, and neuroprotection. Prostaglandins Other Lipid Mediat 2005; 77(1–4):65–76.
30. Frances H, Monier C, Bourre JM. Effects of dietary alpha-linolenic acid deficiency on neuromuscular and cognitive functions in mice. Life Sci 1995; 57(21):1935–1947.
31. Shaldubina A, Nemets B, Bersudsky Y. Lack of effect of eicosapentaenoic acid in the Porsolt forced swimming test model of depression. Acta Neuropsychiatrica 2002; 14:203–206.
32. Carlezon WA, Jr., Mague SD, Parow AM, et al. Antidepressant-like effects of uridine and omega-3 fatty acids are potentiated by combined treatment in rats. Biol Psychiatry 2005; 57(4):343–350.
33. Griebel G, Stemmelin J, Scatton B. Effects of the cannabinoid CB1 receptor antagonist rimonabant in models of emotional reactivity in rodents. Biol Psychiatry 2005; 57(3):261–267.
34. Gobbi G, Bambico FR, Mangieri R, et al. Antidepressant-like activity and modulation of brain monoaminergic transmission by blockade of anandamide hydrolysis. Proc Natl Acad Sci U S A 2005; 102(51):18620–18625.
35. Hill MN, Gorzalka BB. Pharmacological enhancement of cannabinoid CB1 receptor activity elicits an antidepressant-like response in the rat forced swim test. Eur Neuropsychopharmacol 2005; 15(6):593–599.
36. Bortolato M, Campolongo P, Mangieri RA, et al. Anxiolytic-like properties of the anandamide transport inhibitor AM404. Neuropsychopharmacology 2006; 31(12):2652–2659.
37. DeMar JC, Jr., Ma K, Bell JM, et al. One generation of n-3 polyunsaturated fatty acid deprivation increases depression and aggression test scores in rats. J Lipid Res 2006; 47(1):172–180.
38. Raygada M, Cho E, Hilakivi-Clarke L. High maternal intake of polyunsaturated fatty acids during pregnancy in mice alters offsprings' aggressive behavior, immobility in the swim test, locomotor activity and brain protein kinase C activity. J Nutr 1998; 128(12):2505–2511.
39. Onaivi ES, Green MR, Martin BR. Pharmacological characterization of cannabinoids in the elevated plus maze. J Pharmacol Exp Ther 1990; 253(3):1002–1009.
40. Hogg S. A review of the validity and variability of the elevated plus-maze as an animal model of anxiety. Pharmacol Biochem Behav 1996; 54(1):21–30.
41. Crabbe JC, Wahlsten D, Dudek BC. Genetics of mouse behavior: Interactions with laboratory environment. Science 1999; 284(5420):1670–1672.
42. Rodgers RJ, Evans PM, Murphy A. Anxiogenic profile of AM-251, a selective cannabinoid CB1 receptor antagonist, in plus-maze-naive and plus-maze-experienced mice. Behav Pharmacol 2005, 16(5–6):405–413.
43. Haller J, Varga B, Ledent C, et al. CB1 cannabinoid receptors mediate anxiolytic effects: Convergent genetic and pharmacological evidence with CB1-specific agents. Behav Pharmacol 2004; 15(4):299–304.
44. Moreira FA, Aguiar DC, Guimaraes FS. Anxiolytic-like effect of cannabinoids injected into the rat dorsolateral periaqueductal gray. Neuropharmacology 2006; 52(3):958–965.
45. Patel S, Hillard CJ. Pharmacological evaluation of cannabinoid receptor ligands in a mouse model of anxiety: Further evidence for an anxiolytic role for endogenous cannabinoid signaling. J Pharmacol Exp Ther 2006; 318(1):304–311.
46. Roohbakhsh A, Moghaddam AH, Massoudi R, et al. Role of dorsal hippocampal cannabinoid receptors and nitric oxide in anxiety like behaviours in rats using the elevated plus-maze test. Clin Exp Pharmacol Physiol 2007; 34(3):223–229.
47. Chakrabarti A, Ekuta JE, Onaivi ES. Neurobehavioral effects of anandamide and cannabinoid receptor gene expression in mice. Brain Res Bull 1998; 45(1):67–74.
48. Kokare DM, Dandekar MP, Chopde CT, et al. Interaction between neuropeptide Y and alpha-melanocyte stimulating hormone in amygdala regulates anxiety in rats. Brain Res 2005; 1043(1–2):107–114.
49. Hill MN, Gorzalka BB. Increased sensitivity to restraint stress and novelty-induced emotionality following long-term, high dose cannabinoid exposure. Psychoneuroendocrinology 2006; 31(4):526–536.
50. Kathuria S, Gaetani S, Fegley D, et al. Modulation of anxiety through blockade of anandamide hydrolysis. Nat Med 2003; 9(1):76–81.
51. Nakashima Y, Yuasa S, Hukamizu Y, et al. Effect of a high linoleate and a high a-linolenate diet on general behavior and drug sensitivity in mice. J Lipid Res 1993; 34(2):239–247.
52. Belzung C, Leguisquet AM, Barreau S, et al. α-Linolenic acid deficiency modifies distractibility but not anxiety and locomotion in rats during aging. J Nutr 1998; 128(9):1537–1542.
53. Silvestre JS, Fernandez AG, Palacios JM. Effects of 5-HT4 receptor antagonists on rat behaviour in the elevated plus-maze test. Eur J Pharmacol 1996; 309(3):219–222.
54. Matsumoto M, Togashi H, Mori K, et al. Evidence for involvement of central 5-HT4 receptors in cholinergic function associated with cognitive processes: Behavioral, electrophysiological, and neurochemical studies. J Pharmacol Exp Ther 2001; 296(3):676–682.

55. Smriga M, Torii K. l-Lysine acts like a partial serotonin receptor 4 antagonist and inhibits serotonin-mediated intestinal pathologies and anxiety in rats. Proc Natl Acad Sci U S A 2003; 100(26):15370–15375.
56. Hill MN, Sun JC, Tse MT, et al. Altered responsiveness of serotonin receptor subtypes following long-term cannabinoid treatment. Int J Neuropsychopharmacol 2006; 9(3):277–286.
57. Kimura T, Ohta T, Watanabe K, et al. Anandamide, an endogenous cannabinoid receptor ligand, also interacts with 5-hydroxytryptamine (5-HT) receptor. Biol Pharm Bull 1998; 21(3):224–226.
58. Li H, Liu D, Zhang E. Effect of fish oil supplementation on fatty acid composition and neurotransmitters of growing rats. Wei Sheng Yan Jiu 2000; 29(1):47–49.
59. Viollet C, Vaillend C, Videau C, et al. Involvement of sst2 somatostatin receptor in locomotor, exploratory activity and emotional reactivity in mice. Eur J Neurosci 2000; 12(10):3761–3770.
60. Farkas T, Kitajika K, Barceló-Coblijn G, et al. Neurological effects of dietary n-3 fatty acids in rat brain. In: Berger A, Roberts MA, eds. Unraveling lipid metabolism with microarrays. New York: Marcel Dekker, 2005:131–146.
61. Mathai ML, Soueid M, Chen N, et al. Does perinatal omega-3 polyunsaturated fatty acid deficiency increase appetite signaling? Obes Res 2004; 12(11):1886–1894.
62. Lawton CL, Delargy HJ, Brockman J, et al. The degree of saturation of fatty acids influences post-ingestive satiety. Br J Nutr 2000; 83(5):473–482.
63. Flint A, Helt B, Raben A, et al. Effects of different dietary fat types on postprandial appetite and energy expenditure. Obes Res 2003; 11(12):1449–1455.
64. Matias I, Gonthier MP, Petrosino S, et al. Role and regulation of acylethanolamides in energy balance: Focus on adipocytes and beta-cells. Br J Pharmacol 2007; 152(5):676–690.
65. Matias I, Carta G, Murru E, et al. Effect of polyunsaturated fatty acids on endocannabinoid and *N*-acyl-ethanolamine levels in mouse adipocytes. Biochim Biophys Acta 2008; 1781(1–2):52–60.
66. Matias I, Petrosino S, Racioppi A, et al. Dysregulation of peripheral endocannabinoid levels in hyperglycemia and obesity: Effect of high fat diets. Mol Cell Endocrinol 2008; 286(1–2 Suppl 1):S66–S78.
67. Matias I, Vergoni AV, Petrosino S, et al. Regulation of hypothalamic endocannabinoid levels by neuropeptides and hormones involved in food intake and metabolism: Insulin and melanocortins. Neuropharmacology 2008; 54(1):206–212.
68. Fu J, Oveisi F, Gaetani S, et al. Oleoylethanolamide, an endogenous PPAR-alpha agonist, lowers body weight and hyperlipidemia in obese rats. Neuropharmacology 2005; 48(8):1147–1153.
69. Hardardottir I, Kinsella JE. Increasing the dietary (n-3) to (n-6) polyunsaturated fatty acid ratio increases tumor necrosis factor production by murine resident peritoneal macrophages without an effect on elicited peritoneal macrophages. J Nutr 1992; 122(10):1942–1951.
70. Awad AB, Begdache LA, Fink CS. Effect of sterols and fatty acids on growth and triglyceride accumulation in 3T3-L1 cells. J Nutr Biochem 2000; 11(3):153–158.
71. Berger A, Jones PJ, Abumweis SS. Plant sterols: Factors affecting their efficacy and safety as functional food ingredients. Lipids Health Dis 2004; 3:5.
72. Assmann G, Cullen P, Kannenberg F, et al. Relationship between phytosterol levels and components of the metabolic syndrome in the PROCAM study. Eur J Cardiovasc Prev Rehabil 2007; 14(2):208–214.
73. Birecki CJ, Drozdowski LA, Suh M, et al. Dietary gangliosides enhance in vitro lipid uptake in weanling rats. J Pediatr Gastroenterol Nutr 2006; 42(1):59–65.
74. Park EJ, Suh M, Thomson B, et al. Dietary ganglioside inhibits acute inflammatory signals in intestinal mucosa and blood induced by systemic inflammation of *Escherichia coli* lipopolysaccharide. Shock 2007, 28(1):112–117.
75. Berger A, Fleith M, Crozier G. Nutritional implications of replacing bovine milk fat with vegetable oil in infant formulas. J Pediatr Gastroenterol Nutr 2000; 30(2):115–130.
76. Raoult D. Obesity pandemics and the modification of digestive bacterial flora. Eur J Clin Microbiol Infect Dis 2008; 27(8):631–634.
77. Wolowczuk I, Verwaerde C, Viltart O, et al. Feeding our immune system: Impact on metabolism. Clin Dev Immunol 2008; 2008:639803.
78. Goodacre R. Metabolomics of a superorganism. J Nutr 2007; 137(1 Suppl.):259S–266S.
79. Chen Q, Bläckberg L, Nilsson A, et al. Digestion of triacylglycerols containing long-chain polyenoic fatty acids in vitro by colipase-dependent pancreatic lipase and human milk bile salt-stimulated lipase. Biochim Biophys Acta 1994; 1210(2):239–243.
80. Pinto L, Capasso R, Di Carlo G, et al. Endocannabinoids and the gut. Prostaglandins Leukot Essent Fatty Acids 2002; 66(2-3):333–341.
81. Kabara JJ, Vrable R. Antimicrobial lipids: Natural and synthetic fatty acids and monoglycerides. Lipids 1977; 12(9):753–759.
82. Kabara JJ. Antimicrobial agents derived from fatty acids. JAOCS 1984; 61(2):397–403.
83. Colarow L, Turini M, Teneberg S, et al. Characterization and biological activity of gangliosides in buffalo milk. Biochim Biophys Acta 2003; 1631(1):94–106.

27 Endocannabinoid Overactivity and Abdominal Obesity

Vincenzo Di Marzo

Endocannabinoid Research Group, Institute of Biomolecular Chemistry, National Research Council, Pozzuoli, Naples, Italy

Jean-Pierre Després

Québec Heart Institute, Hôpital Laval Research Centre and
Division of Kinesiology, Department of Social and Preventive Medicine, Laval University, Québec, QC, Canada

ENDOCANNABINOID OVERACTIVITY IN OBESITY AND HYPERGLYCEMIA: ANIMAL STUDIES

Although, as outlined in the previous chapters of this book, the functions of the endocannabinoid system in the peripheral control of metabolism under physiologic conditions are still not fully understood, there is increasing evidence for an important role played by endocannabinoids under conditions of unbalanced energy homeostasis, such as obesity and hyperglycemia. Several observations suggest that a dysregulation of endocannabinoid tone at CB_1 receptors occurs during such conditions: (*i*) a given dose of an antagonist at a certain receptor is expected to have higher efficacy in the presence of a higher tone of endogenous agonists of that receptor—this is also true to some extent for CB_1 antagonists like rimonabant (1), even though these compounds have been described to act in vitro as inverse agonists at high doses (and hence also produce effects opposite to those of agonists in the absence of endogenous agonists); (*ii*) blockade of CB_1 receptors inhibits food intake and decreases body weight more efficaciously in obese rodents than in lean animals (2,3); (*iii*) even in lean rodents, CB_1 receptor antagonists appear to be more efficacious in the presence of a demonstrated higher tone of the endocannabinoid system in the brain areas that control food intake, such as following brief periods of food deprivation or when animals are exposed to palatable foods (4). Thus, the higher efficacy against food intake observed in obese versus lean animals with CB_1 antagonists such as rimonabant or AM251 (2,5), and the sensitivity to these agents of obese rodents also in the absence of food deprivation (3), strongly suggest that a higher endocannabinoid tone stimulates food consumption in obesity. Accordingly, hypothalamic endocannabinoid levels are significantly higher in *ob/ob* and *db/db* mice or in Zucker rats (3), as it could have been expected from the fact that these rodents possess defective leptin signaling or levels, and also from the fact that leptin negatively controls EC levels (3). Importantly, daily systemic administration of CB_1 antagonists in obese rodents for several weeks causes a reduction of body weight that outlives the inhibition of food intake, which is significant for only ~1 week after the start of the treatment (6). Thus, it is possible that the part of the endocannabinoid system that controls the peripheral aspects of energy balance becomes more active with obesity and for a longer time as compared to what might happen in the brain.

The hypothesis of a peripherally dysregulated endocannabinoid system in obesity is supported by the observation that, in mice fed a high-fat diet [diet-induced obesity (DIO)], the development not only of obesity but also of its metabolic consequences, such as high triglyceride levels, low high-density lipoprotein cholesterol (HDL-C) levels, low adiponectin levels, hyperglycemia, and hyperinsulinemia, are prevented by congenital blockade of CB_1 receptor expression, as in CB_1-knockout mice, or chronic treatment with CB_1 antagonists (6–8). These effects seem to be largely independent from food intake since they are significantly less strong in wild-type mice undergoing food restriction similar to that observed following CB_1-blockade in pair-feeding experiments. Importantly, when CB_1 receptors are genetically or pharmacologically impaired, the dramatic alterations in the expression of several white and brown adipose tissue enzymes and proteins involved in metabolism and energy expenditure, usually found in DIO mice, are also not observed (9). These latter findings suggest that CB_1 signaling may become overactive in the white and brown adipocytes of obese individuals, thus

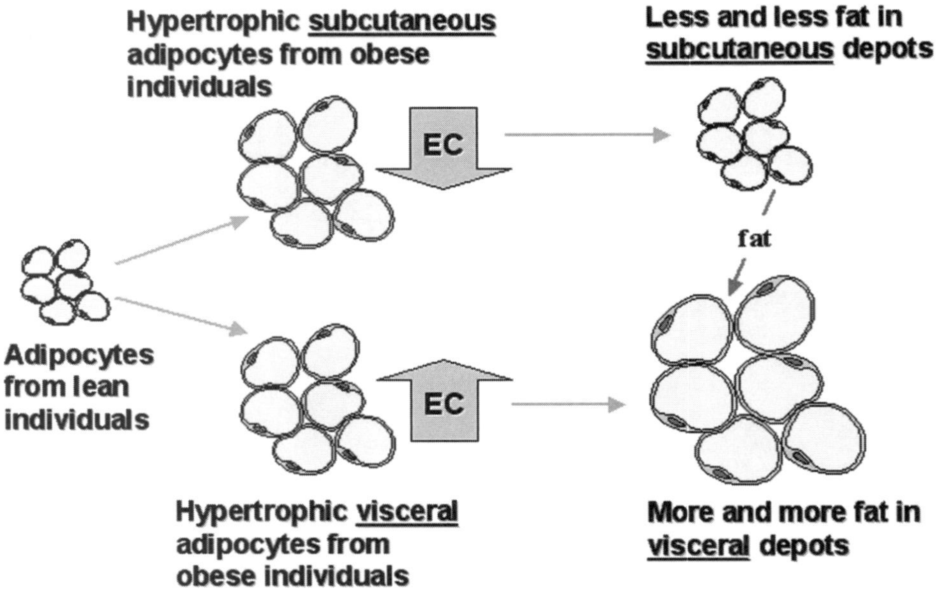

Figure 1 Schematic representation of how, given the proadipogenetic and pro-lipogenetic effects of the endocannabinoids (ECs), the "shift" of EC/CB_1 receptor tone from the subcutaneous to the visceral fat might result in more and more intra-abdominal adiposity, and less and less protective subcutaneous fat, with consequences such as inflamed visceral adipose tissue, reduced adiponectin, increased inflammatory cytokines, increased efflux of free fatty acids to the liver, and ectopic fat formation.

contributing to high-fat-diet–induced changes in the metabolic enzyme expression patterns of these cells. Indeed, a direct evidence of endocannabinoid upregulation has also been reported in the mouse epidydimal adipose tissue and in mouse adipocytes. For example, 3T3-F442A preadipocytes, when treated with a high concentration of insulin, differentiate into mature and eventually hypertrophic and insulin-resistant adipocytes, in which the levels of CB_1 receptors and 2-AG, but not those of anandamide, are significantly higher than in preadipocytes (10–12). The effect on 2-AG levels might result from changes in the regulation of 2-AG biosynthesis by PPAR-γ, occurring when passing from mature to hypertrophic adipocytes (11). Accordingly, enhanced levels of 2-AG, but not anandamide, have been reported in the epididymal fat of DIO mice compared with mice fed a normal diet (11). Overstimulation of CB_1 receptors in hypertrophic adipocytes appears to lead to inhibition of adiponectin expression (10,11). This explains why CB_1 receptor antagonism causes elevation of adiponectin expression in adipocytes more effectively in obese than in lean mice (10), and the expression of several adiponectin-dependent genes, which is strongly dysregulated in the adipose tissue of DIO mice, is restored to that of a lean phenotype following blockade of CB_1 receptors (9). Importantly, unlike the epididymal fat, the subcutaneous fat of DIO mice exhibits lower levels of both anandamide and 2-AG (13). In view of the pro-adipogenetic and pro-lipogenetic effects of CB_1 receptor stimulation (see previous chapters of this book), this "shift" in endocannabinoid activity from the subcutaneous towards the epididymal fat (and intra-abdominal fat in humans, see later) might lead to more and more accumulation of nonsubcutaneous and easily inflamed fat, thus possibly contributing to ectopic fat formation and further insulin resistance (Fig. 1).

Evidence suggests that the levels of either endocannabinoids or CB_1 receptors, or both, are also permanently upregulated in other peripheral organs and tissues of obese animals and humans (14). Increased levels of both CB_1 and anandamide were found in the livers of DIO mice (15). This phenomenon was suggested to underlie in part the occurrence, particularly during overweight and obesity, of hepatosteatosis (fatty liver), which is not only the first step towards the development of nonalcoholic steatohepatitis, but is now also considered an important cardiovascular risk factor accompanying insulin resistance and dyslipoproteinemia and causing. Accordingly, recent data showed that oral treatment of obese Zucker rats with rimonabant 30 mg/kg/day for 8 days abolished obesity-associated hepatic steatosis and related features of metabolic syndrome, including inflammation [elevated plasma levels of tumor necrosis factor-α

(TNF-α)], dyslipidemia, and hypoadiponectinemia, and concomitantly improved dyslipidemia by both decreasing plasma levels of triglycerides, free fatty acids, and total cholesterol, and increasing the HDL-C/low-density lipoprotein cholesterol (LDL-C) ratio (16). CB_1 antagonism also reduced hepatomegaly, elevation of plasma levels of enzyme markers of hepatic damage (alanine aminotransferase, γ-glutamyltransferase, and alkaline phosphatase), and the high levels of circulating TNF-α associated with the eventual development of steatohepatitis. Most of these effects were induced only to a smaller extent by diet restriction, pointing to the existence of direct effects of CB_1 receptor antagonism in the liver (16).

In RIN-m5F rat insulinoma pancreatic β-cells, where both CB_1 and CB_2 receptors are expressed and a high glucose "pulse" elevates both anandamide and 2-AG levels, insulin keeps anandamide and 2-AG levels under negative control when the cells are maintained at a relatively low concentration of glucose. However, under conditions mimicking hyperglycemia, insulin not only does not inhibit glucose-induced endocannabinoid levels per se but it also stimulates these levels (11). Accordingly, enhanced levels of both anandamide and 2-AG were observed in the pancreas of hyperglycaemic DIO mice as compared with mice fed a normal diet (11,13). In view of the preliminary data described in previous chapters of this book, this "pancreatic overactivity" of the endocannabinoid system might impact on insulin and, perhaps, also on glucagon and somatostatin levels, and, hence, on glucose utilization and metabolism.

Very recent data indicate that endocannabinoid upregulation might also occur very early after the beginning of a high-fat diet in the soleus muscle (17). Furthermore, a significant upregulation of CB_1 receptor expression seems to occur in the skeletal muscle of DIO mice (18). This finding, together with the observation that CB_1 receptor blockade in obese mice causes enhanced glucose uptake by the soleus muscle and increases oxygen consumption (19), might suggest that the overstimulation of CB_1 receptors by the elevated endocannabinoid levels found in the skeletal muscle might tonically inhibit insulin sensitivity and glucose uptake and utilization. Whether, however, CB_1 stimulation inhibits insulin sensitivity in the skeletal muscle is yet to be investigated.

These observations in animal models of obesity and hyperglycemia support the existence of a peripherally overactive endocannabinoid system accompanying, and very likely contributing to, the deleterious consequences of obesity, and substantiate the possibility that CB_1 receptor antagonism can be used for the treatment of obesity-associated metabolic disorders with effects that go beyond those obtainable with dietary restriction and weight loss alone.

ENDOCANNABINOID DYSREGULATION IN ABDOMINAL OBESITY AND HYPERGLYCEMIA: HUMAN STUDIES

Data are accumulating to suggest the occurrence of a dysregulation of endocannabinoid signaling also in humans, in association not so much with obesity per se but rather with high visceral adiposity and hyperglycemia. In fact, early findings in women with obesity caused by conditions such as binge-eating disorder (20) or menopause (21), in whom the blood levels of anandamide or anandamide and 2-AG, respectively, were found to be significantly higher than those in age-matched normoweight volunteers, were soon followed by studies that have better defined the phenotype of the overweight/obese subject with altered circulating or adipose tissue levels of endocannabinoids. In agreement with the aforementioned observations in DIO mice, significantly higher of 2-AG, but not anandamide, levels were detected in the visceral, but not in the subcutaneous, fat of obese patients (11). In a recent study by Pagano and coworkers (22), the hypothesis of a dysregulated endocannabinoid system in the adipose tissue was confirmed by showing that, as again observed in mice (13), both the subcutaneous and visceral abdominal fat of obese patients exhibit higher CB_1 receptor expression and endocannabinoid turnover (in terms of the expression of endocannabinoid biosynthetic and degrading enzymes) than that observed in analogous tissues from lean individuals, whereas a reduction was instead observed in the subcutaneous gluteal fat. As mentioned above for the studies in mice, this phenomenon, in view of the prolipogenetic role of the endocannabinoid system in the adipose tissue, might eventually result in more fat being stored in abdominal depots and less in subcutaneous depots, with potential deleterious consequences on cardiometabolic risk factors (23).

Human peripheral endocannabinoid overactivity does not seem to be just a feature of obesity per se. In nonobese [$28\ kg/m^2 <$ body mass index (BMI) $< 32\ kg/m^2$] patients with type 2 diabetes and only partially corrected hyperglycemia, the blood levels of both anandamide and 2-AG were significantly higher than those in age-, BMI-, and gender-matched nondiabetic volunteers (11). It has also been recently shown that obesity and type 2 diabetes appear to be independently associated with high levels of circulating endocannabinoids, since obese subjects with type 2 diabetes exhibit a further elevation of plasmatic 2-AG levels with respect to nonobese patients with this metabolic disorder (L. Van Gaal and V. Di Marzo, unpublished observations).

Two recent independent studies established a direct relationship between intra-abdominal adiposity (IAA) and high circulating 2-AG levels (24,25). When examining two cohorts of obese patients with quite different anthropometric features and past histories of medications, both studies identified a strong direct correlation between the concentration of 2-AG, but not of anandamide, in the blood and the amount of IAA determined by computer tomography. More importantly, high 2-AG levels were also directly correlated with several cardiometabolic risk factors, including low HDL-C levels, high triglyceride levels, and low insulin sensitivity and glucose tolerance and, in one of the two studies (25), also with low plasma adiponectin levels. These findings represent the first direct evidence of a link between IAA-related cardiometabolic risks and peripheral endocannabinoid dysregulation.

One might wonder how the measured plasma levels of endocannabinoids relate to the possible activation state of CB_1 receptors in peripheral organs, since it is known that these mediators are not hormones, and usually act locally in a paracrine or even autocrine manner. It can be suggested that the plasmatic levels of endocannabinoids represent either (*i*) a "spillover" effect, that is, they reflect the overproduction of these compounds in one or more peripheral tissues or (*ii*) an overactivity in blood cells, which do produce and degrade immuno-modulatory endocannabinoids and might play a role in the immune-inflammatory response of obese individuals. The former hypothesis is supported by (*i*) the observation that plasma concentrations of anandamide and, particularly, 2-AG are 1 to 2 orders of magnitude lower than those usually found in tissues and (*ii*) the finding that in cirrhotic individuals in whom an overproduction of endocannabinoids seems to occur in the liver, the levels of 2-AG in the sovra-hepatic vein are almost 3-fold higher than those in peripheral blood (P. Caraceni and V. Di Marzo, unpublished observations), thus suggesting that "spill-over" might occur at least from this organ.

POSSIBLE CAUSES OF ENDOCANNABINOID OVERACTIVITY IN OBESITY AND HYPERGLYCEMIA

What are the causes of the overactive endocannabinoid signaling observed in obesity and hyperglycemia? Is this phenomenon a consequence or a cause of these metabolic disorders, or both? The DIO mice studies by Starowicz et al. (13) and the human studies by Pagano et al. (22), clearly point to the aberrant expression/function of endocannabinoid biosynthetic and degradation enzymes as a possible cause of tissue-specific alterations in endocannabinoid levels. This hypothesis is also supported by studies showing reduction of the activity or expression of the endocannabinoid degrading enzyme, fatty acid amide hydrolase (FAAH), in the liver of DIO mice (15) or in the subcutaneous fat of obese patients (21,24). This can be due, in turn, to the malfunctioning of leptin and/or insulin signaling, which typically accompany obesity and IAA. Indeed, in normoweight and normoglycemic volunteers, the blood concentration of anandamide was found to decrease immediately following a meal (11) in agreement with a possible downregulation by both leptin and insulin on anandamide levels. Accordingly, both leptin and insulin upregulate (26,27), whereas glucocorticoids (the levels of which are also elevated in obesity) downregulate (28) the expression of FAAH. Obesity and hyperglycemia might thus override the negative control exerted by leptin and insulin on endocannabinoid tissue concentrations at the central and peripheral levels, respectively [although a recent study carried out in mice showed how central leptin also controls endocannabinoid levels in the mouse white adipose tissue (29)]. Since endocannabinoid levels are determined not only by the activity of biosynthesising and degrading enzymes but also by the levels of their phospholipid-derived biosynthetic precursors, it is possible also that, as reviewed in another chapter of this book, the presence of certain polyunsaturated fatty acid precursors rather than others in the diet might contribute to the development of aberrant endocannabinoid concentrations in certain tissues.

Genetic predisposition to dysfunctions in endocannabinoid signaling might also be a cause of endocannabinoid dysregulation. A study carried out by Sipe and coworkers pointed to a strong correlation, in white and African-Americans but not Asian-Americans, between a BMI >25 kg/m^2 and a phenotypic missense mutation of FAAH (P129T), which is known to lead to a more rapid FAAH degradation (30). This would suggest that a general malfunctioning of the metabolism of endocannabinoids is a hallmark of visceral obesity. However, Jensen (31) could not confirm these results in a larger population of white Americans. Correlations have also been recently found between CB_1 receptor gene polymorphisms and obesity (32,33) or leanness (34). However, no functional studies have been carried out to assess whether these point mutations in the *Cnr1* gene result in a change of the expression or function (e.g., at the level of G-protein coupling) of the CB_1 receptor.

CONCLUSIONS: CONSEQUENCES OF ENDOCANNABINOID DYSREGULATION IN ABDOMINAL OBESITY

If, as implied in the present article, the dysregulation of endocannabinoid levels and CB_1 receptor activity is not a mere epi-phenomenon accompanying abdominal obesity, but instead contributes to this disorder and its typical metabolic and cardiovascular consequences, one should see, in both animal models of obesity and in abdominally obese humans affected by the metabolic syndrome, an amelioration of these dysfunctions following prolonged treatment with CB_1 receptor antagonists. While the results of preclinical studies aimed at addressing this possibility have been reviewed in some of the previous chapters, and have indeed suggested a causative role for the endocannabinoid system in metabolic disorders in laboratory animals, the next chapters in this book will focus on the current and future uses of CB_1 receptor antagonists in the clinic.

REFERENCES

1. Rinaldi-Carmona M, Barth F, Heaulme M, et al. SR141716A, a potent and selective antagonist of the brain cannabinoid receptor. FEBS Lett 1994; 350:240–244.
2. Chambers AP, Sharkey KA, Koopmans HS. Cannabinoid (CB)1 receptor antagonist, AM 251, causes a sustained reduction of daily food intake in the rat. Physiol Behav 2004; 82:863–869.
3. Di Marzo V, Goparaju SK, Wang L, et al. Leptin-regulated endocannabinoids are involved in maintaining food intake. Nature 2001; 410:822–825.
4. Kirkham TC, Williams CM, Fezza F, et al. Endocannabinoid levels in rat limbic forebrain and hypothalamus in relation to fasting, feeding and satiation: Stimulation of eating by 2-arachidonoyl glycerol. Br J Pharmacol 2002; 136:550–557.
5. McLaughlin PJ, Winston K, Swezey L, et al. The cannabinoid CB1 antagonists SR 141716A and AM 251 suppress food intake and food-reinforced behavior in a variety of tasks in rats. Behav Pharmacol 2003; 14:583–588.
6. Ravinet Trillou C, Arnone M, Delgorge C, et al. Anti-obesity effect of SR141716, a CB1 receptor antagonist, in diet-induced obese mice. Am J Physiol Regul Integr Comp Physiol 2003; 284;345–353.
7. Ravinet Trillou C, Delgorge C, Menet C, et al. CB1 cannabinoid receptor knockout in mice leads to leanness, resistance to diet-induced obesity and enhanced leptin sensitivity. Int J Obes Relat Metab Disord 2004; 28:640–648.
8. Poirier B, Bidouard JP, Cadrouvele C, et al. The anti-obesity effect of rimonabant is associated with an improved serum lipid profile. Diabetes Obes Metab 2005; 7:65–72.
9. Jbilo O, Ravinet-Trillou C, Arnone M, et al. The CB1 receptor antagonist rimonabant reverses the diet-induced obesity phenotype through the regulation of lipolysis and energy balance. FASEB J 2005; 19:1567–1569.
10. Bensaid M, Gary-Bobo M, Esclangon A, et al. The cannabinoid CB1 receptor antagonist SR141716 increases Acrp30 mRNA expression in adipose tissue of obese fa/fa rats and in cultured adipocyte cells. Mol Pharmacol 2003; 63:908–914.
11. Matias I, Gonthier MP, Orlando P, et al. Regulation, function and dysregulation of endocannabinoids in models of adipose and β-pancreatic cells and in obesity and hyperglycemia. J Clin Endocrinol Metab 2006; 91:3171–3180.
12. Roche R, Hoareau L, Bes-Houtmann S, et al. Presence of the cannabinoid receptors, CB1 and CB2, in human omental and subcutaneous adipocytes. Histochem Cell Biol 2006; 4:1–11.
13. Starowicz K, Cristino L, Matias I, et al. Endocannabinoid dysregulation in the pancreas and adipose tissue of mice fed a high fat diet. Obesity 2008; 16:553–565.
14. Di Marzo V, Matias I. Endocannabinoid control of food intake and energy balance. Nat Neurosci 2005; 8:585–589.

15. Osei-Hyiaman D, DePetrillo M, Pacher P, et al. Endocannabinoid activation at hepatic CB1 receptors stimulates fatty acid synthesis and contributes to diet-induced obesity. J Clin Invest 2005; 115:1298–1305.
16. Gary-Bobo M, Elachouri G, Gallas JF, et al. Rimonabant reduces obesity-associated hepatic steatosis and features of metabolic syndrome in obese Zucker fa/fa rats. Hepatology 2007; 46:122–129.
17. Matias I, Petrosino S, Racioppi A, et al. Dysregulation of peripheral endocannabinoid levels in hyperglycemia and obesity: Effect of high fat diets. Mol Cell Endocrinol 2008; 286(1–2 Suppl. 1):S66–S78.
18. Pagotto U, Marsicano G, Cota D, et al. The emerging role of the endocannabinoid system in endocrine regulation and energy balance. Endocr Rev 2006; 27:73–100.
19. Liu YL, Connoley IP, Wilson CA, et al. Effects of the cannabinoid CB1 receptor antagonist SR141716 on oxygen consumption and soleus muscle glucose uptake in Lep(ob)/Lep(ob) mice. Int J Obes (Lond) 2005; 29:183–187.
20. Monteleone P, Matias I, Martiadis V, et al. Blood levels of the endocannabinoid anandamide are increased in anorexia nervosa and in binge-eating disorder, but not in bulimia nervosa. Neuropsychopharmacology 2005; 30:1216–1221.
21. Engeli S, Bohnke J, Feldpausch M, et al. Activation of the peripheral endocannabinoid system in human obesity. Diabetes 2005; 54:2838–2843.
22. Pagano C, Pilon C, Calcagno A, et al. The endogenous cannabinoid system stimulates glucose uptake in human fat cells via phosphatidylinositol 3-kinase and calcium-dependent mechanisms. J Clin Endocrinol Metab 2007; 92:4810–4819.
23. Despres JP, Lemieux I. Abdominal obesity and metabolic syndrome. Nature 2006; 444:881–887.
24. Bluher M, Engeli S, Kloting N, et al. Dysregulation of the peripheral and adipose tissue endocannabinoid system in human abdominal obesity. Diabetes 2006; 55:3053–3060.
25. Cote M, Matias I, Lemieux I, et al. Circulating endocannabinoid levels, abdominal adiposity and related cardiometabolic risk factors in obese men. Int J Obes (Lond) 2007; 31:692–699.
26. Maccarrone M, Di Rienzo M, Finazzi-Agro A, et al. Leptin activates the anandamide hydrolase promoter in human T lymphocytes through STAT3. J Biol Chem 2003; 278:13318–13324.
27. Murdolo G, Kempf K, Hammarstedt A, et al. Insulin differentially modulates the peripheral endocannabinoid system in human subcutaneous abdominal adipose tissue from lean and obese individuals. J Endocrinol Invest 2007; 30(8):RC17–RC21.
28. Waleh NS, Cravatt BF, Apte-Deshpande A, et al. Transcriptional regulation of the mouse fatty acid amide hydrolase gene. Gene 2002; 291:203–210.
29. Buettner C, Muse ED, Cheng A, et al. Leptin controls adipose tissue lipogenesis via central, STAT3-independent mechanisms. Nat Med 2008; 14:667–675.
30. Sipe JC, Waalen J, Gerber A, et al. Overweight and obesity associated with a missense polymorphism in fatty acid amide hydrolase (FAAH). Int J Obes (Lond) 2005; 29:755–759.
31. Jensen MD. Potential role of new therapies in modifying cardiovascular risk in overweight patients with metabolic risk factors. Obesity (Silver Spring) 2006; 14(Suppl. 3):143S–149S.
32. Russo P, Strazzullo P, Cappuccio FP, et al. Genetic variations at the endocannabinoid type 1 receptor gene (CNR1) are associated with obesity phenotypes in men. J Clin Endocrinol Metab 2007; 92:2382–2386.
33. Peeters A, Beckers S, Mertens I, et al. The G1422A variant of the cannabinoid receptor gene (CNR1) is associated with abdominal adiposity in obese men. Endocrine 2007; 31:138–141.
34. Gazzerro P, Caruso MG, Notarnicola M, et al. Association between cannabinoid type-1 receptor polymorphism and body mass index in a southern Italian population. Int J Obes (Lond) 2007; 31:908–912.

28 CB_1 Antagonism in the Management of Abdominal Obesity

Luc F. Van Gaal
Department of Endocrinology, Diabetology and Metabolism, Antwerp University Hospital, Antwerp, Belgium

INTRODUCTION

Over the last few decades, an epidemic growth in the prevalence of obesity has been experienced with an estimation of over 1 billion cases (1). Obesity, in particular abdominal obesity, is a well-established risk predictor to the development of more life-threatening diseases such as type 2 diabetes and cardiovascular disease (CVD), due to its close association with multiple cardiometabolic risk factors including insulin resistance, hyperglycemia, dyslipidaemia, alterations in haemostasis and fibrinolysis, and inflammation (2–7). Recent evidence from INTERHEART, the Nurses Health, the Heart Outcomes Protection Evaluation (HOPE), the Paris Prospective, and the IDEA survey studies has shown abdominal obesity to be an independent risk factor for CVD and type 2 diabetes (8–12). The current health threat posed by abdominal obesity is largely due to excess intra-abdominal adipose tissue, a highly metabolically active endocrine organ. Intra-abdominal adiposity (IAA), through the secretion of excess free fatty acids and altered adipokine release, provides an indirect link to the progression of atherosclerosis and CVD (13–15).

CVD continues to be the leading cause of global mortality, highlighting a significant shortfall in current treatment options (16). Despite the well-known potent effects of statin therapy, it has been shown that there exists an important residual risk among diabetics, in particular. New therapies are therefore desperately needed in order to improve cardiovascular outcomes and stop or delay the growing impact on health issues. Obesity as such also contributes significantly to the global economic health burden.

Lifestyle changes such as improved diet and increased physical exercise continue to be the primary treatment option for patients at risk aiming for 5% to 10% weight loss (17). However, in the face of the growing epidemic of abdominal obesity, diabetes, and the metabolic syndrome, recently highlighted (12) in a large worldwide survey (the IDEA study), the current clinical challenge is to discover new treatments that focus on early intervention and tackle multiple cardiometabolic risk factors, associated with intra-abdominal obesity. Cannabinoid receptor $(CB)_1$ antagonism is one such option and operates by regulating overactivity of the endocannabinoid system, which is commonly observed in those with abdominal obesity and associated risk factors. The endocannabinoid system, under normal conditions, plays an important role in the central regulation of the rewarding properties of food and the control of energy balance (18), and in the peripheral activity of adipocytes, hepatocytes, and β cells (18,19). It has recently been shown that diabetic patients are also characterized by abdominal fat accumulation (Table 1) (20) and an overstimulated endocannabinoid system.

The activity of the endocannabinoid system has been under investigation since the 1960s and a number of comprehensive reviews have been published over recent years describing its location, activity, and therapeutic potential (21–22). This chapter summarizes the evidence supporting CB_1 antagonism of the overactive endocannabinoid system as an effective treatment option for abdominal obesity and its related cardiometabolic risk factors, mainly in patients at risk, such as type 2 diabetic patients with the metabolic syndrome.

ENDOCANNABINOID RECEPTORS: A KEY TARGET FOR ABDOMINAL OBESITY

The endocannabinoid system is a lipid signaling system which plays a key role in the central and peripheral regulation of energy balance and abdominal fat accumulation, as well as in lipid and glucose metabolism (22–25). The system comprises endocannabinoids, which

Table 1 Abdominal Fat Accumulation in Diabetic Patients

	Nondiabetic women ($n = 30$)	Diabetic women ($n = 30$)	p-Value
Age (yr)	62 ± 7	63 ± 7	0.458
Weight (kg)	82.5 ± 10.8	82.6 ± 10.7	0.958
BMI (kg/m^2)	32.4 ± 4.0	32.4 ± 3.7	0.968
Total fat mass (%)	47.0 ± 5.5	45.1 ± 7.9	0.275
Total abdominal fat (cm^2)	706 ± 120	684 ± 151	0.526
Subcutaneous fat (cm^2)	519 ± 109	490 ± 217	0.524
Visceral fat (cm^2)	188 ± 51	227 ± 76	0.022

For comparable values of age, weight, BMI, total fat-mass percentage, total abdominal fat, and subcutaneous fat, visceral fat was significantly higher in the diabetic subjects ($p < 0.05$). *Source*: Adapted from Ref. 20.

are endogenous lipids derived from arachidonic acid, for example, anandamide (AEA) and 2-arachidonoylglycerol (2-AG), and CB_1 and CB_2 receptors (26–28). Endocannabinoids are synthesized on demand from lipid precursors in postsynaptic cells, inhibit neurotransmitter release by activating presynaptically located cannabinoid receptors, and are then rapidly inactivated by hydrolysis (27,29).

Until recently, the majority of data available surrounding the existence of the overactive endocannabinoid system in obesity was derived from experimental studies in animals. Research has therefore provided the definitive link between the endocannabinoid system and obesity, highlighting a need to prove this link in humans. The findings have now been expanded to include the discovery of a peripheral endocannabinoid system which becomes overactive in the obese state in humans (30). Engeli et al. showed that CB_1 receptor expression was evident in human adipose tissue, as well as in other organs relating to the pathogenesis of obesity and obesity-associated metabolic disorders such as reproductive and gastrointestinal (GI) tract tissue (30). Furthermore, Matias et al. demonstrated that circulating levels of AEA and 2-AG were elevated in obese patients compared with lean patients ($p < 0.05$ vs. lean) (31), while higher levels were found in patients with type 2 diabetes compared with healthy patients ($p < 0.01$ and $p < 0.005$ vs. controls for AEA and 2-AG, respectively) (31). Obese patients were found to have significantly higher endocannabinoid levels in their visceral fat compared with their subcutaneous fat ($p < 0.01$ vs. visceral), underlining the potential health implications associated with this particular fat distribution (31). Additional evidence supporting a correlation between visceral fat accumulation and the dysregulation of the endocannabinoid system has recently been provided by Blüher and colleagues (32). Among other findings, the authors reported that circulating 2-AG levels were significantly higher in viscerally obese patients ($p < 0.05$ vs. subcutaneous, $p < 0.01$ vs. lean) and that CB_1 mRNA expression was higher in visceral compared with subcutaneous adipose tissue in all patients ($p < 0.05$) (32).

CB_1 ANTAGONISM REDUCES ABDOMINAL OBESITY AND ASSOCIATED RISK FACTORS

The relationship between endocannabinoid system overactivity and obesity has indicated a potential therapeutic target for addressing abdominal obesity and its associated risk factors. Extensive animal studies have shown the beneficial effects of CB_1 antagonism in reducing food intake and body weight.

The rimonabant-induced body-weight loss reported in obese mice is also accompanied by normalization of insulin resistance and of plasma leptin, insulin and free fatty acid levels (25,33).

In contrast to the central effects of CB_1, in the periphery, selective CB_1 antagonism has a marked effect on adipocytes. CB_1 antagonism with rimonabant improves lipolysis, increases energy expenditure and improves the regulation of glucose homeostasis through its effects in adipose tissue (18,34). Rimonabant also impacts on adipokine levels in adipose tissue. Increased adiponectin mRNA levels in both obese (*fa/fa*) and lean rats (35), and $CB_1^{+/+}$ mice, but not in $CB_1^{-/-}$ mice, following treatment with rimonabant, confirm that this effect is CB_1-receptor mediated (35). In animal studies, a selective reduction in abdominal fat accumulation was found along with other peripheral effects in CB_1 knockout mice (18).

CB_1 ANTAGONISM IN THE CLINICAL SETTING

The cardiometabolic benefits of CB_1 antagonism have also been examined in clinical trials with the first selective CB_1 blocker, rimonabant. At present, rimonabant is the only CB_1 blocker to have reached late-stage clinical development with results derived from the Phase III Rimonabant in Obesity (RIO) program, the SERENADE, STRADIVARIUS, and ADAGIO trial.

The RIO program effects of rimonabant on multiple cardiometabolic risk factors including abdominal obesity, HDL-cholesterol, triglycerides, blood pressure, and HbA_{1C} (in diabetic patients) were evaluated in four large-scale studies (RIO-Diabetes, RIO-Lipids, RIO-Europe, and RIO-North America), which randomized more than 6600 patients for up to 2 years. The RIO-Diabetes study (36) investigated the efficacy and safety of rimonabant in overweight/obese patients with type 2 diabetes suboptimally controlled by metformin or sulphonylurea monotherapy [HbA_{1C} 6.5–10.0%, FPG 5.6–15.0 mmol/L (100–270 mg/dL)] and the RIO-Lipids study (37) investigated rimonabant in overweight/obese patients with untreated dyslipidaemia as defined by fasting triglycerides [1.7–7.9 mmol/L (150–700 mg/dL), and total-cholesterol:HDL-cholesterol ratio >4.5 (women) or >5.0 (men)]. Two other studies, RIO-Europe (38) and RIO-North America (39), investigated rimonabant in overweight/obese patients with or without hypertension and/or dyslipidaemia. The primary endpoint of all the four studies was the change in body weight at 1 year (Table 2; Figs. 1 and 2).

Table 2 presents a summary of the key results from the RIO trial program. In all the four studies, patients achieved significant improvements in body weight, abdominal fat reduction expressed by changes in waist circumference, and lipid parameters (all $p < 0.001$ vs. placebo) following 1 year of treatment with rimonabant 20 mg/day.

Improvements in cardiometabolic risk parameters were maintained during the second year of the RIO-Europe and RIO-North America trials (39).

Patients in the RIO-Diabetes study population achieved less reduction in waist circumference than those in the other three studies (36). This is not surprising in light of previous reports which state that weight loss and maintenance of weight loss in type 2 diabetic patients are generally more difficult than in nondiabetic individuals due, in part, to the concomitant weight gain produced by most antidiabetic medications (sulfonylureas, thiazolidinediones, and insulin, in particular) (40–42). However, the placebo subtracted findings are close to the results achieved in nondiabetic subjects; this finding was confirmed in the SERENADE study in therapy naive type 2 diabetic patients.

Improvements were also reported in a number of other metabolic parameters following treatment with rimonabant 20 mg/day. In the RIO-Diabetes trial, rimonabant evoked a significant reduction in HbA_{1c} from a baseline of 7.3% [$-0.6 \pm 0.8\%$; $p < 0.001$ vs. placebo (0.1 ± 1.0)] and in the RIO-Lipids trial, significant reductions were reported in C-reactive protein [-0.9 mg/L; $p = 0.02$ vs. placebo (-0.4)]. Systolic blood pressure was significantly reduced in the RIO-Diabetes and RIO-Lipids trials ($p < 0.05$ vs. placebo) (36,37), while fasting insulin levels ($p < 0.05$ vs. placebo) were reduced in nondiabetic patients and insulin resistance (HOMA-IR; $p < 0.05$ vs. placebo) improved in all the four trials. The RIO-Lipids trial also reported a significant shift towards a less atherogenic low-density lipoprotein (LDL) subclass profile and a 46% increase in levels of adiponectin (37). Rimonabant has been shown to produce consistent improvements in lipid and glucose parameters irrespective of concomitant statin treatment (43).

The rimonabant-induced effects beyond those attributable to weight loss alone were assessed using standard regression methodology, in which weight loss was introduced as a covariate (analysis of covariance, ANCOVA). Approximately half of the improvements seen with rimonabant on cardiometabolic risk factors often associated with visceral fat accumulation such as HDL-cholesterol, triglycerides, adiponectin, and HbA_{1C} are a direct result of antagonism of peripheral CB_1 receptors in metabolically active tissues such as the liver, adipose tissue and skeletal muscle (37–40).

Table 2 Rimonabant Significantly Improves Key Cardiometabolic Parameters After 1 Year of Treatment[a]

Change from baseline	RIO-Diabetes Placebo ($n = 348$)	RIO-Diabetes Rimonabant 20 mg ($n = 339$)	RIO-Lipids Placebo ($n = 342$)	RIO-Lipids Rimonabant 20 mg ($n = 346$)	RIO-Europe Placebo ($n = 305$)	RIO-Europe Rimonabant 20 mg ($n = 599$)	RIO-North America Placebo ($n = 607$)	RIO-North America Rimonabant 20 mg ($n = 1219$)
Body weight (kg)	−1.4 ± 3.6	−5.3 ± 5.2[b]	−1.5 ± 5.0	−6.9 ± 6.1[b]	−1.8 ± 6.4	−6.6 ± 7.2[b]	−1.6 ± 5.7	−6.3 ± 7.1[b]
Waist circumference (cm)	−1.9 ± 5.5	−5.2 ± 6.1[b]	−2.4 ± 5.7	−7.1 ± 6.8[b]	−2.4 ± 6.9	−6.5 ± 7.4[b]	−2.5 ± 6.9	−6.1 ± 7.1[b]
HDL-cholesterol (%)	+7.1 ± 13.5	+15.4 ± 17.4[b]	+11.0 ± 15.8	+19.1 ± 20.9[b]	+13.4 ± 18.3	+22.3 ± 20.7[b]	+5.4 ± 15.4	+12.6 ± 17.2[b]
Triglycerides (%)	+7.3 ± 43.0	−9.1 ± 44.3[b]	−0.2 ± 38.7	−12.6 ± 41.2[b]	+8.3 ± 43.0	−6.8 ± 34.4[b]	+7.9 ± 45.2	−5.3 ± 39.8[b]

[a]Data presented are from the ITT population [ANOVA of 1 year (LOCF method) (SD)]

[b]$p < 0.001$ vs. placebo.

Abbreviations: HDL, high-density lipoprotein; ITT, intention-to-treat; LOCF, last observation carried forward; SD, standard deviation (36–39).

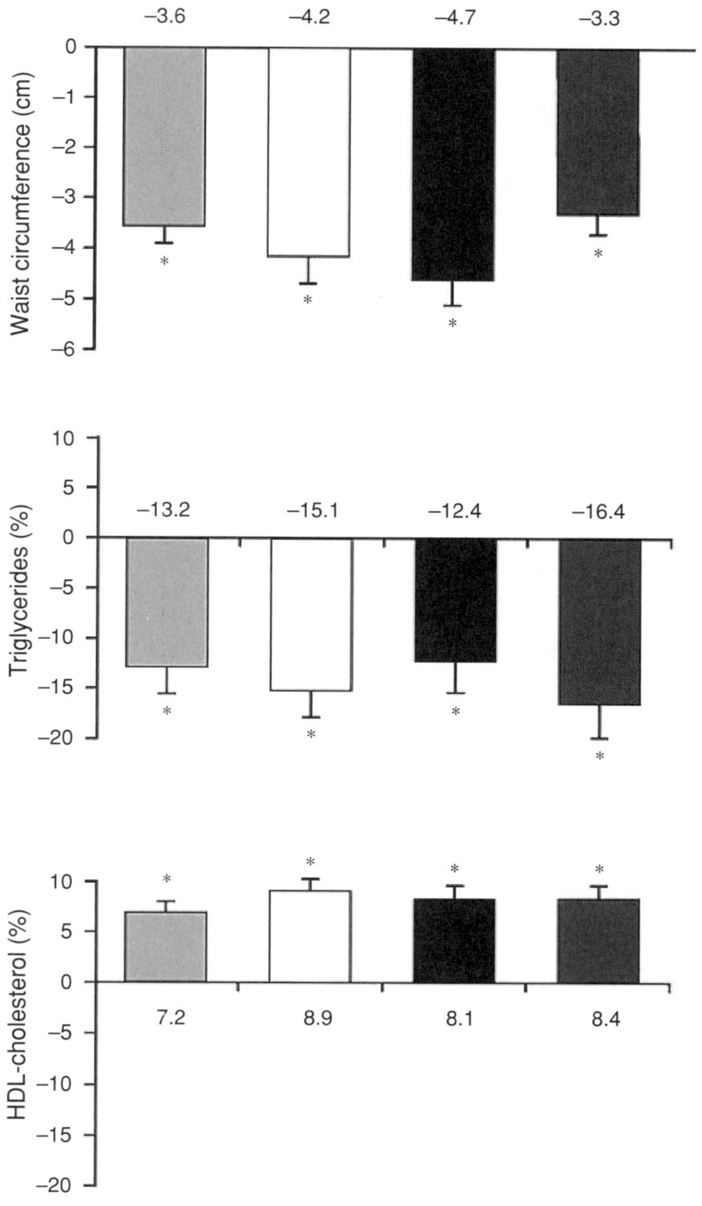

Figure 1 RIO-Program: placebo-subtracted mean change in cm and % for metabolic parameters at 1 year. Data presented from the ITT population [ANOVA of 1-year data (LOCF method)] (36–39); mean (±SEM); HDL-cholesterol, high-density lipoprotein-cholesterol. $^{*}p > 0.001$, $^{**}p > 0.05$.

Preliminary data from SERENADE were released at the International Diabetes Federation Meeting in December 2006 (44). Rimonabant 20 mg/day was reported to improve glycaemic control with the additional benefits of reducing weight and improving the levels of other metabolic risk factors such as HDL-cholesterol and triglycerides in treatment-naive type 2 diabetes patients. Results from SERENADE (44) and RIO-Diabetes (36), taken together, support a potential role for rimonabant in the future management of type 2 diabetes.

Safety

Rimonabant was shown to be generally safe and well tolerated in the RIO program with the majority of adverse events (AE) being mild and transient and occurring early in the treatment

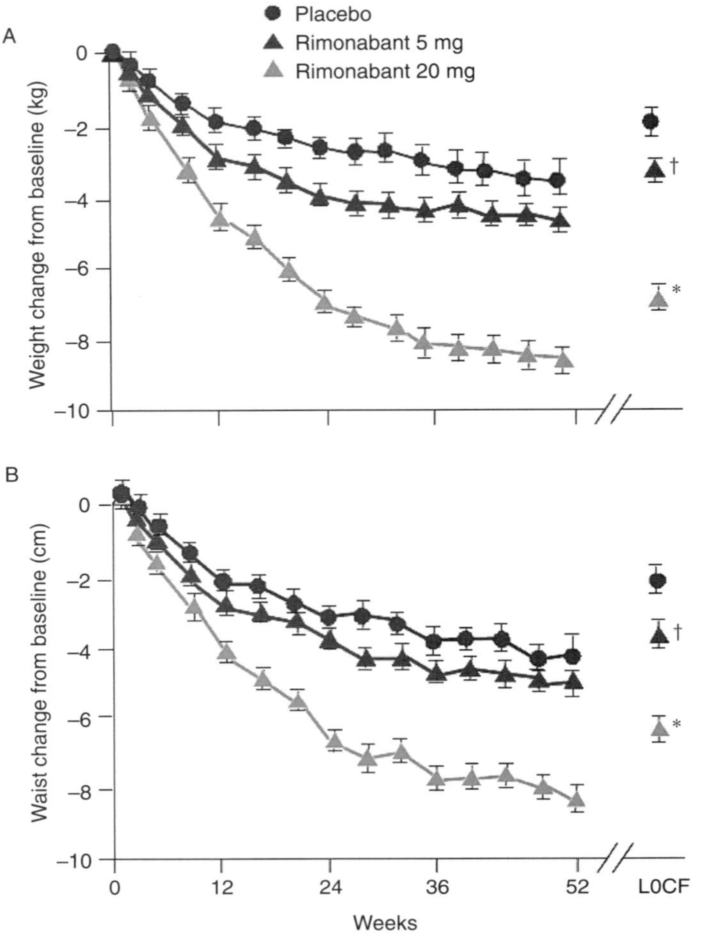

Figure 2 Rio-Program: changes from baseline in bodyweight and waist circumference after 1 year. Changes from baseline in bodyweight **(A)** and waist circumference **(B)**. Data are mean (SE) values for patients completing each scheduled visit, and LOCF (values for the full ITT population with the last observations carried forward). $^{*}p > 0.001$ versus placebo. $^{**}p = 0.002$ versus placebo (38).

period. The most common AEs affecting more than 5% of patients receiving rimonabant 20 mg were nausea, dizziness, diarrhoea, anxiety, and insomnia. AEs resulting in discontinuation across all the four trials during year 1 of treatment were depressive disorders, nausea, mood alterations with depressive symptoms, anxiety, and dizziness. These AE's were lees frequent during the second year of observation and not different from placebo (39,45).

Can CB_1 Antagonism Selectively Reduce Abdominal Obesity?

The question arises whether visceral fat as a target for cannabinoid blockade can be substantiated by hard outcome data. The RIO program data show the important reduction in waist circumference, later confirmed in the SERENADE and STRADIVARIUS study (46). Recently, the ADAGIO study was presented (http://www.sanofi-aventis.se/live/se/sv/layout.jsp?cnt=52DC240C-CD09–4B62–87DC-C3FDD0B8AA43). An imaging substudy using computed tomography (CT) for visceral fat estimation was performed to test whether rimonabant could induce a preferential loss of visceral fat. The study was conducted in patients with high abdominal obesity and dyslipidemia. After 12 months of treatment, the results confirmed the consistent effects of rimonabant on several markers of cardiometabolic risk, such as HDL-cholesterol, triglyceride, and adiponectin improvement. In the CT analysis, treatment with rimonabant led to preferential mobilization of visceral adipose tissue compared to placebo (reduction of 10.1% vs. placebo), which was greater than the loss of subcutaneous fat (decrease of 5.1% vs. placebo). Although very suggestive for a specific abdominal fat effect, the changes between both body fat compartments did not seem to be significant. Further studies are needed to explore this interesting issue and its subsequent effect on diabetes and CVD.

CONCLUSIONS

CB_1 blockade of the overactive endocannabinoid system is emerging as a strong therapeutic candidate in the fight to reduce the global health and economic threat of abdominal obesity and ultimately to reduce the progression to CVD.

Data from experimental studies have uncovered associations between endocannabinoid system overactivity and the development of obesity and its associated risk factors. CB_1 receptor expression is widespread throughout the body and is found in several central and peripheral locations relating to the pathogenesis of obesity including the brain, adipose tissue, skeletal muscle, the gut, the liver, and potentially the pancreas. CB_1 blockade with rimonabant and AM-251 in animal models of obesity and CB_1 knockout mice reduces adiposity, inhibits lipogenesis, increases glucose uptake, and increases secretion of adiponectin.

Normalizing the overactive endocannabinoid system with CB_1 antagonists to address abnormalities in energy balance, fat accumulation, and lipid and glucose metabolism could help to prevent both the development and the maintenance of obesity and associated cardiometabolic risk factors.

Robust data from the RIO program of Phase III trials have demonstrated the value of the first selective CB_1 blocker rimonabant in improving multiple risk factors in more than 6600 overweight or obese patients with diabetes, dyslipidaemia, or other comorbidities. Rimonabant (20 mg/day) evoked clinically meaningful reductions in body weight and abdominal fat reduction, HbA_{1c} levels, C-reactive protein, and improvements in lipid parameters. The reduction of 8 to 10 cm of the waist circumference is roughly equivalent to 30% to 33% of visceral fat (measured by CT), as we could demonstrate in another clinical study. The tolerability and safety of rimonabant confirms its suitability as an adjunct to diet and exercise for the management of patients with elevated cardiometabolic risk.

In light of this information, patients most likely to benefit from treatment with rimonabant have multiple cardiometabolic risk factors that are known to be improved by the drug, such as abdominal obesity, and type 2 diabetes, or dyslipidaemia (low HDL-cholesterol and/or high triglycerides). An early indication of patients who could benefit from treatment with rimonabant is the presence of abdominal obesity (assessed by a simple measure of waist circumference) (47). However, as with all obesity-reduction plans, patients would have to be willing to embrace long-term treatment and concomitant lifestyle changes to gain maximum benefit from the treatment.

Both preclinical and clinical evidences support CB_1 blockade as a comprehensive therapeutic strategy to reduce obesity and related cardiovascular outcomes. Ongoing and future studies with rimonabant aim to explore further the benefits of CB_1 blockade on a range of cardiometabolic parameters including cardiovascular endpoints and outcomes, atherosclerosis, visceral fat volume, and pre-diabetes (48).

REFERENCES

1. WHO. Obesity and overweight. Available at: http://www.who.int/dietphysicalactivity/media/en/gsfs_obesity.pdf. Accessed on October 16, 2006.
2. Despres JP, Moorjani S, Lupien PJ, et al. Regional distribution of body fat, plasma lipoproteins, and cardiovascular disease. Arteriosclerosis 1990; 10(4):497–511.
3. Pouliot MC, Despres JP, Nadeau A, et al. Visceral obesity in men. Associations with glucose tolerance, plasma insulin, and lipoprotein levels. Diabetes 1992; 41(7):826–834.
4. Kissebah AH, Freedman DS, Peiris AN. Health risks of obesity. Med Clin North Am 1989; 73(1):111–138.
5. Carey VJ, Walters EE, Colditz GA, et al. Body fat distribution and risk of non-insulin-dependent diabetes mellitus in women. The Nurses' Health Study. Am J Epidemiol 1997; 145(7):614–619.
6. Van Gaal L, Mertens I, De Block. Mechanisms linking obesity to cardiovascular disease. Nature 2006; 444:875–880.

7. Mertens I, Considine RV, Van Der Planken M, et al. Hemostasis and fibrinolysis in non-diabetic overweight and obese men and women. Is there still a role for leptin? Eur J Endocrinol 2006; 155(3):477–484.
8. Yusuf S, Hawken S, Ounpuu S, et al. Effect of potentially modifiable risk factors associated with myocardial infarction in 52 countries (the INTERHEART study): Case-control study. Lancet 2004; 364(9438):937–952.
9. Rexrode KM, Carey VJ, Hennekens CH, et al. Abdominal adiposity and coronary heart disease in women. JAMA 1998; 280(21):1843–1848.
10. Dagenais GR, Yi Q, Mann JF, et al. Prognostic impact of body weight and abdominal obesity in women and men with cardiovascular disease. Am Heart J 2005; 149(1):54–60.
11. Empana JP, Ducimetiere P, Charles MA, et al. Sagittal abdominal diameter and risk of sudden death in asymptomatic middle-aged men: The Paris Prospective Study I. Circulation 2004; 110(18):2781–2785.
12. Balkau B, Deanfield JE, Després JP, et al. International Day for the Evaluation of Abdominal obesity (IDEA): A study of waist circumference, cardiovascular disease and diabetes mellitus in 168000 primary care patients in 63 countries. Circulation 2007; 116(17):1942–1951.
13. Kershaw EE, Flier JS. Adipose tissue as an endocrine organ. J Clin Endocrinol Metab 2004; 89(6):2548–2556.
14. Lee YH, Pratley RE. The evolving role of inflammation in obesity and the metabolic syndrome. Curr Diab Rep 2005; 5(1):70–75.
15. Boden G, Shulman GI. Free fatty acids in obesity and type 2 diabetes: Defining their role in the development of insulin resistance and beta-cell dysfunction. Eur J Clin Invest 2002; 32(Suppl. 3):14–23.
16. Yusuf S, Reddy S, Ounpuu S, et al. Global burden of cardiovascular diseases: Part I: General considerations, the epidemiologic transition, risk factors, and impact of urbanization. Circulation 2001; 104(22):2746–2753.
17. Van Gaal LF, Wauters MA, De Leeuw IH. The beneficial effects of modest weight loss on cardiovascular risk factors. Int J Obes Relat Metab Disord 1997; 21(Suppl. 1):S5–S9.
18. Cota D, Marsicano G, Tschop M, et al. The endogenous cannabinoid system affects energy balance via central orexigenic drive and peripheral lipogenesis. J Clin Invest 2003; 112(3):423–431.
19. Osei-Hyiaman D, DePetrillo M, Pacher P, et al. Endocannabinoid activation at hepatic CB1 receptors stimulates fatty acid synthesis and contributes to diet-induced obesity. J Clin Invest 2005; 115(5):1298–1305.
20. Mertens I, Van der Planken M, Corthouts B, et al. Visceral fat is a determinant of PAI-1 activity in diabetic and non-diabetic overweight and obese women. Horm Metab Res 2001; 33(10):602–607.
21. Pagotto U, Pasquali R. Endocannabinoids and energy metabolism. J Endocrinol Invest 2006; 29(3 Suppl.):66–76.
22. Di Marzo V, Bifulco M, De Petrocellis L. The endocannabinoid system and its therapeutic exploitation. Nat Rev Drug Discov 2004; 3(9):771–784.
23. Gomez R, Navarro M, Ferrer B, et al. A peripheral mechanism for CB1 cannabinoid receptor-dependent modulation of feeding. J Neurosci 2002; 22(21):9612–9617.
24. Cota D, Genghini S, Pasquali R, et al. Antagonizing the cannabinoid receptor type 1: A dual way to fight obesity. J Endocrinol Invest 2003; 26(10):1041–1044.
25. Ravinet Trillou C, Arnone M, Delgorge C, et al. Anti-obesity effect of SR141716, a CB1 receptor antagonist, in diet-induced obese mice. Am J Physiol Regul Integr Comp Physiol 2003; 284(2):R345–R353.
26. Sugiura T, Kondo S, Sukagawa A, et al. 2-Arachidonoylglycerol: A possible endogenous cannabinoid receptor ligand in brain. Biochem Biophys Res Commun 1995; 215(1):89–97.
27. De Petrocellis L, Cascio MG, Di Marzo V. The endocannabinoid system: A general view and latest additions. Br J Pharmacol 2004; 141(5):765–774.
28. Howlett AC, Barth F, Bonner TI, et al. International Union of Pharmacology (XXVII). Classification of cannabinoid receptors. Pharmacol Rev 2002; 54(2):161–202.
29. Kirkham TC, Tucci SA. Endocannabinoids in appetite control and the treatment of obesity. CNS Neurol Disord Drug Targets 2006; 5(3):272–292.
30. Engeli S, Bohnke J, Feldpausch M, et al. Activation of the peripheral endocannabinoid system in human obesity. Diabetes 2005; 54(10):2838–2843.
31. Matias I, Gonthier MP, Orlando P, et al. Regulation, function, and dysregulation of endocannabinoids in models of adipose and beta-pancreatic cells and in obesity and hyperglycemia. J Clin Endocrinol Metab 2006; 91(8):3171–3180.
32. Blüher M, Engeli S, Kloting N, et al. Dysregulation of the peripheral and adipose tissue endocannabinoid system in human abdominal obesity. Diabetes 2006; 55(11):3053–3060.
33. Poirier B, Bidouard JP, Cadrouvele C, et al. The anti-obesity effect of rimonabant is associated with an improved serum lipid profile. Diabetes Obes Metab 2005; 7(1):65–72.

34. Jbilo O, Ravinet-Trillou C, Arnone M, et al. The CB1 receptor antagonist rimonabant reverses the diet-induced obesity phenotype through the regulation of lipolysis and energy balance. Faseb J 2005; 19(11):1567–1569.
35. Bensaid M, Gary-Bobo M, Esclangon A, et al. The cannabinoid CB1 receptor antagonist SR141716 increases Acrp30 mRNA expression in adipose tissue of obese fa/fa rats and in cultured adipocyte cells. Mol Pharmacol 2003; 63(4):908–914.
36. Scheen AJ, Finer N, Hollander P, et al. Efficacy and tolerability of rimonabant in overweight or obese patients with type 2 diabetes: A randomised controlled study. Lancet 2006; 368(9548):1660–1672.
37. Despres JP, Golay A, Sjostrom L. Effects of rimonabant on metabolic risk factors in overweight patients with dyslipidemia. N Engl J Med 2005; 353(20):2121–2134.
38. Van Gaal LF, Rissanen AM, Scheen AJ, et al. Effects of the cannabinoid-1 receptor blocker rimonabant on weight reduction and cardiovascular risk factors in overweight patients: 1-Year experience from the RIO-Europe study. Lancet 2005; 365(9468):1389–1397.
39. Pi-Sunyer FX, Aronne LJ, Heshmati HM, et al. Effect of rimonabant, a cannabinoid-1 receptor blocker, on weight and cardiometabolic risk factors in overweight or obese patients: RIO-North America: A randomized controlled trial. JAMA 2006; 295(7):761–775.
40. Scheen AJ. Current management strategies for coexisting diabetes mellitus and obesity. Drugs 2003; 63(12):1165–1184.
41. Wing RR, Marcus MD, Epstein LH, et al. Type II diabetic subjects lose less weight than their overweight nondiabetic spouses. Diabetes Care 1987; 10(5):563–566.
42. Guare JC, Wing RR, Grant A. Comparison of obese NIDDM and nondiabetic women: Short- and long-term weight loss. Obes Res 1995; 3(4):329–335.
43. Despres JP, Van Gaal LF, Scheen AJ, et al. Rimonabant improves cardiometabolic risk factors in overweight/obese patients irrespective of treatment with statins: Pooled data from the RIO program. Presented at the XIV International Symposium on Atherosclerosis 2006, Rome, Italy.
44. Iranmanesh A, Rosenstock J, Hollander P. SERENADE: Rimonabant monotherapy for treatment of multiple cardiometabolic risk factors in treatment-naïve patients with type 2 diabetes. Diabet Med 2006; 23(Suppl. 4):230.
45. Van Gaal LF. 2-Year data from the RIO-Europe study: Metabolic effects of rimonabant in overweight/obese patients. J Am Coll Cardiol 2005; 45(3 Suppl. A):1A–446A.
46. Nissen SE, Nicholls SJ, Wolski K, et al. For the STRADIVARIUS investigators. Effect of rimonabant on progression of atherosclerosis in patients with abdominal obesity and coronary artery disease: The STRADIVARIUS Randomized Controlled Trial. JAMA 2008; 299(13):1547–1560.
47. Pouliot MC, Despres JP, Lemieux S, et al. Waist circumference and abdominal sagittal diameter: Best simple anthropometric indexes of abdominal visceral adipose tissue accumulation and related cardiovascular risk in men and women. Am J Cardiol 1994; 73(7):460–468.
48. ClinicalTrials.gov. Available at: http://www.clinicaltrials.gov. Accessed on October 18, 2006.

29 Abdominal Obesity and the Endocannabinoid System CB_1 Blockade, Insulin Resistance, and Type 2 Diabetes

André J. Scheen

Division of Diabetes, Nutrition and Metabolic Disorders, CHU Sart Tilman, University of Liege, Liege, Belgium

INTRODUCTION

Type 2 diabetes mellitus (T2DM) is associated with excess morbidity and mortality, and is considered as one of the most costly and burdensome chronic diseases of our time (1). T2DM frequently coexists with a cluster of other cardiovascular and metabolic risk factors including abdominal obesity, low high-density lipoprotein-cholesterol (HDL-C), high triglycerides (TG), elevated blood pressure, and silent inflammation (elevated C-reactive protein), all of them being more or less closely related to insulin resistance and the so-called metabolic syndrome (2,3). T2DM increases the risk of cardiovascular disease (CVD) by 2 to 4 times and may be considered as a "cardiovascular risk equivalent" (4). Therefore, treatment of multiple cardiovascular and metabolic risk factors is central to the management of T2DM (5,6). The importance of weight management is well recognized in T2DM (7–9), although affected patients often have more difficulty in losing weight than nondiabetic obese individuals and experience weight gain associated with most antidiabetic medications (7,9).

Huge amount of evidences accumulated during recent years have shown that endocannabinoid system (ECS) plays a significant role not only in appetite drive and associated behaviors, but also in endocrine and metabolic regulation and energy balance, essentially via CB_1 receptors (10). Remarkably, while antagonism of CB_1 receptors acutely reduces food intake, the long-term effects on weight reduction and metabolic regulation rather appear to be mediated by stimulation of energy expenditure and by peripheral effects related to adipose tissue, liver, skeletal muscle, and pancreas physiology, all organs where the presence of CB_1 receptors is now recognized (11). Such observations extend the potential use of CB_1 antagonists for the management of overweight/obese individuals with insulin resistance and multiple cardiometabolic risk factors (12), especially those with T2DM (13,14) (Fig. 1).

The aim of the present review is to analyze the rationale for use and the potential role of CB_1 receptor antagonists, especially rimonabant, the first commercialized selective CB_1 blocker, in the management of overweight/obese patients with T2DM and other cardiometabolic risk factors.

RATIONALE FOR USE OF CB_1 INHIBITORS IN TYPE 2 DIABETES

Overactivity of EC System in Abdominal Obesity and T2DM

There is increasing evidence in humans for ECS overactivity during conditions of unbalanced energy homeostasis, that is, obesity (especially abdominal obesity) and T2DM, and for its causative role in these disorders (15). Circulating 2-acylglycerol (2-AG) levels were significantly correlated with body fat, visceral fat mass, and fasting plasma insulin concentrations, but negatively correlated to glucose infusion rate during clamp, a measure of insulin sensitivity (16). In untreated asymptomatic men, plasma 2-AG levels correlated positively with body mass index (BMI), waist girth, intra-abdominal adiposity, fasting TG and insulin levels, and negatively with HDL-C and adiponectin concentrations (17). All together, these findings suggest that intra-abdominal fat accumulation is a critical correlate of peripheral ECS dysregulation and that ECS may represent a primary target for the treatment of abdominal obesity and associated metabolic changes, including T2DM (12–14).

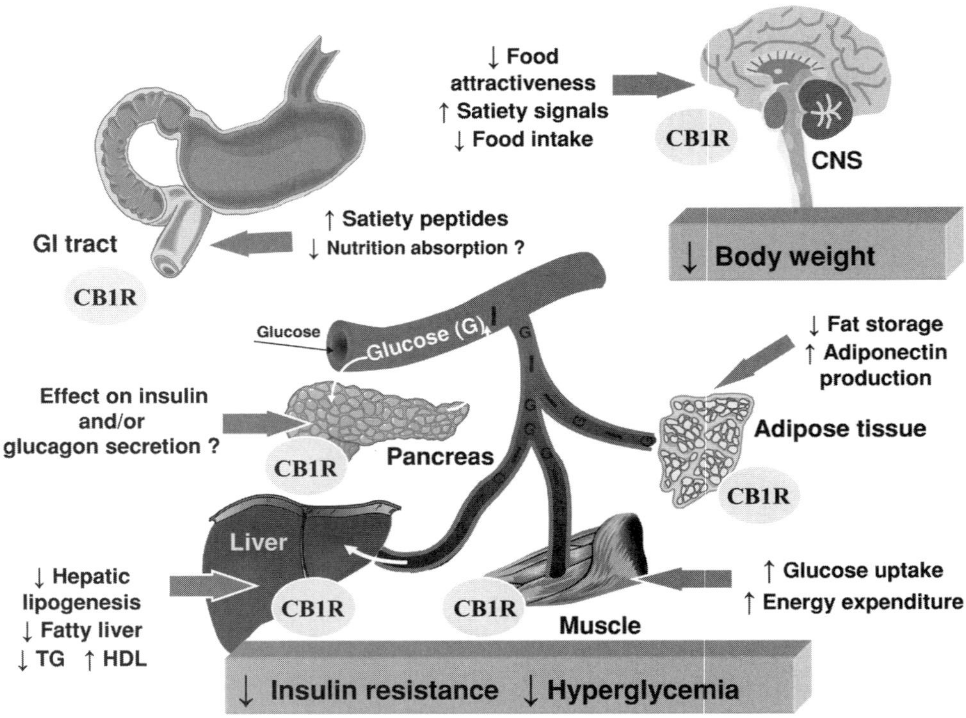

Figure 1 Potential mechanisms of action of rimonabant, a selective cannabinoid type 1 receptor (CB_1R) antagonist, in the improvement of glucose control and other cardiometabolic risk factors in overweight/obese patients with type 2 diabetes. *Abbreviations*: CNS, central nervous system; TG, triglycerides; HDL, high-density lipoprotein; GI tract, gastrointestinal tract. *Source*: Adapted from Ref. 14.

EFFECTS OF RIMONABANT IN OVERWEIGHT/OBESE NONDIABETIC PATIENTS

The phase III RIO (Rimonabant in Obesity) program comprised three large placebo-controlled randomized clinical trials (RCTs) evaluating rimonabant in overweight/obese nondiabetic patients—two 2-year RCTs (RIO-Europe and RIO-North America) (18–20) and one 1-year RCT (RIO-Lipids), specifically devoted to patients with untreated dyslipidemia (21). After 1 year of followup, rimonabant 20 mg has been shown to produce consistent and significant weight loss (−4.7 to −5.4 kg) and waist circumference reduction (−3.6 to −4.7 cm) as compared to placebo, when combined with diet and exercise advices. In addition, improvements in multiple cardiovascular and metabolic risk factors were noticed, including a significant improvement of the HOMA-insulin resistance index. In particular, consistent significant reductions in TG levels (−12.4% to −15.1%) and increases in HDL-C levels (+7.2% to +8.9%) were observed in patients treated with rimonabant 20 mg. These improvements persisted after 2 years (19,20). Remarkably, almost half (between 45% and 57%) of the overall treatment effect at year 1 on HDL-C, TG, fasting insulin, and insulin resistance was due to a direct effect not attributable to weight loss. Weight-loss adjusted improvements in all factors were significantly better with rimonabant than placebo ($p \leq 0.001$ for HDL-C and TG, $p \leq 0.02$ for fasting insulin and HOMA-IR insulin resistance index).

Pooled analysis from these three trials was conducted on 1-year data from a subgroup of patients identified with prediabetes as defined by impaired fasting glucose (≥5.5 to ≤7 mmol/L) (22). Rimonabant 20 mg reduced fasting insulin levels (−2.7 μIU/mL, $p \leq 0.001$ vs. placebo) and HOMA-IR (−0.8%, $p = 0.002$ vs. placebo) with a trend to reverse or retard the progression of impaired fasting glucose as suggested by a numerically greater percentage of patients converting to normal fasting plasma glucose and a lesser proportion of patients progressing to T2DM.

To determine whether rimonabant improves glucose tolerance in overweight/obese nondiabetic patients, data were pooled from the two studies involving oral glucose tolerance tests (OGTTs) at baseline and 1 year RCT (RIO-Lipids and RIO-Europe) (23,24). After 1 year, rimonabant 20 mg produced significantly greater reductions than placebo in plasma glucose (−0.64 vs. −0.37 mmol/L, $p \leq 0.01$) and insulin (−15.2 vs. −1.8 μIU/mL, $p \leq 0.001$) levels at 120 minutes post-OGTT. Both glucose and insulin areas under the plasma concentration–time curve values were also reduced ($p \leq 0.001$). Furthermore, rimonabant 20 mg significantly improved the distribution of glucose tolerance status at 1 year in the pooled intention-to-treat population ($p \leq 0.01$), with an increased proportion of patients with normal glucose tolerance and a decreased proportion of patients with impaired glucose tolerance or diabetes. Favorable effects on glucose tolerance status persisted after 2 years, despite a weight stabilization from year 1 to year 2 (19). These results demonstrate that rimonabant 20 mg can prevent or reverse progression of fasting and post-glucose load dysglycemia in overweight/obese patients, suggesting a potential to prevent T2DM in those patients. This potential is currently evaluated in a prospective trial in overweight/obese patients with impaired glucose tolerance (RAPSODI trial).

CLINICAL TRIALS WITH RIMONABANT IN TYPE 2 DIABETES

RIO-Diabetes in Metformin- or Sulfonylurea-Treated Patients

The RIO-Diabetes trial investigated the efficacy and safety of rimonabant in overweight/obese patients with T2DM (25). Therefore, 1047 overweight/obese type 2 diabetes patients (BMI 27–40kg/m^2) with an HbA1c from 6.5% to 10.0% (mean ± SD 7.3 ± 0.9% at baseline) already on metformin or sulfonylurea monotherapy were given a mild hypocaloric diet and randomized to placebo or rimonabant (5 or 20 mg) for 1 year. The primary endpoint was weight change from baseline after 1 year of treatment. Secondary endpoints included changes in waist circumference, HbA1c, HDL-C, and TG levels. Almost two-thirds of the diabetic population received metformin as monotherapy, the oral antidiabetic drug considered as first choice in the management of type 2 diabetes.

Weight loss in the intention-to-treat population was significantly greater after 1 year with rimonabant 20 mg (−5.3 ± 5.2 kg, $p \leq 0.001$) than with placebo (−1.4 ± 3.6 kg). These weight differences compared favorably with those previously reported with orlistat and sibutramine in overweight/obese T2DM patients (26–28). Rimonabant 20 mg improved HbA1c (−0.6 ± 0.8% vs. +0.1 ± 1.0% for placebo, $p \leq 0.001$) in patients with mean baseline HbA1c of 7.3%. Therefore, a greater number of patients attained the HbA1c ADA target (HbA1c ≤7%, 67.9% vs. 47.6% with placebo) and the HbA1c IDF target (HbA1c ≤6.5%, 42.9% vs. 20.8% with placebo). HbA1c improvements were almost similar in patients treated with metformin or sulfonylurea at baseline. In patients with higher HbA1c levels (≥8%) at baseline, reductions of 0.3% and 1.1% were observed in the placebo and rimonabant 20 mg treatment groups, respectively ($p = 0.001$).

Waist circumference, HDL-C, TG, fasting glucose levels, HOMA-estimated insulin resistance, systolic blood pressure, metabolic syndrome prevalence, and C-reactive protein levels also improved significantly with rimonabant 20 mg versus placebo (Fig. 2). A significant reduction of liver enzymes was also observed (29), suggesting a reduction of liver fat content. This finding is in agreement with the intimate relationship between liver steatosis, insulin resistance, and abdominal obesity, especially in patients with T2DM, and the favorable impact of weight loss on these parameters (30,31). In contrast to what was reported with sibutramine, rimonabant was associated with a significant reduction in arterial blood pressure, especially in diabetic patients with elevated values at baseline, and this effect appeared to be entirely explained by the greater weight loss observed with rimonabant 20 mg (32). These favorable effects on multiple cardiovascular risk factors, similar to those previously observed in the nondiabetic population, are important in order to improve the overall CVD prognosis in patients with T2DM (33). The 0.7% observed reduction in HbA1c levels with rimonabant 20 mg versus placebo appears to be greater than the corresponding reduction observed with orlistat or sibutramine (26,27). Such HbA1c reduction is clinically relevant according to the United Kingdom Prospective Diabetes Study (UKPDS), which showed that each 1% reduction in HbA1c was significantly associated with a reduction in risk of 21% for any endpoint related to diabetes (34).

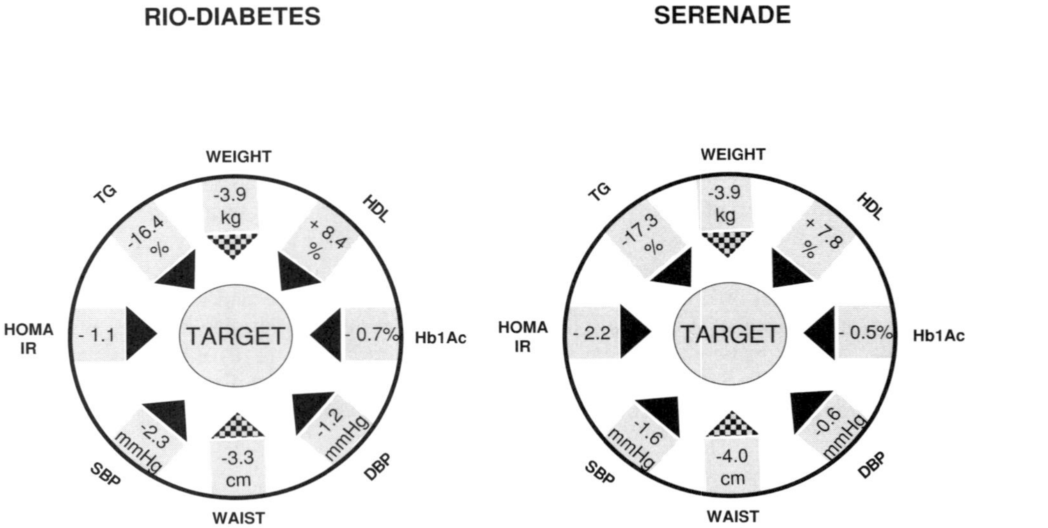

Figure 2 Multiple consistent effects of rimonabant 20 mg on various parameters considered as CVD risk factors in T2DM patients. Results are expressed as placebo-subtracted differences after 1 year in RIO-Diabetes (*left panel*) and after 6 months in SERENADE (*right panel*). *Abbreviations*: SBP, systolic blood pressure; DBP, diastolic blood pressure.

SERENADE IN DRUG-NAIVE PATIENTS

The favorable effects of rimonabant in T2DM have been recently confirmed in SERENADE (Study Evaluating Rimonabant Efficacy in drug-NAive DiabEtic patients), a 6-month placebo-controlled trial in overweight/obese with recent-onset diabetes treated with diet alone (35). The attrition rate was lower in this trial than in RIO-Diabetes (15% dropouts after 6 months). HbA1c (primary endpoint in SERENADE, mean baseline HbA1c 7.9%) decreased by 0.8% in the group receiving rimonabant 20 mg compared to 0.3% in the group receiving placebo ($p = 0.0002$). These differences were almost similar to those observed after 6 months in RIO-Diabetes (25). In patients with higher HbA1c levels (≥8.5%) at baseline, reductions of 0.7% and 1.9% were observed in the placebo and rimonabant 20 mg treatment groups, respectively ($p \leq 0.001$). Similar to the changes observed in RIO-Diabetes, significant reductions in body weight, waist circumference, and TG levels were observed, whereas a significant increase in HDL-C was noticed with rimonabant (Fig. 2). Rimonabant also decreased HOMA-IR insulin resistance index and significantly increased plasma adiponectin levels (+1.8 μg/mL, $p \leq 0.0001$), confirming previous observations in the nondiabetic population of RIO-Lipids (21). Knowing the favorable effect of adiponectin on insulin sensitivity (36), this increase in adiponectin may contribute to the improvement in glucose control induced by rimonabant 20 mg. As in RIO-Diabetes (24) and in other RIO trials (18–21), almost half of the metabolic improvement observed in SERENADE occurred beyond weight loss (57% for HbA1c reduction) (35).

OTHER CLINICAL TRIALS WITH RIMONABANT

In STRADIVARIUS performed in patients with coronary heart disease, abdominal obesity and the metabolic syndrome and treatment with rimonabant 20 mg for 18 months reduced body weight and waist circumference and improved lipid profiles, glycemic measures (changes from baseline 6.7% HbA1c level in the diabetic subgroup: −0.30% in the rimonabant group versus +0.37% in the placebo group; $p = 0.0003$), and CRP levels, thus confirming the results of the RIO program (37). However, rimonabant did not significantly reduce coronary atherosclerosis (assessed by intravascular ultrasonography or IVUS) for the primary efficacy parameter, that is, change in percent atheroma volume (+0.25% with rimonabant vs. +0.57% with placebo; $p = 0.13$). Nevertheless, rimonabant treatment did show a statistically significant favorable effect for a secondary IVUS endpoint (total atheroma volume; $p = 0.02$) and an additional exploratory endpoint (maximum atheroma thickness; $p = 0.01$). In the recent ADAGIO trial, which essentially investigated the effects of rimonabant 20 mg on lipid profile and visceral adipose tissue, diabetes was not an exclusion criterion and 17% of the randomized patients had T2DM. This study confirmed the positive effect of rimonabant 20 mg on waist reduction and on HDL-C and TG levels, and demonstrated a significant reduction in visceral adipose tissue and liver fat content (38). This finding is important in T2DM because fatty liver has been shown to be strongly associated with insulin resistance and profound glucose metabolism dysregulation (30).

The effect of rimonabant 20 mg is currently evaluated in several RCTs specifically devoted to patients with T2DM. The "ARPEGGIO" trial recently reported the effect of rimonabant 20 mg in overweight/obese patients already treated with exogenous insulin (39). In the intention-to-treat population, mean baseline HbA1c level (9.1%) was reduced significantly more with rimonabant than with placebo (−0.89 vs −0.24%; $p > 0.0001$) at 48 weeks of follow up. This insulin-requiring T2DM population is interesting to evaluate, as one major problem of insulin therapy in T2DM is weight gain and its associated multiple disturbances (7–9). In all new trials in T2DM, HbA1c reduction has been chosen as a primary endpoint. These studies will broaden the spectrum of combined therapy with rimonabant in T2DM and, if conclusive, may support the role of rimonabant as a possible new antidiabetic agent (13,14).

Considering the high CVD risk associated with T2DM (4), it is of major interest to demonstrate that rimonabant is able to improve the overall CVD prognosis of such high-risk patients. Weight management (9), especially correction of abdominal obesity (2,3), is crucial to obtain a global cardiovascular risk reduction, and previous studies have shown that intentional weight loss is able to reduce overall and CVD mortality in T2DM patients (40). Furthermore, rimonabant may exert several pleiotropic effects, independent of weight loss, which could contribute to reduce global CVD risk (41). The ongoing "CRESCENDO" (Comprehensive Rimonabant Evaluation Study of Cardiovascular ENDpoints and Outcomes) RCT will assess whether rimonabant 20 mg can reduce the incidence of major CVD events in 17,000 abdominally obese patients with clustering risk factors (at least half with type 2 diabetes) followed for 5 years (42).

SAFETY ISSUES WITH RIMONABANT IN T2DM PATIENTS

The overall safety profile of rimonabant was similar in patients with T2DM as in overweight/obese nondiabetic individuals (41). In RIO-Diabetes, although overall discontinuation rates were similar, discontinuations due to adverse events (AEs) were more frequent in the rimonabant 20 mg (15.0%) compared with placebo (5.5%) (25). The most common AEs leading to premature study discontinuation in the rimonabant 20 mg group were depressed mood disorders, nausea, and dizziness. These AEs were almost similar to those reported in nondiabetic overweight/obese individuals of the RIO program. No serious AEs linked to psychiatric disorders were recorded in the rimonabant 20 mg group in RIO-Diabetes. Hypoglycemia symptoms were uncommon, although slightly more frequent in the rimonabant-treated group than in the placebo group, essentially in diabetic patients receiving sulfonylureas. Overall, the safety profile of rimonabant 20 mg in SERENADE (35) was comparable to that previously reported in RIO-Diabetes and in other RIO trials. The overall safety of rimonabant in the RIO program and other clinical trials has been extensively reviewed elsewhere (43), especially the effects on central nervous system and psychological status (44).

RIMONABANT IN CLINICAL PRACTICE

Rimonabant (Acomplia®, 20 mg), the first of this new class of CB_1 receptor antagonists, has been approved by the Committee for Medicinal Products for human Use of the European Medicines Agency (EMEA) "as an adjunct to diet and exercise for the treatment of obese patients (BMI $\geq 30\,kg/m^2$), or overweight patients (BMI $\geq 27\,kg/m^2$) with associated risk factor(s), such as type 2 diabetes or dyslipidemia". Furthermore, the committee recognized that almost half of the observed improvements in several metabolic parameters (HbA1c, HDL-C, and TG) in patients who received 20 mg rimonabant was beyond that expected from weight loss, in agreement with direct peripheral metabolic effects.

Patients most likely to benefit from rimonabant are those with multiple cardiometabolic risk factors, such as insulin resistance and related metabolic disturbances, known to be improved by the drug. In this context, patients with T2DM are good candidates for being prescribed a drug like rimonabant, especially when abdominal obesity is a crucial issue and contribute to drug failure with other glucose-lowering agents (13,14).

Because patients with antecedent of depression or receiving antidepressant agents were excluded from the RIO program and because mood disorders were more frequently observed with rimonabant than with placebo in all RCTs, rimonabant is contraindicated in patients with uncontrolled serious psychiatric illness such as major depression, or patients receiving antidepressant medication (43,44). Monitoring for on-treatment anxiety and depression will be necessary in the future to ensure the safe use of rimonabant.

CONCLUSIONS

CB_1 receptor blockade is a novel therapeutic strategy that addresses the underlying mechanisms of abdominal obesity, insulin resistance, and cardiometabolic risk, all being strongly associated with T2DM. Even if lifestyle intervention is essential, the potential role of rimonabant in overweight/obese patients with T2DM and high-risk cardiovascular disease has been demonstrated in both RIO-Diabetes and SERENADE randomized controlled trials. Most metabolic improvements, especially the reduction in HbA1c, the increase in HDL-C, and the diminution in TG levels, were almost twice that expected from the weight loss alone. These observations are consistent with direct peripheral metabolic effects of the drug, via CB_1 blockade in various organs playing a key role in the pathophysiology of T2DM such as adipose tissue, liver, skeletal muscle, gut, and possibly pancreas. These findings support the use of rimonabant 20 mg as a new approach to improve glucose control and reduce multiple cardiovascular and metabolic risk factors in overweight/obese patients with T2DM, in addition to diet and exercise, provided that psychiatric contraindications are respected. Further ongoing studies should confirm the long-term efficacy and safety of rimonabant, the first selective CB_1 receptor antagonist, particularly in T2DM.

REFERENCES

1. Zimmet P. Global and societal implications of the diabetes epidemic. Nature 2001; 414:782–787.
2. Després JP, Lemieux I. Abdominal obesity and metabolic syndrome. Nature 2006; 444:881–887.
3. Van Gaal LF, Mertens IL, De Block CE. Mechanisms linking obesity with cardiovascular disease. Nature 2006; 444:875–880.
4. Task force on diabetes and cardiovascular diseases of the European Society of Cardiology (ESC) and the European Society for the Study of Diabetes (EASD). Guidelines on diabetes, prediabetes and cardiovascular diseases: Executive summary. Eur Heart J 2007; 28:88–136.
5. American Diabetes Association. Clinical practice recommendations 2008. Diabetes Care 2008; 31(Suppl. 1):S1–S104.
6. IDF Clinical Guidelines Task force. Global guideline for type 2 diabetes: Recommendations for standard, comprehensive, and minimal care. Diabet Med 2006; 23:579–593.
7. Scheen AJ. Current management strategies for coexisting diabetes mellitus and obesity. Drugs 2003; 63:1165–1184.
8. Anderson JW, Kendall CWC, Jenkins DJA. Importance of weight management in type 2 diabetes: Review with meta-analysis of clinical studies. J Am Coll Nutr 2003; 22:331–339.
9. Lee M, Aronne LJ. Weight management for type 2 diabetes mellitus: Global cardiovascular risk reduction. Am J Cardiol 2007; 99(Suppl.):68B–79B.
10. Pagotto U, Marsicano G, Cota D, et al. The emerging role of the endocannabinoid system in endocrine regulation and energy balance. Endocr Rev 2006; 27:73–100.
11. Matias I, Di Marzo V. Endocannabinoids and the control of energy balance. Trends Endocrinol Metab 2007; 18:27–37.
12. Di Marzo V, Bifulco M, De Petrocellis L. The endocannabinoid system and its therapeutic exploitation. Nat Rev Drug Discov 2004; 3:771–784.

13. Lafontan M, Piazza PV, Girard J. Effects of CB_1 antagonist on the control of metabolic functions in obese type 2 diabetic patients. Diabetes Metab 2007; 33:85–95.
14. Scheen AJ. Cannabinoid receptor-1 antagonists in type-2 diabetes. Best Pract Res Clin Endocrinol Metab 2007; 21:535–553.
15. Matias I, Gonthier MP, Orlando P, et al. Regulation, function, and dysregulation of endocannabinoids in models of adipose and β-pancreatic cells and in obesity and hyperglycemia. J Clin Endocrinol Metab 2006; 91:3171–3180.
16. Bluher M, Engeli S, Kloting N, et al. Dysregulation of the peripheral and adipose tissue endocannabinoid system in human abdominal obesity. Diabetes 2006; 55:3053–3060.
17. Cote M, Matias I, Lemieux I, et al. Circulating endocannabinoid levels, abdominal adiposity and related cardiometabolic risk factors in obese men. Int J Obesity 2007; 31:692–699.
18. Van Gaal LF, Rissanen AM, Scheen AJ, et al. Effects of the cannabinoid-1 receptor blocker rimonabant on weight reduction and cardiovascular risk factors in overweight patients: 1-year experience from the RIO-Europe study. Lancet 2005; 365:1389–1397.
19. Van Gaal LF, Scheen AJ, Rissanen AM, et al. Long-term effect of CB_1 blockade with rimonabant on cardiometabolic risk factors: 2-year results from the RIO-Europe Study. Eur Heart J 2008; 29:1761–1771.
20. Pi-Sunyer FX, Aronne LJ, Heshmati HM, et al. Effect of rimonabant, a cannabinoid-1 receptor blocker, on weight and cardiometabolic risk factors in overweight or obese patients. RIO-North America: A randomized controlled trial. JAMA 2006; 295:761–775.
21. Després JP, Golay A, Sjöström L. Rimonabant in Obesity-Lipids Study Group. Effects on metabolic risk factors in overweight patients with dyslipidemia. N Engl J Med 2005; 353:2121–2134.
22. Rosenstock J. The potential of rimonabant in prediabetes: Pooled 1-year results from the RIO-Lipids, RIO-Europe and RIO-North America studies (Abstract). Diabetologia 2005; 48(Suppl. 1):A16.
23. Després JP, Van Gaal L, Golay A, et al. Rimonabant improves oral glucose tolerance in non-diabetic overweight/obese patients with/without comorbidities (Abstract). Diabetes 2006; 55(Suppl. 1):A80–A81.
24. Scheen A, Van Gaal L, for the RIO-Europe Study Group. Long-term efficacy of rimonabant in improving glucose tolerance in overweight/obese non-diabetic patients: 2-year results from RIO-Europe (Abstract). Diabetes 2008; 57(Suppl 1):A1,101-OR.
25. Scheen AJ, Finer N, Hollander P, et al. For the RIO-Diabetes Study Group. Efficacy and tolerability of rimonabant in overweight or obese patients with type 2 diabetes: A randomised controlled study. Lancet 2006; 368:1660–1672.
26. Scheen AJ, Ernest Ph. Antiobesity treatment in type 2 diabetes: Results of clinical trials with orlistat and sibutramine. Diabetes Metab 2002; 28:437–445.
27. Norris SL, Zhang X, Avenell A, et al. Efficacy of pharmacotherapy for weight loss in adults with type 2 diabetes mellitus: A meta-analysis. Arch Intern Med 2004; 164;395–404.
28. Padwal RS, Majumdar SR. Drug treatments for obesity: Orlistat, sibutramine, and rimonabant. Lancet 2007; 369:71–77.
29. Scheen A, Van Gaal L. The CB_1 blocker rimonabant reduces liver enzyme levels in overweight/obese people with type 2 diabetes: The RIO Diabetes study (Abstract). Diabetic Med 2006; 23(Suppl. 4):251–252.
30. Yk-Järvinen H. Fat in the liver and insulin resistance. Ann Med 2005; 37:347–356.
31. Luyckx FH, Scheen AJ, Lefèbvre PJ. Non-alcoholic steatohepatitis: Association with obesity and insulin resistance, and influence of weight loss. Diabetes Metab 2000; 26;98–106.
32. Ruilope LM, Després JP, Scheen A, et al. Effect of rimonabant on blood pressure in overweight/obese patients with/without co-morbidities: Analysis of pooled Rimonabant in Obesity (RIO) study results. J Hypertens 2007; 26:357–367.
33. Gaede P, Vedel P, Larsen N, et al. Multifactorial intervention and cardiovascular disease in patients with type 2 diabetes. N Engl J Med 2003; 348:383–393.
34. Stratton IM, Adler AI, Neil HA, et al. Association of glycaemia with macrovascular and microvascular complications of type 2 diabetes (UKPDS 35): Prospective observational study. BMJ 2000; 321;405–412.
35. Iranmanesh A, Rosenstock J, Hollander P. SERENADE-Study-Group. SERENADE: Rimonabant monotherapy for treatment of multiple cardiometabolic risk factors in treatment-naïve patients with type 2 diabetes (Abstract). Diabet Med 2006; 23(Suppl. 4):230.
36. Lihn AS, Pedersen SB, Richelsen B. Adiponectin: Action, regulation and association to insulin sensitivity. Obes Rev 2005; 6:13–21.
37. Nissen SE, Nicholls SJ, Wolski K, et al. Effect of rimonabant on progression of atherosclerosis in patients with abdominal obesity and coronary artery disease. The STRADIVARIUS randomized controlled trial. JAMA 2008; 299:1547–1560.
38. Després JP. Results of ADAGIO trial (personal communication).
39. Hollander PA, Amod A, Litwak LE. Rimonabant improves glycemic control in insulin-treated type 2 diabetes: The ARPEGGIO trial (Abstract). Diabetes 2008; 57(Suppl 1):A95.
40. Williamson DF, Thompson TJ, Thun M, et al. Intentional weight loss and mortality among overweight individuals with diabetes. Diabetes Care 2000; 23;1499–1504.

41. Bifulco M, Grimaldi C, Gazzerro P, et al. Rimonabant: Just an antiobesity drug? Current evidence on its pleiotropic effects. Mol Pharmacol 2007; 71:1445–1456.
42. CRESCENDO: Comprehensive Rimonabant Evaluation Study of Cardiovascular ENDpoints and Outcomes. http://www.clinicaltrials.gov/ct/show/NCT00263042?order=2. Accessed February 1, 2007.
43. Van Gaal L, Pi-Sunyer X, Després JP, et al. Efficacy and safety of rimonabant for improvement of multiple cardiometabolic risk factors in overweight/obese patients: Pooled 1-year data from the RIO program. Diabetes Care 2008; 31(Suppl 2):S229–S240.
44. Christensen R, Kristensen PK, Bartels EM, et al. Efficacy and safety of the weight-loss drug rimonabant: A meta-analysis of randomised trials. Lancet 2007; 370:1706–1713.

30 Abdominal Obesity As a Therapeutic Target to Manage the Atherogenic Dyslipidemia and Related Metabolic Abnormalities

Jean-Pierre Després

Québec Heart Institute, Hôpital Laval Research Centre and
Division of Kinesiology, Department of Social and Preventive Medicine, Université Laval,
Québec City, QC, Canada

INTRODUCTION

In the "lipid world," the reduction of plasma cholesterol (particularly LDL-cholesterol) concentrations is widely and appropriately emphasized in the management of the patient at high risk of coronary heart disease (CHD). However, patients and physicians also need to be aware that abdominal obesity, especially when accompanied by markers of metabolic abnormalities such as elevated triglyceride concentrations or other features of the metabolic syndrome, is characterized by an atherogenic dyslipidemia which CHD risk is not often captured by LDL-cholesterol levels (1,2). For instance, the typical high triglyceride–low HDL-cholesterol, small dense LDL dyslipidemia, which is frequently found in patients with abdominal obesity, further increases the risk of CHD assumed from the presence of classical risk factors including a given LDL-cholesterol level (3–6). Thus, even optimal management of traditional risk factors is unlikely to normalize the level of CHD risk found in patients who have the additional athero-thrombotic–inflammatory abnormalities of abdominal obesity.

TARGETING ABDOMINAL OBESITY: THE SECRET OF A SUCCESSFUL WEIGHT (WAIST) LOSS PROGRAM

The National Cholesterol Education Program—Adult Treatment Panel III (NCEP-ATP III) guidelines recommend therapeutic lifestyle changes for patients who are at risk for cardiovascular disease and who have lifestyle-related factors such as obesity, and the International Diabetes Federation has issued a statement emphasizing the central role of abdominal obesity as the prevalent form of the metabolic syndrome (7,8). Thus, in addition to aiming at blood pressure and LDL-cholesterol lowering, a pharmacological approach to target the excess visceral/ectopic fat, which most of the time accompanies the features of the metabolic syndrome, could be relevant to consider as a complementary approach if lifestyle modification is not sufficient to normalize the atherogenic and diabetogenic profile of the abdominally obese patient.

As reviewed in this book, there is evidence that the endocannabinoid system is specifically activated in patients with abdominal obesity (Fig. 1) (9,10). Furthermore, elevated plasma concentrations of an abundant endocannabinoid, 2-arachidonoylglycerol (2-AG), have been shown to be predictive of several features of the metabolic syndrome including increased plasma triglyceride and reduced HDL-cholesterol levels (Fig. 1) (9,10).

Therefore, it would appear reasonable to assume that antagonism of the endocannabinoid system would be particularly beneficial for patients with an overactivated endocannabinoid system. In this regard, published results from the phase III program conducted using the first cannabinoid 1 (CB_1) antagonist developed, rimonabant, have provided evidence that such an approach could be useful for the management of abdominal obesity and related abnormalities (11–14). Not only does rimonabant act centrally to reduce food intake through antagonism of the CB_1 receptor, there is now evidence that it also has peripheral effects in key tissues involved in carbohydrate and lipid metabolism such as the liver (15) and adipose tissue (16). CB_1 antagonism with rimonabant in animals has been shown to reduce liver lipogenesis (15) and to stimulate adiponectin gene expression and the secretion of this important adipose tissue–derived

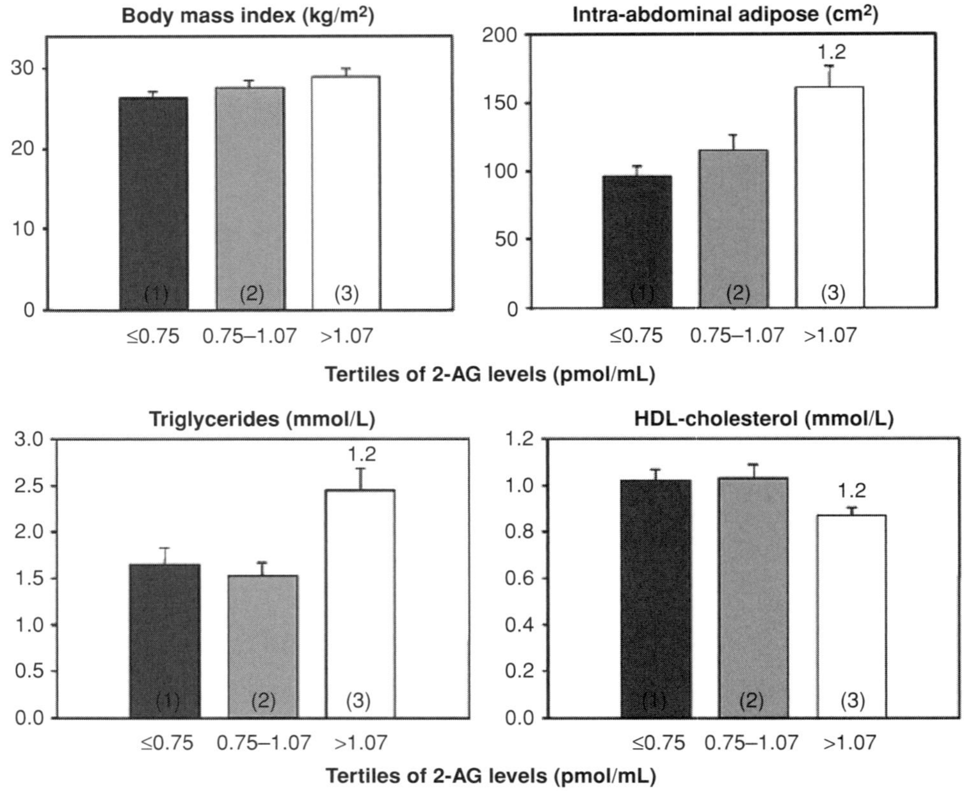

Figure 1 Relationships between tertiles of plasma 2-arachidonoylglycerol (2-AG) levels and adiposity indices (*top panels*) or lipoprotein–lipid variables (*bottom panels*). 1.2, significantly different from the corresponding tertiles. *Source*: Adapted from Ref. 10.

cytokine by fat cells (17). Since one of the key features of visceral obesity is deposition of fat in undesired sites such as the liver, the heart, the skeletal muscle, and the pancreas (18,19), antagonism of the endocannabinoid system may limit such ectopic fat deposition, including visceral fat. Thus, targeting the endocannabinoid system may represent a preferred therapeutic option to target patients with an unfavorable pattern of regional fat deposition. This issue will be examined later on in this chapter.

PUBLISHED STUDIES ON THE EFFECTS OF THE CB_1 ANTAGONIST RIMONABANT ON PLASMA LIPOPROTEIN–LIPID LEVELS

Four phase III studies (RIO program for Rimonabant In Obesity) have been published with rimonabant (11–14), which is the first CB_1 antagonist available in clinical practice in some countries. Treatment with rimonabant (20 mg/day) has been shown to decrease body weight and induce a significant reduction in waist circumference (a crude index of abdominal fat) (11–14). Rimonabant has also been shown to improve insulin sensitivity (indices of plasma glucose–insulin homeostasis), decrease plasma triglyceride and increase HDL-cholesterol levels, decrease the proportion of small LDL particles, reduce inflammation C-reactive protein (CRP), and increase plasma adiponectin concentrations (11–14).

Comparison of changes in metabolic parameters across subgroups with different levels of weight loss achieved revealed that for any given weight loss, rimonabant-treated patients had a more substantial reduction in triglyceride levels and a further increase in plasma HDL-cholesterol concentration compared to that of placebo-treated patients achieving the same weight loss (12–14). Additional multivariate analyses revealed that about one half of the effect of rimonabant on triglycerides, HDL-cholesterol, indices of insulin sensitivity, and adiponectin

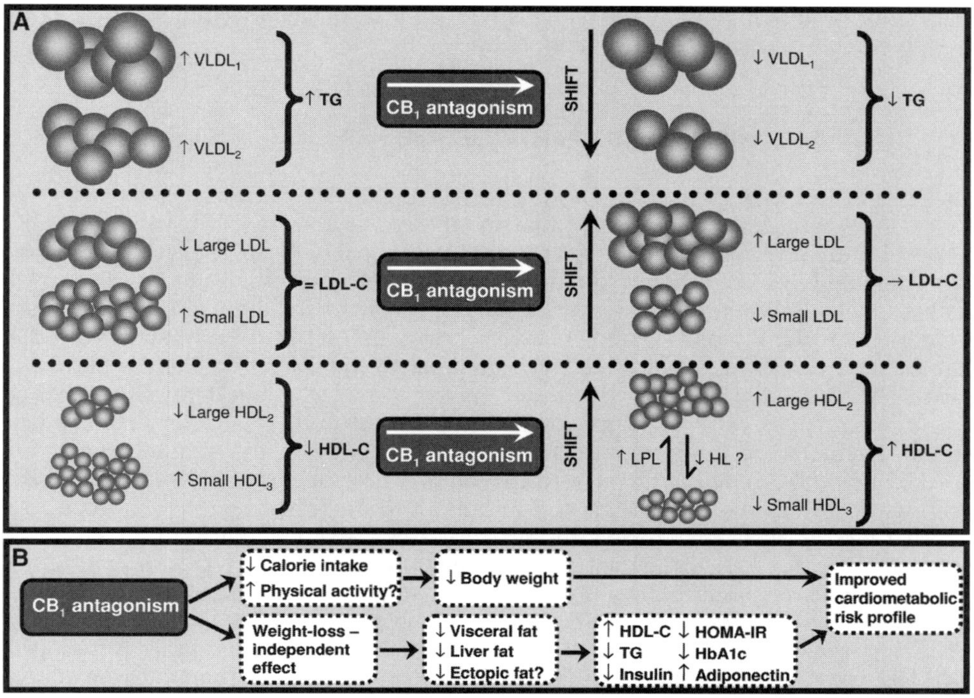

Figure 2 (*Panel A*): Schematic representation of the atherogenic lipoprotein–lipid profile of patients with visceral obesity. Viscerally obese, insulin-resistant patients have increased fasting triglyceride (TG) levels because of an overproduction of large, TG-rich $VLDL_1$ particles. Plasma LDL-cholesterol (LDL-C) levels are generally in a normal range in viscerally obese patients, a potentially misleading information for clinicians as these individuals are often characterized by an increased proportion of small, dense LDL particles. Plasma HDL-cholesterol (HDL-C) levels are also reduced in viscerally obese patients, particularly the concentration of the large, cholesteryl-ester–rich HDL_2 subfraction, leading to a reduced HDL particle size. Decreases in $VLDL_1$ and $VLDL_2$ with rimonabant generate a reduction in TG concentrations. Moreover, rimonabant treatment induces changes not only in lipoprotein–lipid concentrations but also in particle size. It is important to point out that the shift in LDL particle size (increase) reported with rimonabant cannot be appreciated by LDL-C concentrations, which show no change. Finally, increases in HDL-C noted with CB_1 antagonism seem to be the consequence of an increased HDL_2 subfraction. (*Note*: differences in particle size between the VLDL (very large), LDL (intermediate), and HDL (small) could not be appropriately scaled in this oversimplified illustration). (*Panel B*): Two mechanisms have been proposed to explain the cardiometabolic improvements produced by CB_1 antagonism with rimonabant: (1) body weight loss–related effects; (2) body weight loss–independent effect through loss of visceral fat, liver fat, and other ectopic fat depots. The weight loss–independent effect of the CB_1 antagonist rimonabant on several features of the cardiometabolic risk profile has been reported in Ref. (64) and is as follows: 45% for HDL-C, 46% for TG, 49% for fasting insulin, 49% for homeostasis model assessment for insulin resistance (HOMA-IR), 55% for glycated haemoglobin (HbA1c) and 57% for adiponectin. *Abbreviations*: HL, hepatic lipase; LPL, lipoprotein lipase.

could not be attributed to the magnitude of weight loss (11–14), suggesting a direct effect of CB_1 antagonism on metabolic processes affecting these markers (Fig. 2). One trial in which liver fat and visceral adiposity were directly measured by computed tomography (ADAGIO-Lipids) recently reported that rimonabant induced a preferential mobilization of visceral compared to subcutaneous fat which was also accompanied by a reduction in liver-fat content (20). These changes in markers of ectopic fat are fully consistent with the documented presence of CB_1 receptors in tissues such as the visceral adipose tissue and in the liver, and with the effect of CB_1 antagonism on adipose tissue and liver lipogenesis and metabolism. It is also important to point out that intervention studies have shown that moderate weight loss in viscerally obese patients is generally associated with a greater loss of visceral than subcutaneous abdominal adipose tissue (21–26). For instance, the greater the initial level of visceral adiposity, the more likely that the relative loss of visceral fat will be substantial in response to any interventions aiming at weight loss. Thus, it is not clear at this stage whether the same caloric deficit produced by rimonabant versus a hypocaloric diet would produce the same loss of visceral adipose tissue, and further studies will have to test this hypothesis. However, for the time being, it appears certain that high-risk abdominally obese patients with an atherogenic dyslipidemia lose both visceral and liver fat in response to rimonabant therapy (20).

EFFECT OF CB_1 ANTAGONISM ON LDL PARTICLE SIZE

Rimonabant has been reported to have no effect on LDL-cholesterol concentrations (Fig. 2) (11,13,14). It is important to stress that abdominal obesity is not associated with increased LDL-cholesterol levels but rather with an increased proportion of small LDL particles (1). Weight loss and exercise training have been shown to induce a shift in LDL particle size in the absence of major changes in the LDL-cholesterol concentration (27–30). Therefore, the shift in LDL particle size observed in the RIO-Lipids (11) and ADAGIO-Lipids (20) trials are consistent with the notion that therapies lowering triglyceride levels are likely to have a favorable effect on LDL particles (31). Furthermore, clinicians should not only rely on LDL-cholesterol to appreciate the impact of weight loss or of CB_1 antagonism on LDL quantity/quality in abdominally obese patients. An increased proportion of small LDL has been shown to be predictive of an increased CHD risk (32–36), although such relationship is no longer significant after control for triglycerides and HDL-cholesterol. It is also important to stress that no intervention study has shown that increasing LDL particle size as a target for therapy could reduce CHD risk. However, the finding that LDL size is not an independent predictor of CHD after control for triglycerides and HDL-cholesterol does not imply that small LDL particles are not directly involved in atherosclerosis. For instance, several basic investigations have provided evidence that small LDL particles could contribute to the accelerated atherosclerotic process (reduced affinity for LDL receptor, increased susceptibility to oxidation, etc.) (31). Therefore, the added value of antagonism of the endocannabinoid system with rimonabant on abdominal obesity and on additional metabolic risk markers beyond LDL-cholesterol should be considered for the management of the residual CHD risk of these patients.

EFFECT OF CB_1 ANTAGONISM ON TRIGLYCERIDE LEVELS

It is well documented that abdominally obese patients have increased plasma triglyceride levels (37,38). Triglyceride molecules are not atherogenic by themselves (39–41). However, hypertriglyceridemia accompanied by abdominal obesity is predictive of a markedly increased probability of finding patients with the whole cluster of athero-thrombotic–inflammatory abnormalities linked to insulin resistance which is often called the metabolic syndrome (42). Therefore, the reduction in triglyceride levels and waist circumference observed in the RIO studies suggests that CB_1 antagonism with pharmacological agents like rimonabant could have a significant impact on the cluster of metabolic abnormalities of the metabolic syndrome by treating the culprit causes of this condition (Fig. 2). Thus, the reduction in triglyceride levels produced by rimonabant is of course explained to a certain extent by weight loss and the loss of abdominal fat, but the reduced hepatic lipid content produced by rimonabant is also a key phenomenon which has been shown to be associated with a reduced production rate of large $VLDL_1$ particles by the liver (43). Thus, losses of visceral and hepatic fat produced by rimonabant are probably key factors responsible for the triglyceride lowering effect of this CB_1 antagonist.

EFFECT OF CB_1 ANTAGONISM ON INFLAMMATION

Abdominal obesity has been shown to be an important correlate of elevated CRP concentration (a marker of inflammation) (44,45). On that basis, one should expect that the loss of abdominal fat produced with rimonabant therapy would reduce plasma CRP levels (46,47). Several trials have now documented significant reduction in plasma CRP levels with rimonabant (11,13,20,48). For the time being, it appears that the loss of abdominal fat produced by rimonabant is probably the key factor responsible for the reduction in CRP but additional mechanistic studies are needed to test whether antagonism of the endocannabinoid system could have direct effects on processes affecting inflammation.

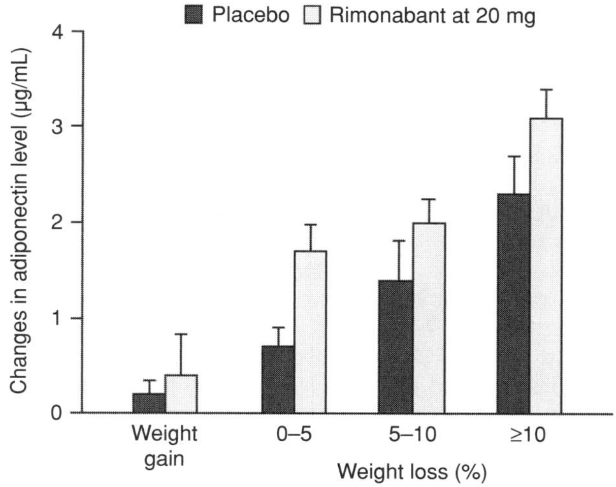

Figure 3 Changes in adiponectin levels according to categories of body weight changes observed in response to rimonabant (20 mg/day) or placebo therapy for 1 year among dyslipidemic overweight/obese patients of the RIO-Lipids trial. *Source*: Adapted from Ref. 11.

EFFECT OF CB_1 ANTAGONISM ON ADIPOSE CELL METABOLISM

Adipose tissue is more than a lipid storage/mobilization organ and it has now become clear that it also plays important endocrine functions (49). Hypertrophied abdominal adipose tissue is infiltrated with macrophages which contribute to the increased production of inflammatory cytokines (50). Some of these cytokines [such as tumor necrosis factor (TNF)-α] have a significant effect on the production of an abundant adipose tissue–derived cytokine, adiponectin (51,52), whereas interleukin-6 is well known to stimulate the production of CRP by the liver (53). Plasma adiponectin levels are markedly reduced in patients with visceral obesity, type 2 diabetes, and CHD (54–56). Clinical studies with rimonabant have shown that this CB_1 antagonist could increase plasma adiponectin levels beyond what could be expected from the magnitude of weight loss (Fig. 3) (11). Approximately more than one half of the increase in adiponectin levels cannot be explained by weight loss, an observation fully consistent with studies which have documented the presence of CB_1 receptors on adipose tissue cells (57,58). Indeed, animal studies have previously shown that agonists for the CB_1 receptor decreased adiponectin gene expression and protein secretion by adipose tissue and that rimonabant stimulates adiponectin production by fat cells (17). Adiponectin has numerous potentially important metabolic effects (such as major effects on liver metabolism, on the insulin signaling pathway, on insulin sensitivity, and on processes affecting HDL-cholesterol concentrations) (59,60). We have proposed that such an effect of rimonabant of adipose tissue adiponectin secretion could be one of the mechanisms by which this CB_1 antagonist could improve the cardiometabolic risk profile beyond what could be explained by its weight-loss properties. Studies are underway to further clarify this issue.

EFFECTS OF CB_1 ANTAGONISM ON LIVER FAT AND FUNCTION

Excess liver fat is a feature of ectopic fat deposition for which excess visceral adiposity is an excellent marker (19). As a consequence of increased hepatic lipid content, liver enzyme levels are elevated in abdominally overweight/obese patients with dyslipidemia (61,62). In clinical studies with rimonabant, it was found that this CB_1 antagonist could significantly reduce alanine aminotransferase (ALT), a crude but useful marker of fatty liver disease whose level has been shown to be predictive of insulin resistance and of the features of the metabolic syndrome (63). Such an effect of rimonabant on liver function is fully consistent with the recently reported effect of this CB_1 antagonist on liver-fat content estimated by computed tomography (20). Therefore, through its effect on liver fat, rimonabant could improve liver function and related metabolic abnormalities.

ANTAGONISM OF THE ENDOCANNABINOID SYSTEM: WHO IS THE RIGHT PATIENT?

Because of its comprehensive cardiometabolic effects, targeting the endocannabinoid system appears as a promising option for the treatment of visceral obesity/ectopic fat and related metabolic abnormalities. Unfortunately, as soon as results of the phase III program with the first CB_1 antagonism developed, rimonabant, became available, this drug was announced with great hype in the media as a possible miracle drug for the treatment of obesity. With the moderate weight loss produced by this agent and with its well-documented side effect profile which includes nausea, dizziness, anxiety, mood changes, and increased susceptibility to depressive symptoms (64), it has become quite evident that this drug should not be prescribed to patients with a history of depression. When such patients have been included in trials such as in the STRADIVARIUS study, high absolute prevalence rates of depressive symptoms were reported in both rimonabant and placebo arms with even greater prevalence numbers in the rimonabant arm (48). In contrast, when patients with history of severe or recurrent depression episodes were excluded such as in the recently reported ADAGIO-Lipids trial (20), lower incidence rates of depressive symptoms were found, although a slightly higher prevalence was nevertheless reported in the rimonabant than in the placebo group. These results should be seriously considered in the analysis of the benefit/risk ratio of CB_1 antagonists. Because of the risk of depression in susceptible individuals, patients with a history of depression should not be treated with this class of drugs. In addition, there is a low but clear "signal" that a greater incidence of depressive symptoms is found with rimonabant compared to placebo. Although it is uncertain whether this is related to rimonabant or to weight loss per se, it would be prudent to re-evaluate patients treated with rimonabant at the early once beginning of treatment with regular follow-ups. Finally, it is unlikely that targeting the endocannabinoid system is the solution to the management of overall obesity. Rather, because of the link between an overactivated endocannabinoid system and visceral obesity and ectopic fat deposition, CB_1 antagonism may represent a useful pharmacological approach to treat ectopic fat (including excess visceral fat) and related metabolic abnormalities. Patients with type 2 diabetes (at least 80–85% of them) have some excess of visceral/ectopic fat and represent the subpopulation of choice for the use of a CB_1 antagonist, provided that patients at high risk of depression are excluded. Furthermore, visceral obesity/excess ectopic fat is associated with insulin resistance and with an atherogenic dyslipidemic state which includes elevated triglyceride and apolipoprotein B levels, small dense LDL particles, and low HDL-cholesterol concentrations (19). This is another group of patients likely to considerably benefit from targeting their overactivated endocannabinoid system. As a very significant proportion of these viscerally obese patients with the atherogenic dyslipidemia of insulin resistance are also often dysglycemic and at increased risk of type 2 diabetes, there could also be a window of opportunity to prevent their conversion from impaired glucose tolerance to type 2 diabetes by loss of visceral/ectopic fat and related improvements in indices of plasma glucose–insulin homeostasis. Irrespective of the mechanism of action of rimonabant, the weight loss and loss of abdominal adipose tissue have been shown to reduce the risk of type 2 diabetes by almost 60%, a remarkable finding (65,66). Whether the weight loss–independent properties of rimonabant could further reduce risk of developing diabetes in these high-risk prediabetic patients is under investigation.

CONCLUSION

Visceral obesity more than subcutaneous obesity is a form of overweight/obesity associated with elevated concentrations of inflammatory cytokines, a depressed adiponectin production by fat cells, insulin resistance, and with an atherogenic dyslipidemia. Smoking, hypertension, and elevated LDL-cholesterol levels are well-established targets for the management of

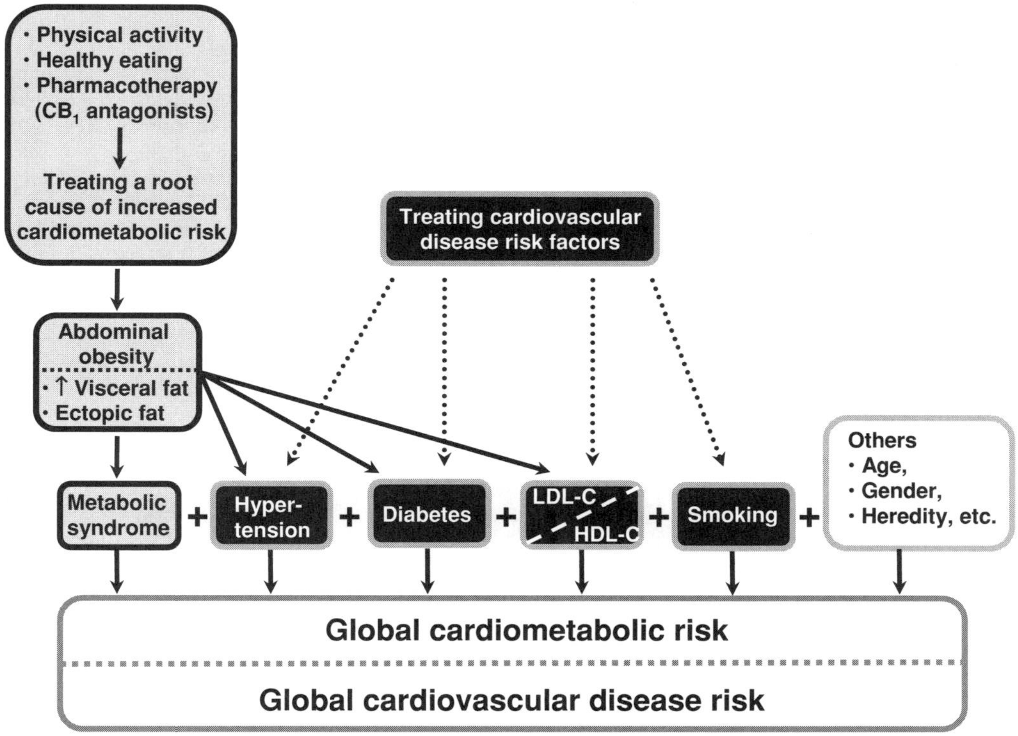

Figure 4 Added value of targeting excess visceral fat/ectopic fat by healthy eating, physical activity, and, if required, pharmacotherapy aimed at the endocannabinoid system in order to optimally manage global cardiometabolic risk markers/factors. The model also recognizes the importance of targeting "traditional" risk factors.

elevated cardiovascular risk. On the basis of the evidence published over almost three decades, it is proposed that abdominal obesity should be evaluated and managed in clinical practice. In this regard, results from preclinical and clinical studies have indicated that targeting the overactivated endocannabinoid system may represent a new and potentially interesting approach for the optimal management of the elevated cardiometabolic risk of patients with abdominal obesity (Fig. 4). CB_1 antagonism not only reduces weight and waist circumference, but more importantly has been shown to also induce favorable changes in several markers of cardiometabolic risk beyond what could be attributed to weight loss alone. Antagonism of the endocannabinoid system appears to target some central determinants of a cluster of metabolic abnormalities often referred to as the metabolic syndrome which are the results of a sedentary affluent lifestyle combined to a genetic predisposition. Thus, to describe CB_1 antagonists as "weight loss drugs" is not fair. This class of drugs will not be the "quick fix" to the overall obesity epidemic but a useful and welcome addition to the pharmacological arsenal currently available to manage the elevated cardiovascular disease risk of an expanding proportion of patients for whom visceral obesity appears to represent a new and important modifiable risk factor. The challenge ahead in clinical practice will be to make sure that this class of drugs is prescribed to the right patient for whom the benefit/risk ratio is overwhelmingly favorable.

ACKNOWLEDGMENTS

The work of the author has been supported by research grants from the Canadian Institutes of Health Research, the Canadian Diabetes Association, the Heart and Stroke Foundation, and by the Foundation of the Québec Heart Institute. Dr. Després is the Scientific Director of the International Chair on Cardiometabolic Risk, which is supported by an unrestricted grant from Sanofi-Aventis awarded to Université Laval.

REFERENCES

1. Tchernof A, Lamarche B, Prud'homme D, et al. The dense LDL phenotype. Association with plasma lipoprotein levels, visceral obesity, and hyperinsulinemia in men. Diabetes Care 1996; 19(6):629–637.
2. Després JP, Moorjani S, Ferland M, et al. Adipose tissue distribution and plasma lipoprotein levels in obese women. Importance of intra-abdominal fat. Arteriosclerosis 1989; 9(2):203–210.
3. Lamarche B, Tchernof A, Mauriège P, et al. Fasting insulin and apolipoprotein B levels and low-density lipoprotein particle size as risk factors for ischemic heart disease. JAMA 1998; 279(24):1955–1961.
4. Secondary prevention by raising HDL cholesterol and reducing triglycerides in patients with coronary artery disease: The Bezafibrate Infarction Prevention (BIP) study. Circulation 2000; 102(1):21–27.
5. Jeppesen J, Hein HO, Suadicani P, et al. Relation of high TG–low HDL cholesterol and LDL cholesterol to the incidence of ischemic heart disease. An 8-year follow-up in the Copenhagen Male Study. Arterioscler Thromb Vasc Biol 1997; 17(6):1114–1120.
6. Manninen V, Tenkanen L, Koshinen P, et al. Joint effects of serum triglyceride and LDL cholesterol and HDL cholesterol concentrations on coronary heart disease risk in the Helsinki Heart Study: Implications for treatment. Circulation 1992; 85:37–45.
7. Alberti KG, Zimmet P, Shaw J. The metabolic syndrome—A new worldwide definition. Lancet 2005; 366(9491):1059–1062.
8. Expert Panel on Detection, Evaluation, and Treatment of High Blood Cholesterol in Adults. Executive summary of the third report of the National Cholesterol Education Program (NCEP) Expert Panel on detection, evaluation, and treatment of high blood cholesterol in adults (Adult Treatment Panel III). JAMA 2001; 285(19):2486–2497.
9. Bluher M, Engeli S, Kloting N, et al. Dysregulation of the peripheral and adipose tissue endocannabinoid system in human abdominal obesity. Diabetes 2006; 55(11):3053–3060.
10. Côté M, Matias I, Lemieux I, et al. Circulating endocannabinoid levels, abdominal adiposity and related cardiometabolic risk factors in obese men. Int J Obes 2007; 31:692–699.
11. Després JP, Golay A, Sjöström L. Effects of rimonabant on metabolic risk factors in overweight patients with dyslipidemia. N Engl J Med 2005; 353(20):2121–2134.
12. Pi-Sunyer FX, Aronne LJ, Heshmati HM, et al. Effect of rimonabant, a cannabinoid-1 receptor blocker, on weight and cardiometabolic risk factors in overweight or obese patients: RIO-North America: A randomized controlled trial. JAMA 2006; 295(7):761–775.
13. Scheen AJ, Finer N, Hollander P, et al. Efficacy and tolerability of rimonabant in overweight or obese patients with type 2 diabetes: A randomised controlled study. Lancet 2006; 368(9548):1660–1672.
14. Van Gaal LF, Rissanen AM, Scheen AJ, et al. Effects of the cannabinoid-1 receptor blocker rimonabant on weight reduction and cardiovascular risk factors in overweight patients: 1-year experience from the RIO-Europe study. Lancet 2005; 365(9468):1389–1397.
15. Osei-Hyiaman D, DePetrillo M, Pacher P, et al. Endocannabinoid activation at hepatic CB_1 receptors stimulates fatty acid synthesis and contributes to diet-induced obesity. J Clin Invest 2005; 115(5):1298–1305.
16. Di Marzo V, Bifulco M, De Petrocellis L. The endocannabinoid system and its therapeutic exploitation. Nat Rev Drug Discov 2004; 3(9):771–784.
17. Bensaid M, Gary-Bobo M, Esclangon A, et al. The cannabinoid CB_1 receptor antagonist SR141716 increases Acrp30 mRNA expression in adipose tissue of obese fa/fa rats and in cultured adipocyte cells. Mol Pharmacol 2003; 63(4):908–914.
18. Després JP, Lemieux I. Abdominal obesity and metabolic syndrome. Nature 2006; 444(7121):881–887.
19. Després JP, Lemieux I, Bergeron J, et al. Abdominal obesity and the metabolic syndrome: Contribution to global cardiometabolic risk. Arterioscler Thromb Vasc Biol 2008; 28(6):1039–1049.
20. Després JP, Ross R, Boka G, et al. For the ADAGIO-Lipids investigators. Rimonabant reduces both intra-abdominal adiposity and liver fat and improves cardiometabolic risk factors: The ADAGIO-Lipids trial. Presented at the late breaking session of the 77th European Atherosclerosis Society meeting, Istanbul, 2008.
21. Chaston TB, Dixon JB. Factors associated with percent change in visceral versus subcutaneous abdominal fat during weight loss: Findings from a systematic review. Int J Obes (Lond) 2008; 32(4):619–628.
22. Paré A, Dumont M, Lemieux I, et al. Is the relationship between adipose tissue and waist girth altered by weight loss in obese men? Obes Res 2001; 9(9):526–534.
23. Goodpaster BH, Kelley DE, Wing RR, et al. Effects of weight loss on regional fat distribution and insulin sensitivity in obesity. Diabetes 1999; 48:839–847.
24. Després JP, Lamarche B. Effects of diet and physical activity on adiposity and body fat distribution: Implications for the prevention of cardiovascular disease. Nutr Res Rev 1993; 6:137–159.
25. Zamboni M, Armellini F, Turcato E, et al. Effect of weight loss on regional body fat distribution in premenopausal women. Am J Clin Nutr 1993; 58(1):29–34.
26. Leenen R, van der Kooy K, Deurenberg P, et al. Visceral fat accumulation in obese subjects: Relation to energy expenditure and response to weight loss. Am J Physiol 1992; 263:E913–E919.

27. Kraus WE, Houmard JA, Duscha BD, et al. Effects of the amount and intensity of exercise on plasma lipoproteins. N Engl J Med 2002; 347(19):1483–1492.
28. Baumstark MW, Frey I, Berg A. Acute and delayed effects of prolonged exercise on serum lipoproteins. II. Concentration and composition of low-density lipoprotein subfractions and very low-density lipoproteins. Eur J Appl Physiol Occup Physiol 1993; 66(6):526–530.
29. Houmard JA, Bruno NJ, Bruner RK, et al. Effects of exercise training on the chemical composition of plasma LDL. Arterioscler Thromb Vasc Biol 1994; 14(3):325–330.
30. Williams PT, Krauss RM, Vranizan KM, et al. Effects of exercise-induced weight loss on low density lipoprotein subfractions in healthy men. Arterioscler Thromb Vasc Biol 1989; 9:623–632.
31. Lamarche B, Lemieux I, Després JP. The small, dense LDL phenotype and the risk of coronary heart disease: Epidemiology, patho-physiology and therapeutic aspects. Diabetes Metab 1999; 25(3):199–211.
32. Lamarche B, Tchernof A, Moorjani S, et al. Small, dense low-density lipoprotein particles as a predictor of the risk of ischemic heart disease in men. Prospective results from the Québec Cardiovascular Study. Circulation 1997; 95:69–75.
33. St-Pierre AC, Ruel IL, Cantin B, et al. Comparison of various electrophoretic characteristics of LDL particles and their relationship to the risk of ischemic heart disease. Circulation 2001; 104(19):2295–2299.
34. Stampfer MJ, Krauss RM, Ma J, et al. A prospective study of triglyceride level, low-density lipoprotein particle diameter, and risk of myocardial infarction. JAMA 1996; 276:882–888.
35. Gardner CD, Fortmann SP, Krauss RM. Association of small low-density lipoprotein particles with the incidence of coronary artery disease in men and women. JAMA 1996; 276:875–881.
36. Arsenault BJ, Lemieux I, Després JP, et al. Cholesterol levels in small LDL particles predict the risk of coronary heart disease in the EPIC-Norfolk prospective population study. Eur Heart J 2007; 28(22):2770–2777.
37. Després JP, Moorjani S, Lupien PJ, et al. Regional distribution of body fat, plasma lipoproteins, and cardiovascular disease. Arteriosclerosis 1990; 10(4):497–511.
38. Pouliot MC, Després JP, Nadeau A, et al. Visceral obesity in men. Associations with glucose tolerance, plasma insulin, and lipoprotein levels. Diabetes 1992; 41(7):826–834.
39. Austin MA, McKnight B, Edwards KL, et al. Cardiovascular disease mortality in familial forms of hypertriglyceridemia: A 20-year prospective study. Circulation 2000; 101(24):2777–2782.
40. Nordestgaard BG, Benn M, Schnohr P, et al. Nonfasting triglycerides and risk of myocardial infarction, ischemic heart disease, and death in men and women. JAMA 2007; 298:299–308.
41. Bansal S, Buring JE, Rifai N, et al. Fasting compared with nonfasting triglycerides and risk of cardiovascular events in women. JAMA 2007; 298:309–316.
42. Lemieux I, Pascot A, Couillard C, et al. Hypertriglyceridemic waist. A marker of the atherogenic metabolic triad (hyperinsulinemia, hyperapolipoprotein B, small dense LDL) in men? Circulation 2000; 102:179–184.
43. Adiels M, Westerbacka J, Soro-Paavonen A, et al. Acute suppression of VLDL1 secretion rate by insulin is associated with hepatic fat content and insulin resistance. Diabetologia 2007; 50(11):2356–2365.
44. Hak AE, Stehouwer CD, Bots ML, et al. Associations of C-reactive protein with measures of obesity, insulin resistance, and subclinical atherosclerosis in healthy, middle-aged women. Arterioscler Thromb Vasc Biol 1999; 19(8):1986–1991.
45. Lemieux I, Pascot A, Prud'homme D, et al. Elevated C-reactive protein: Another component of the atherothrombotic profile of abdominal obesity. Arterioscler Thromb Vasc Biol 2001; 21(6):961–967.
46. Tchernof A, Nolan A, Sites CK, et al. Weight loss reduces C-reactive protein levels in obese postmenopausal women. Circulation 2002; 105(5):564–569.
47. Heilbronn LK, Noakes M, Clifton PM. Energy restriction and weight loss on very-low-fat diets reduce C-reactive protein concentrations in obese, healthy women. Arterioscler Thromb Vasc Biol 2001; 21(6):968–970.
48. Nissen SE, Nicholls SJ, Wolski K, et al. Effect of rimonabant on progression of atherosclerosis in patients with abdominal obesity and coronary artery disease: The STRADIVARIUS randomized controlled trial. JAMA 2008; 299(13):1547–1560.
49. Flier JS. The adipocyte: Storage depot or node on the energy information superhighway? Cell 1995; 80(1):15–18.
50. Weisberg SP, McCann D, Desai M, et al. Obesity is associated with macrophage accumulation in adipose tissue. J Clin Invest 2003; 112(12):1796–1808.
51. Fasshauer M, Klein J, Neumann S, et al. Hormonal regulation of adiponectin gene expression in 3T3-L1 adipocytes. Biochem Biophys Res Commun 2002; 290(3):1084–1089.
52. Kern PA, Di Gregorio GB, Lu T, et al. Adiponectin expression from human adipose tissue: Relation to obesity, insulin resistance, and tumor necrosis factor-alpha expression. Diabetes 2003; 52(7):1779–1785.
53. Yudkin JS, Stehouwer CD, Emeis JJ, et al. C-reactive protein in healthy subjects: Associations with obesity, insulin resistance, and endothelial dysfunction: A potential role for cytokines originating from adipose tissue? Arterioscler Thromb Vasc Biol 1999; 19(4):972–978.

54. Côté M, Mauriège P, Bergeron J, et al. Adiponectinemia in visceral obesity: Impact on glucose tolerance and plasma lipoprotein and lipid levels in men. J Clin Endocrinol Metab 2005; 90(3):1434–1439.
55. Pischon T, Girman CJ, Hotamisligil GS, et al. Plasma adiponectin levels and risk of myocardial infarction in men. JAMA 2004; 291(14):1730–1737.
56. Spranger J, Kroke A, Mohlig M, et al. Adiponectin and protection against type 2 diabetes mellitus. Lancet 2003; 361(9353):226–228.
57. Engeli S, Bohnke J, Feldpausch M, et al. Activation of the peripheral endocannabinoid system in human obesity. Diabetes 2005; 54(10):2838–2843.
58. Roche R, Hoareau L, Bes-Houtmann S, et al. Presence of the cannabinoid receptors, CB_1 and CB_2, in human omental and subcutaneous adipocytes. Histochem Cell Biol 2006; 126(2):177–187.
59. Ukkola O, Santaniemi M. Adiponectin: A link between excess adiposity and associated comorbidities? J Mol Med 2002; 80(11):696–702.
60. Hotta K, Funahashi T, Arita Y, et al. Plasma concentrations of a novel, adipose-specific protein, adiponectin, in type 2 diabetic patients. Arterioscler Thromb Vasc Biol 2000; 20:1595–1599.
61. Church TS, Kuk JL, Ross R, et al. Association of cardiorespiratory fitness, body mass index, and waist circumference to nonalcoholic fatty liver disease. Gastroenterology 2006; 130(7):2023–2030.
62. Yamada J, Tomiyama H, Yambe M, et al. Elevated serum levels of alanine aminotransferase and gamma glutamyltransferase are markers of inflammation and oxidative stress independent of the metabolic syndrome. Atherosclerosis 2006; 189(1):198–205.
63. Després JP, Golay A, Sjöström L. Evidence that rimonabant has beneficial effects on liver enzymes in overweight/obese patients with dyslipidemia—RIO-Lipids Trial (abstract). Circulation 2006; 114(18):II-223.
64. Van Gaal L, Pi-Sunyer X, Després JP, et al. Efficacy and safety of rimonabant for improvement of multiple cardiometabolic risk factors in overweight/obese patients: Pooled 1-year data from the Rimonabant in Obesity (RIO) program. Diabetes Care 2008; 31(Suppl. 2):S229–S240.
65. Knowler WC, Barrett-Connor E, Fowler SE, et al. Reduction in the incidence of type 2 diabetes with lifestyle intervention or metformin. N Engl J Med 2002; 346(6):393–403.
66. Tuomilehto J, Lindstrom J, Eriksson JG, et al. Prevention of type 2 diabetes mellitus by changes in lifestyle among subjects with impaired glucose tolerance. N Engl J Med 2001; 344(18):1343–1350.

31 CB_1 Blockade and Hypertension

Luis M. Ruilope

Hypertension Unit, Hospital 12 de Octubre, Madrid, Spain

The term metabolic syndrome refers to a common pattern of multiple risk factors facilitating the development of cardiovascular (CV) disease and type 2 diabetes that has emerged recently, and is largely but not completely driven by obesity (1). An adequate stratification of global CV risk must then contemplate the presence of traditional CV risk factors and emerging markers found in individuals with excess intra-abdominal adiposity and a "dysfunctional" adipose tissue phenotype. This global risk is defined as cardiometabolic risk (2) and is particularly elevated in the hypertensive population (3–4). More than two-thirds of the hypertensive population present with overweight and obesity, and 40% to 60% can be classified as having metabolic syndrome according to ATP III criteria (3–4). On the other hand, arterial hypertension is number one killer in the general population in developed as well as in developing countries, as is demonstrated in recently published data from WHO (5), and the association of elevated blood pressure and diabetes is the most devastating for the CV and the renal systems (6). The need to consider cardiometabolic risk in the risk stratification of hypertensive patients as well as the need to consider its treatment is nowadays totally required. In fact, this situation has forced the recognition by the Guidelines of the European Society of Hypertension and European Society of Cardiology (7) of metabolic syndrome as a situation of high added risk as soon as BP is above 130 and/or 85 mmHg (high-normal BP and above) (Fig. 1).

On the other hand, an enhanced global CV risk due to the presence of cardiometabolic components is simultaneously accompanied by an increased prevalence of chronic kidney disease (albuminuria and/or a diminished estimated glomerular filtration rate). In fact, the higher the number of components present in the definition of metabolic syndrome, the higher is the possibility of developing either microalbuminuria and/or an estimated GFR value $\leq$60 mL/min/1.73 m^2 (8).

ABOUT THE DEVELOPMENT OF DIABETES MELLITUS IN A HYPERTENSIVE POPULATION

The development of diabetes and its relevance in hypertensive patients has been widely considered recently (9–10). Beyond lifestyle changes, both dietetic and related to physical activity, the type of antihypertensive therapy used, alone or in combination, has been shown to be relevant to prevent or accelerate the appearance of diabetes. A recent network meta-analysis (11) has shown that the best protection is obtained when angiotensin receptor blockers or converting enzyme inhibitors are used, while diuretics and betablockers are occupying the last position in particular when used in combination. Some authors have denied the fact that the development of diabetes contributes to worsen the short-term (3–5 years) prognosis of hypertensive patients; according to the data of studies like SHEP (Systolic Hypertension in the Elderly Program) (12) and ALLHAT (Antihypertensive and Lipid-Lowering Treatment to Prevent Heart Attack Trial) (13), it seems clear that becoming a diabetic must be relevant for the long-term prognosis of patients. In fact, it has been shown that with two and a half years of follow-up above that in ALLHAT, the risk of new diabetics was equal to that of patients entering the study as declared diabetics (14).

On the other hand, different studies have shown the capacity of orally active antidiabetic drugs like metformin (15), acarbose (16), and rosiglitazone (17), as well as antiobesity drugs like orlistat, (18) to prevent the development of diabetes. Moreover, prevention of the development of established arterial hypertension has been shown to occur in the STOP-NIDDM (Study To Prevent Non-Insulin-Dependent Diabetes Mellitus) study that tested acarbose (16).

Other risk factors, OD or disease	Blood pressure (mmHg)				
	Normal SBP 120–129 or DBP 80–84	High normal SBP 130-139 or DBP 85–89	Grade 1 HT SBP 140–159 or DBP 90–99	Grade 2 HT SBP 160–179 or DBP 100–109	Grade 3 HT SBP ≥ 159 or DBP ≥ 110
No other risk factors	Average risk	Average risk	Low added risk	Moderate added risk	High added risk
1-2 risk factors	Low added risk	Low added risk	Moderate added risk	Moderate added risk	Very high added risk
3 or more risk factors, MS, OD or diabetes	Moderate added risk	High added risk	High added risk	High added risk	Very high added risk
Established CV or renel diseas	Very high added risk	Very high added risk	Very high added risk	Very high added risk	Very high added risk

Stratification of CV risk in four categories. SBP; systolic blood pressure; DBP diastolic blood pressure; CV: cardiovascular; HT: hypertension. Low, moderat, high and very high risk refer to 10 year of a CV fatal or non-fatal event. The term " added" indicates that in all categories risk is greater than average. OD: subclinical organ damage; MS: metabolic syndrome. The dashed line indicates how definition of hypertension may be variable, depending on the level of total CV risk.

Figure 1 Stratification of CV risk in four categories. Low, moderate, high, and very high risk refer to 10-year risk of a CV fatal or nonfatal event. The term "added" indicates that in all categories, risk is greater than average. The dashed line indicates how definition of hypertension may be variable, depending on the level of fatal CV risk. *Abbreviations*: SBP, systolic blood pressure; DBP, diastolic blood pressure; CV, cardiovascular; HT, hypertension; OD, subclinical organ damage; MS, metabolic syndrome.

MANAGEMENT OF PATIENTS WITH ESSENTIAL HYPERTENSION AND CARDIOMETABOLIC RISK

Long-term adherence to lifestyle modifications, obviously constitutes the first-step therapy when considering the correction of an increased cardiometabolic risk, including an adequate diet accompanied by physical activity. This will facilitate a fall in body weight in intra-abdominal adiposity and an improvement in insulin resistance. Hypertensive patients presenting with an elevated cardiometabolic risk require a tight BP control (≤130/80 mmHg). The inclusion of a suppressor of renin–angiotensin system (7) and if possible the avoidance of drugs facilitate metabolic alterations, in particular the development of diabetes. This must be accompanied by an adequate correction of dyslipidemia and insulin resistance. In this sense, new guidelines contemplate the addition of a statin to every hypertensive patient in a situation of high or very high added risk, even in the presence of normal values of total and LDL-cholesterol (7). Dyslipidemia accompanying cardiometabolic risk is charactherized by the presence of elevated levels of triglycerides and low levels of HDL-cholesterol. Some data indicate that considering the use of nicotinic acid or fibrates can have a beneficial effect in patients with metabolic syndrome, insulin resistance, or diabetes (19–20).

Antiobesity drugs can also be considered in hypertensive patients presented with a body mass index (BMI) above 30, and two different pharmacological approaches are available. The first is represented by sibutramine, a drug acting on monoaminergic systems currently approved for the long-term control of obesity. Several clinical trials have demonstrated the superiority of sibutramine with respect to placebo in reducing weight and waist circumference (median at one year: 4.5 kg). However, in hypertensive patients, sibutramine slightly increases blood pressure and heart rate and should be used with caution (21). A recent trial suggests that the effects of sibutramine in hypertensive patients under antihypertensive treatment largely depend on the type of the antihypertensive drugs used (22). The second approach is represented by orlistat, an inhibitor of gastrointestinal lipases. Its efficacy in producing a superior weight loss with respect to placebo has also been proven, although the weight loss is usually less than that obtained with sibutramine. Orlistat has a favorable influence on lipids and glycemic control, especially in diabetics, although gastrointestinal tolerance is poor.

THE ROLE OF CB_1 BLOCKADE IN ARTERIAL HYPERTENSION

The link between obesity (particularly abdominal obesity) and hypertension and other cardiometabolic risk factors is well established (23,24). Indeed, data from the Framingham Heart Study estimate that 75% and 65% of the cases of hypertension in men and women, respectively, are directly attributable to overweight and obesity (25). The attributable risk of hypertension induced by abdominal obesity has been estimated to range from 21% to 57% depending on gender and ethnicity (26). Body weight change is itself a potent modulator of hypertension risk: in the Nurses Health Study, after adjusting for BMI, weight gain in adulthood of as little as 2.1 to 4.9 kg increased the risk of hypertension by 29%, whereas weight loss of 5 kg was associated with a 15% reduction in hypertension risk (27). A meta-analysis of randomized, controlled trials showed that weight loss is important for the prevention and treatment of hypertension: blood pressure reductions were −1.05 mmHg for systolic blood pressure (SBP) and −0.92 mmHg for diastolic blood pressure (DBP) when expressed per kilogram of weight loss (28). While short-term interventions to produce weight loss effectively lower blood pressure, long-term maintenance of a reduced body weight is a difficult objective to achieve.

The recently discovered endocannabinoid system (ECS) plays a role in energy balance, and glucose and lipid metabolism through central and peripheral actions (29–30). Recently, an association between the overactivation of the ECS, the abdominal obesity phenotype characterized by high visceral or intra-abdominal fat, and the different cardiometabolic risk factors has been described (31–32). While this association with abdominal obesity suggests the overactive ECS as a potential target for addressing blood pressure, current evidence indicates that in rodent models of hypertension, inhibition of the overactive ECS using cannabinoid type 1 receptor (CB_1) blockade evoked sustained further increases in blood pressure (33).

Rimonabant, the first selective CB_1 receptor blocker, has been shown to improve multiple cardiometabolic risk factors, such as abdominal obesity, dyslipidaemia, glycaemic control, and insulin resistance in overweight/obese patients (34–37). About 50% of the effects of rimonabant on lipid and glycaemic variables has been shown to be independent of weight loss and may reflect direct metabolic effects of CB_1 blockade in peripheral tissues (29,30,36).

The effect on blood pressure of CB_1 blockade has been recently reviewed (38) by assessing the impact of rimonabant on blood pressure in overweight/obese patients with dyslipidaemia, type 2 diabetes, and high blood pressure (SBP $\geq$ 130 and/or DBP $\geq$ 85 mmHg in patients with type 2 diabetes and SBP $\geq$ 140 and/or DBP $\geq$ 90 mmHg in patients without diabetes) using pooled and individual study data from the four large Rimonabant-In-Obesity (RIO) multicentre, randomized controlled trials. The pooled 1-year intention-to-treat (ITT) population consisted of $N = 1602$ patients and $N = 2503$ patients randomized to placebo and rimonabant 20 mg, respectively. Overall, the RIO studies represent an at-risk population of overweight/obese patients with an elevated waist circumference (86–97%) and a high rate of cardiometabolic risk factors. In total, 37% of the pooled population had previously diagnosed hypertension, comprising 61% of patients in RIO-Diabetes (BP $\geq$ 130/85 mmHg) and 27% of RIO-Lipids and 30% and 41% of RIO-North America and RIO-Europe, respectively (BP $\geq$ 140/90 mmHg). Of the patients previously diagnosed with hypertension, 71% of the pooled patients were receiving antihypertensive medication and during the treatment period most patients had no changes in anti-hypertensive medications (approximately 94% of patients) and the distribution of changes in anti-hypertensive medication was not significantly different in the two treatment arms.

As can be seen in Table 1 (A), in the overall population during the run-in period (before randomization to placebo or rimonabant treatment), there was a substantial mean (SD) decrease in SBP [−2.9 (11.3) mmHg] and DBP [−1.3 (7.8) mmHg] [Table 1 (A)]. This decrease was even more marked in those patients with high blood pressure, at the beginning of the placebo run-in period: SBP −7.4 (11.9) mmHg, and DBP −3.7 (8.0) mmHg [Table 1 (A)]. During the run-in period, body weight and waist circumference decreased by −1.8 (2.1) kg and −1.9 (3.8) cm, respectively, in the overall pooled population, and by −2.0 (2.1) kg and −1.8 (3.6) cm, respectively, in the subgroup with high blood pressure at baseline. The effect of 1-year treatment with rimonabant 20 mg/day on blood pressure in the pooled ITT population is shown in Table 1 (B).

Body weight loss and the reductions in waist circumference at 1 year were significantly greater in the rimonabant 20 mg group compared with placebo. In the overall pooled ITT population receiving rimonabant 20 mg/day, mean weight loss from baseline at 1 year was

Table 1 Change in Blood Pressure During Run-In **(A)** and After 1 Year (**B**) (Four Pooled Studies[a])

(A) Change in blood pressure during placebo run-in period at screening (4 weeks; ITT population)

	Overall population	**High blood pressure[b] at screening**
N	6625	1987
Supine SBP (mmHg)		
Start of run-in	127.5 (13.9)	142.5 (9.5)
End of run-in	124.6 (13.5)	135.1 (12.3)
Change	−2.9 (11.3)	−7.4 (11.9)
Supine DBP (mmHg)		
Start of run-in	79.8 (8.7)	87.0 (7.8)
End of run-in	78.5 (8.3)	83.3 (7.9)
Change	−1.3 (7.8)	−3.7 (8.0)

(B) Change in blood pressure after 1 year (ITT population, LOCF)

	Overall population		**High blood pressure[b] at baseline**	
	Placebo	**Rimonabant 20 mg**	**Placebo**	**Rimonabant 20 mg**
N	1570	2466	396	526
Supine SBP (mmHg)				
Mean baseline (SD)	124.7 (13.4)	124.6 (13.4)	140.7 (9.3)	141.7 (9.8)
Year 1	125.0 (13.8)	123.8 (13.6)	136.0 (13.5)	134.3 (13.0)
Mean change from baseline (SD)	0.3 (12.0)	−0.8 (12.4)	−4.7 (13.2)	−7.5 (13.2)
LS mean change vs. placebo (SE)	-	−1.1 (0.4)	-	−2.5 (0.9)
p Value (20 mg vs. placebo)	-	($p = 0.007$)	-	($p = 0.005$)
Supine DBP (mmHg)				
Mean baseline (SD)	78.6 (8.1)	78.4 (8.3)	85.5 (7.4)	86.5 (7.6)
Year 1	78.3 (8.4)	77.5 (8.2)	82.5 (8.7)	81.3 (8.0)
Mean change from baseline (SD)	−0.3 (8.2)	−0.8 (8.4)	−3.0 (8.8)	−5.2 (8.1)
LS mean change vs. placebo (SE)	-	−0.6 (0.3)	-	−2.0 (0.6)
p Value (20 mg vs. placebo)	-	$p = 0.029$	-	($p \leq 0.001$)

[a] Pooled group comprises patients undergoing the first year of treatment in the RIO-North America, RIO-Europe, RIO-Lipids, and RIO-Diabetes studies.
[b] BP ≥140/90 mmHg (RIO-North America, RIO-Europe, and RIO-Lipids) or ≥130/85 mmHg (RIO-Diabetes).
Abbreviations: ITT, intention-to-treat; LOCF, last observation carried forward.

−6.3 (6.8) kg ($p \leq 0.001$ vs. placebo). Similar reductions in body weight were found in patients with normal and high blood pressure at baseline (38). As expected, there was a strong linear relationship between degree of weight loss and blood pressure reductions. However, this relationship was similar in the two treatment arms. After adjusting the observed changes in blood pressure for weight changes in the analysis of covariance, the residual treatment effect on blood pressure was not significant. Thus, the effect of rimonabant 20 mg/day is consistent with that seen for placebo in patients matched for the same degree of weight loss. This suggests that rimonabant 20 mg/day does not have an additional effect on blood pressure beyond that attributable to weight loss.

Figures 2 and 3 represent the changes in BP observed for normo and hypertensive patient with diabetes (RIO-Diabetes) and with hyperlipidemia (RIO-Lipids). The data reflect similar changes as in the pooled population with more significant changes in hypertensive patients.

In summary, the individual RIO trials and the pooled data, small but consistent decrease in both SBP and DBP, were observed following 1 year of treatment with rimonabant 20 mg/day. This relatively small reduction was observed despite normal mean blood pressure at baseline. However, in the subset of patients with elevated blood pressure at baseline, more pronounced reductions in both SBP and DBP were noted and both were reduced significantly—more by rimonabant 20 mg compared with placebo treatment. It is also relevant to note that the total blood pressure lowering effect does not include the 1 to 4 mmHg reductions in blood pressure observed during the 4-week run-in period in these trials. These results are consistent with the body weight reductions observed in hypertension prevention trials in patients with normal or high blood pressure (38) and favor the utilization of rimonabant in hypertensive patients with an

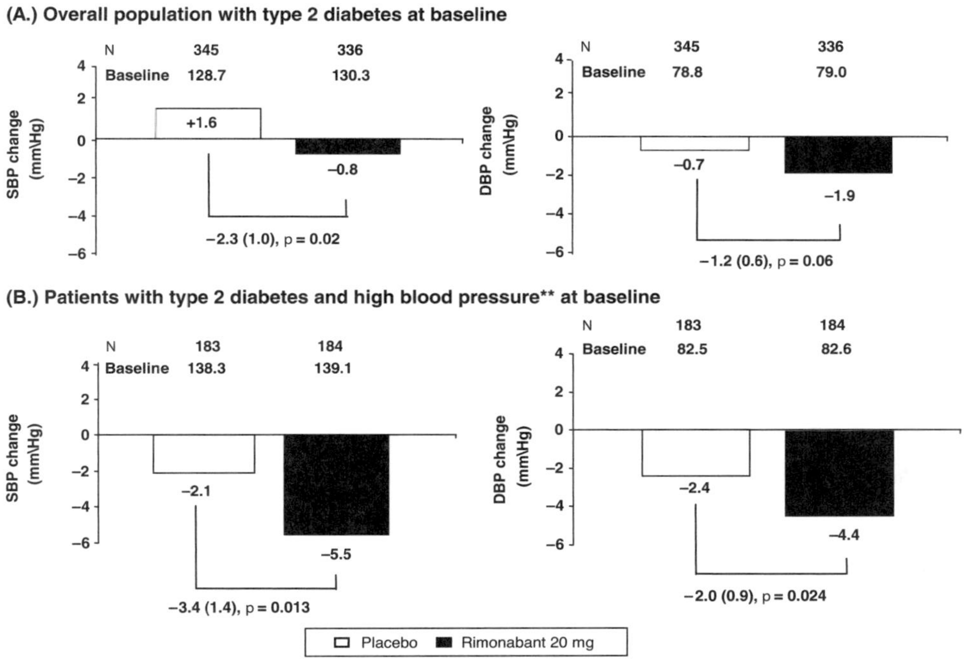

*Type 2 diabetes (RIO-Diabetes): defined as haemoglobin A_{1c} 6.5–10.0% and fasting glucose concentration 5.55–15.04 mmol/L as per protocol.

**High blood pressure: SBP ≥ 130 and/or DBP ≥ 85 mm/Hg in patients with type 2 diabetes.

Figure 2 **(A)** Changes in SBP (*left panel*) and DBP (*right panel*) at 1 year in the subset of patients with type 2 diabetes at baseline. Data are mean from the ITT population. Between-group comparisons are least-squares mean differences (SEM) (*p* vs. placebo). **(B)** Changes in SBP (*left panel*) and DBP (*right panel*) at 1 year in the subset of patients with type 2 diabetes and high blood pressure at baseline.

increased global cardiometabolic risk. In fact, the positive effect can contribute to diminish the observed enhanced need of antihypertensive therapy observed in hypertensive patients with metabolic syndrome when compared to those without (4). Last but not the least, tolerability of rimonabant was similar between normo and hypertensive patients (38).

Current clinical evidence indicates that blood pressure elevation above optimal levels (i.e., ≥115/75 mmHg) will increase an individual's risk of developing CV diseases (39). Thus, even small reductions in blood pressure from above optimal levels should impart a health benefit, especially in the overweight/obese population (40). Among the individual trials, the reductions in blood pressure were somewhat more evident in the studies which specifically enrolled patients at higher cardiometabolic risk (e.g., patients with dyslipidaemia or type 2 diabetes). The small antihypertensive effect in the overall patient population adds to the other, previously reported, cardiometabolic benefits of rimonabant; namely, reduced body weight and waist circumference, improved lipid profile (higher HDL-C and lower TG), reduced C-reactive protein, and improved glycaemic control (34–37). Since risk factors tend to cluster within individuals, improvements in multiple interrelated parameters is a reasonable approach to reduce overall cardiometabolic risk (41).

CV outcomes trials of anti-hypertension therapy have established that small differences in SBP reductions (2–4 mmHg) are associated with large reductions (10–20%) in major CV events (42). It is also interesting to note that in the Anglo-Scandinavian Cardiac Outcomes Trial (ASCOT), for example, in which two anti-hypertensive regimens were compared (amlodipine plus perindopril as required vs. atenolol plus bendroflumethiazide and potassium as required), differential systolic reductions in SBP and DBP of 2.8 and 1.9 mmHg, respectively, were associated with a 14% reduction in risk of fatal CHD, nonfatal myocardial infarction, and coronary revascularizations (43). This effect applied to the data obtained with rimonabant indicates that the use of this drug in hypertensive patients could be really preventive for the consequences

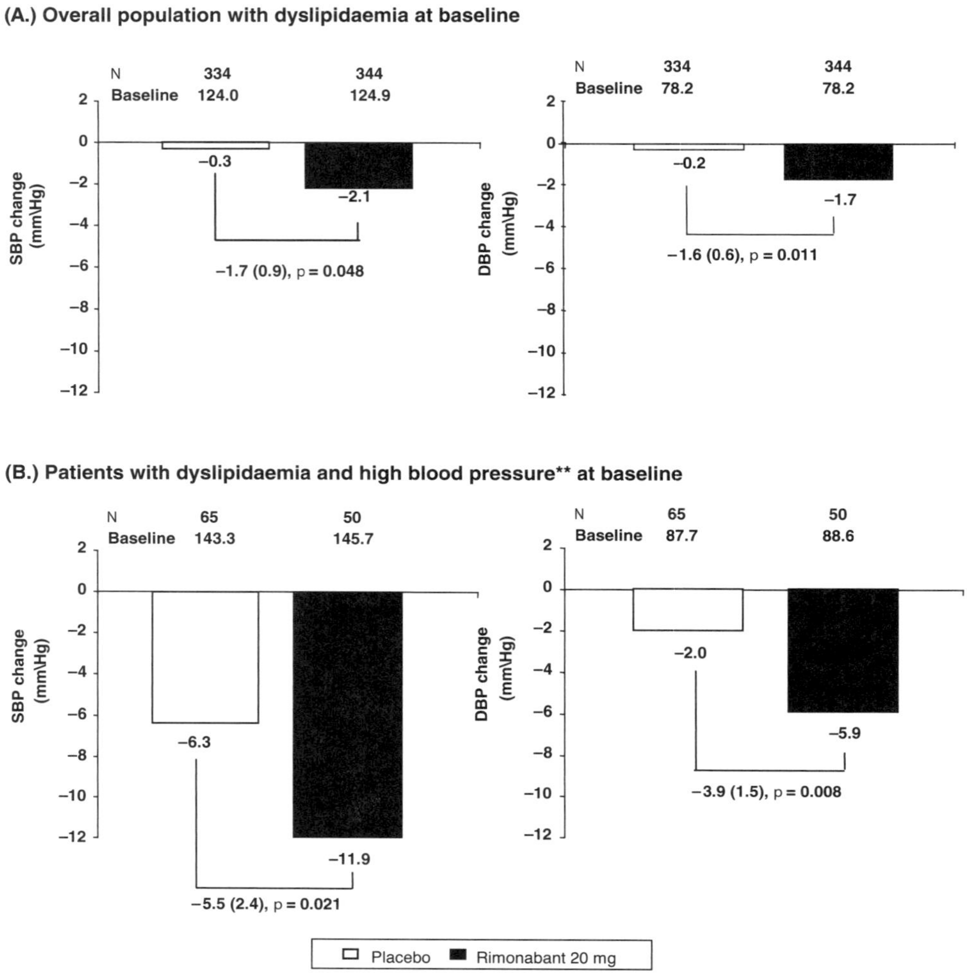

*Dyslipidaemia (RIO-Lipids): defined as TG levels ≥ 1.69 mmol (150 mg/dL) and/or total cholesterol/HDL-C ratio > 4.5 in women or > 5 in men as per protocol.

**High blood pressure: SBP ≥ 140 and/or DBP ≥ 90 mm/Hg in patients.

Figure 3 **(A)** Changes in SBP (*left panel*) and DBP (*right panel*) at 1 year in the subset of patients with untreated dyslipidaemia at baseline. Data are mean from the ITT population. Between-group comparisons are least-squares mean differences (SEM) (*p* vs. placebo). **(B)** Changes in SBP (*left panel*) and DBP (*right panel*) at 1 year in the subset of patients with untreated dyslipidaemia and high blood pressure at baseline following abdominal obesity (waist circumference) ≥102 cm for men and ≥88 cm for women; triglycerides level ≥1.695 mmol (150 mg/dL); HDL-C level ≤1.036 mmol (40 mg/dL) for men and ≤1.295 mmol (50 mg/dL) for women; systolic blood pressure ≥130 mmHg or diastolic blood pressure ≥85 mm Hg; and fasting glucose level ≥6.1 mmol (110 mg/dL).

of CV disease, added on top of the potential effects for prevention due to the correction of cardiometabolic risk including HDL-C, TG, HbA1 c, and fasting blood glucose (44).

The effect of rimonabant 20 mg/day on blood pressure seems to be mediated by weight loss, with rimonabant having no apparent direct effect on blood pressure at the dose of 20 mg/day beyond that attributable to weight loss. In contrast, approximately half of the improvements in HDL-C, TG, and HbA1c levels produced by rimonabant therapy over 1 year was beyond those expected by weight loss alone, as previously reported (36–39). It is difficult to separate the effect of weight loss from concomitant benefits of weight loss, such as reductions in visceral fat, hyperinsulinaemia, and insulin resistance (23–24), all of which may contribute to the observed blood pressure lowering effect of rimonabant therapy. Substantial evidence implicates visceral obesity in the pathophysiology of obesity-related hypertension (23–24). The visceral adipose tissue is an intriguing potential site for the effects of CB_1 blockade, as recent studies in humans have shown increased CB_1 receptor expression in visceral compared with subcutaneous adipose tissue and higher endocannabinoid levels in obese patients with a predominance of visceral compared with subcutaneous excess adipose tissue (31–32). In the RIO trials, reductions in abdominal obesity (as measured by waist circumference) paralleled body weight loss (34–37).

Preclinical studies have shown that endogenous cannabinoids exert a hypotensive effect, particularly in rodent models of hypertension or under conditions of endotoxic or hemorrhagic shock (33). In spontaneously hypertensive rats (SHR), CB_1 agonists lower blood pressure much more in SHR than in normotensive Wistar-Kyoto rats, while CB_1 blockade prevented this effect in SHR but had no effect on blood pressure in normotensive rats (45). These results suggest a role of the ECS in the regulation of blood pressure. However, it is important to note that the blood pressure lowering effect of endocannabinoids in these hypertensive animal models is primarily accounted for by tonic suppression of cardiac contractility in hypertension, and that a pressor effect of CB_1 blockade has only been noted in animal models of hypertension with supraphysiological doses and in anesthetized but not conscious animals (33). There is no evidence of any pressor effect of rimonabant in any clinical studies. Our data demonstrate that rimonabant treatment does not counteract the favorable effects of weight loss and of mobilization of abdominal fat on blood pressure in overweight/obese humans (30). On the contrary, the RIO clinical data showed reductions in blood pressure with rimonabant therapy, which are more pronounced in patients with high blood pressure at baseline.

In summary, treatment with rimonabant at 20 mg/day can lower the blood pressure of overweight/obese patients in addition to its effect on other cardiometabolic risk factors, such as abdominal obesity, dyslipidaemia, inflammation, dysglycaemia, and insulin resistance. While the overall blood pressure lowering effect of rimonabant was relatively small and was entirely attributable to the concomitant body weight loss, there was no evidence of blood pressure increases with rimonabant treatment. In patients with high blood pressure at baseline, improvements in SBP and DBP were more pronounced than in the overall pooled population. Taken collectively, the effects on blood pressure, plus the previously demonstrated improvements in lipid profile, glycaemic control, and abdominal obesity, support the use of selective CB_1 blockade with rimonabant as a novel approach to the management of multiple cardiometabolic risk factors.

REFERENCES

1. Grundy S. A changing paradigm for prevention of cardiovascular disease: Emergence of the metabolic syndrome as a multiple risk factor. Eur Heart J 2008; 10(Suppl. B):B16–B23.
2. Despres JP, Poirier P, Bergeron J, et al. From individual risk factors and the metabolic syndrome to global cardiometabolic risk. Eur Heart J 2008; 10(Suppl. B):B24–B33.
3. Romero R, Bonet J, de la Sierra A, et al. Undiagnosed obesity in hypertension: Clinical and therapeutic implications. Blood Press 2007; 16:347–353.
4. Segura J, Banegas JR, Garcia-Donaire JA, et al. Should hypertension guidelines be changed for hypertensive patients with metabolic syndrome?. J Clin Hypertens 2007; 9:595–600.
5. Ezzati M, Lopez AD, Rodgers A, et al. Comparative Risk Assesment Collaborating Group. Selected major risk factors and global and regional burden of disease. Lancet 2002; 360:1347–1360.
6. Stamler J, Vaccaro O, Neaton JD, et al. Diabetes, other risk factors and 12-yr cardiovascular mortality for men screened in the Multiple Risk Factor Intervention Trial. Diabetes Care 1993; 16:434–444.
7. The task Force for the Management of Arterial Hypertension of the European Society of Hypertension (ESH) and the European Society of Cardiolody. 2007 Guidelines for the management of arterial hypertension. J Hypertens 2007; 25:1105–1187.
8. Kurella M, Lo JC, Chertow GM. Metabolic syndrome and the risk for chronic kidney disease among nondiabetic adults. J Am Soc Nephrol 2005; 16:2134–2140.
9. Samuelsson O, Pennert K, Andersson O, et al. Diabetes mellitus and raised serum triglyceride concentration in treated hypertension: Are they of prognostic importance. Observational study. BMJ 1996; 314:660–663.
10. Verdecchia P, Reboldi G, Angeli F, et al. Adverse prognostic significance of new diabetes in treated hypertensive subjects. Hypertension 2004; 43:963–969.
11. Elliott WJ, Meyer PM. Incident diabetes in clinical trials of antihypertensive drugs: A network meta-analysis. Lancet 2007; 369:201–207.

12. Kostis JB, Wilson AC, Freudenberger RS, et al. Long-term effect of diuretic-based therapy on fatal outcomes in subjects with isolated systolic hypertension with and without diabetes. Am J Cardiol 2005; 95:29–35.
13. Barzilay JI, Davis BR, Cutler JA, et al. Fasting glucose levels and incident diabetes mellitus in older nondiabetic adults randomized to receive 3 different classes of antihypertensive treatment: A report from the Antihypertensive and Lipid-Lowering Treatment to Prevent Heart Attack Trial (ALLHAT). Arch Intern Med 2006; 166:2191–2201.
14. Alderman MH, Cohen H, Madhavan S. Diabetes and cardiovascular events in hyperetensive patients. Hypertension 1999; 33:1130–1134.
15. Knowler WC, Barrett-Connor E, Fowler SE, et al. Reduction in the incidence of type 2 diabetes with lifestyle intervention or metformin. N Engl J Med 2002; 346:393–403.
16. Chiasson JL, Josse RG, Gomis R, et al. Acarbose for prevention of type 2 diabetes mellitus: The STOP-NIDDM randomised trial. Lancet 2002; 359:2072–2077.
17. The DREAM (Diabetes Reduction Assessment with ramipril and rosiglitazone Medication) Trial Investigators. Effect of rosiglitazone on the frequency of diabetes in patients with impaired glucose tolerance or impaired fasting glucose: A randomised controlled trial. Lancet 2006; 368:1096–1105.
18. Hutton B, Fergusson D. Changes in body weight and serum lipid profile in obese patients treated with orlistat in addition to a hypocaloric diet: A systematic review of randomized clinical trials. Am J Clin Nutr 2004; 80:1461–1468.
19. Canner PL, Furberg CD, McGovern ME. Benefits of niacin in patients with versus without the metabolic syndrome and healed myocardial infarction (from the Coronary Drug Project). Am J Cardiol 2006; 97:477–479.
20. Keech A, Simes RJ, Barter P, et al. Effects of long-term fenofibrate therapy on cardiovascular events in 9795 people with type 2 diabetes mellitus (the FIELD study): Randomised controlled trial. Effects of long-term fenofibrate therapy on cardiovascular events in 9795 people with type 2 diabetes mellitus (the FIELD study): Randomised controlled trial. Lancet 2005; 366:1849–1861.
21. Arterburn DE, Crane PK, Veenstra DL. The efficacy and safety of sibutramine for weight loss: A systematic review. Arch Intern Med 2004; 164:994–1003.
22. Scholze J, Grimm E, Hermann D, et al. Optimal treatment of obesity-related hypertension: The hypertension–obesity–sibutramine (HOS) study. Circulation 2007; 115:1991–1998.
23. Després J-P, Lemieux I. Abdominal obesity and metabolic syndrome. Nature 2006; 444:881–887.
24. Van Gaal L, Mertens IL, De Block CE. Mechanisms linking obesity with cardiovascular disease. Nature 2006; 444:875–880.
25. Garrison R, Kannel W, Stokes Jr, et al. Incidence and precursors of hypertension in young adults: The Framingham Off-spring Study. Prev Med 1987; 16:235–251.
26. Okosun IS, Prewitt TE, Cooper RS. Abdominal obesity in the United States: Prevalence and attributable risk of hypertension. J Hum Hypertens 1999; 13:425–430.
27. Huang Z, Willett WC, Manson JE, et al. Body weight, weight change, and risk for hypertension in women. Ann Intern Med 1998; 128:81–88.
28. Neter JE, Stam BE, Kok FJ, et al. Influence of weight reduction on blood pressure: A meta-analysis of randomized controlled trials. Hypertension 2003; 42:878–884.
29. Osei-Hyiaman D, DePetrillo M, Pacher P, et al. Endocannabinoid activation at hepatic CB1 receptors stimulates fatty acid synthesis and contributes to diet-induced obesity. J Clin Invest 2005; 115:1298–1305.
30. Cota D, Marsicano G, Tschop M, et al. The endogenous cannabinoid system affects energy balance via central orexigenic drive and peripheral lipogenesis. J Clin Invest 2003; 112:423–431.
31. Blüher M, Engeli S, Kloting N, et al. Dysregulation of the peripheral and adipose tissue endocannabinoid system in human abdominal obesity. Diabetes 2006; 55:3053–3060.
32. Cote M, Matias I, Lemieux I, et al. Circulating endocannabinoid levels, abdominal adiposity and related cardiometabolic risk factors in obese men. Int J Obes (Lond) 2007; 31:692–699.
33. Batkai S, Pacher P, Osei-Hyiaman D, et al. Endocannabinoids acting at cannabinoid-1 receptors regulate cardiovascular function in hypertension. Circulation 2004; 110:1996–2002.
34. Després J-P, Golay A, Sjöström L, et al. Effects of rimonabant on metabolic risk factors in overweight patients with dyslipidemia. N Engl J Med 2005; 353:2121–2134.
35. Pi-Sunyer FX, Aronne LJ, Heshmati HM, et al. Effect of rimonabant, a cannabinoid-1 receptor blocker, on weight and cardiometabolic risk factors in overweight or obese patients: RIO-North America: a randomized controlled trial. JAMA 2006; 295:761–775.
36. Scheen AJ, Finer N, Hollander P, et al. Efficacy and tolerability of rimonabant in overweight or obese patients with type 2 diabetes: A randomised controlled study. Lancet 2006; 368:1660–1672.
37. Van Gaal LF, Rissanen AM, Scheen AJ, et al. Effects of the cannabinoid-1 receptor blocker rimonabant on weight reduction and cardiovascular risk factors in overweight patients: 1-year experience from the RIO-Europe study. Lancet 2005; 365:1389–1397.

38. Ruilope LM, Despres JP, Scheen A, et al. Effect of rimonabant on blood pressure in overweight/obese patients with/without co-morbidities: Analysis of pooled RIO study results. J Hypertens 2008, 26:357–367.
39. Lewington S, Clarke R, Qizilbash N, et al. Age-specific relevance of usual blood pressure to vascular mortality: A meta-analysis of individual data for one million adults in 61 prospective studies. Lancet 2002; 360:1903–1913.
40. Klein S, Burke LE, Bray GA, et al. Clinical implication of obesity with specific focus on cardiovascular disease: A statement for professionals from the American Heart Association Council on Nutrition, Physical Activity and Metabolism: endorsed by the American College of Cardiology Foundation. Circulation 2004; 110:2952–2967.
41. Gaede P, Vedel P, Larsen N, et al. Multifactorial intervention and cardiovascular disease in patients with type 2 diabetes. N Engl J Med 2003; 348:383–393.
42. Blood Pressure Lowering Treatment Trialists' C. Effects of different blood-pressure-lowering regimens on major cardiovascular events: Results of prospectively-designed overviews of randomised trials. Lancet 2003; 362:1527–1535.
43. Poulter NR, Wedel H, Dahlöf B, et al. Role of blood pressure and other variables in the differential cardiovascular event rates noted in the Anglo-Scandinavian Cardiac Outcomes Trial-Blood Pressure.
44. Ahmed MH. Rimonabant as a potential new treatment for an emerging epidemic of obesity-related glomerulopathy? Expert Opin Emerging Drugs 2006; 11:563–565.
45. Wagner JA, Jarai Z, Batkai S, et al. Hemodynamic effects of cannabinoids: Coronary and cerebral vasodilation mediated by cannabinoid CB(1) receptors. Eur J Pharmacol 2001; 423:203–210.

32 Future Developments 1: CB_1 Blockade for Weight Gain Subsequent to Smoking Cessation

Jaimee L. Heffner and Robert M. Anthenelli

Department of Psychiatry, Tri-State Tobacco and Alcohol Research Center, University of Cincinnati College of Medicine, Cincinnati, Ohio, U.S.A.

INTRODUCTION

The individual and societal costs of cigarette smoking are considerable, including over 5 million deaths per year worldwide (1). Because of the spreading tobacco epidemic in developing nations, projections of tobacco-attributable deaths may get double within the next 25 years (1). Although the prevalence of smoking has been increasing globally, some developed nations such as the United States have seen declining rates of tobacco use in recent years (2). The availability of new pharmacotherapies to aid smoking cessation has likely contributed to this decrease in the prevalence of smoking, but with the long-term success rates of quit attempts bordering on 5% (3), it is clear that there are many challenges still remaining in the effort to help current smokers quit.

One such challenge is the weight gain that frequently accompanies smoking cessation. The vast majority of smokers who quit smoking successfully will gain weight (4), with estimates of average body weight increase ranging from 3 to 10 kg (5–7). Concerns about postcessation weight gain have the potential to interfere with quit attempts, perhaps through an increased likelihood of prematurely abandoning plans for cessation (8,9) or, when a quit attempt is initiated, being less likely to successfully abstain from smoking (10). The evidence regarding the influence of weight concerns on smoking cessation is somewhat mixed, however, possibly as a result of varying definitions of weight concern and differing sets of covariates utilized in predictive models (11).

Concerns about weight gain following smoking cessation are not necessarily limited to aesthetics. Although postcessation weight gain is, in the majority of cases, self-limiting (12,13) and not of a magnitude to rival the negative health effects of continued smoking (14,15), there is a subgroup of smokers for whom success at quitting appears to initiate a large increase in body weight. Epidemiologic data from NHANES III, for example, showed that 16% of men and 21% of women who indicated that they quit smoking during the 10-year interval between data collection points reported a weight gain of 15 kg or more in that time period (16). Such large gains may contribute to increased risk for weight-related health problems, particularly among the growing number of smokers who were overweight, obese, or diabetic prior to quitting.

Given that actual or expected postcessation weight gain may have a number of negative consequences for smokers who are attempting to quit, the development of interventions with long-term efficacy in preventing or attenuating postcessation weight gain would represent a significant step forward in the treatment of nicotine dependence. In this chapter, we discuss theoretical and clinical support for the potential utility of cannabinoid CB_1 receptor antagonists to modulate postcessation weight gain. As a backdrop to this discussion, we first review (1) the hypothesized mechanisms of postcessation weight gain, with a focus on the physiological underpinnings of this phenomenon and (2) the efficacy of other interventions that have been investigated for the purpose of preventing or reducing postcessation weight gain, including behavioral interventions, pharmacological interventions, and the combination of these two.

WHAT CAUSES POSTCESSATION WEIGHT GAIN?

Put simply, the precise answer to this question is unknown. This is due, in large part, to the complex mechanisms governing feeding behavior and the vast interconnectivity among numerous neural and nonneural mediators of energy balance, many of which are influenced by nicotine (17). Although beyond the scope of this chapter (see Ref. 16 for a more comprehensive review), nicotine's appetite-suppressing and weight-lowering effects clearly involve its actions at peripheral nonneural (i.e., adipocytes, hepatocytes), neural (e.g., autonomic, sensory, and enteric neurons), and central autonomic neurons located in portions of the hypothalamus including the arcuate nucleus and the lateral hypothalamus (17). Regarding the peripheral nonneural targets, nicotine decreases triglyceride uptake and net storage in adipocytes by inhibiting lipoprotein lipase activity. It may also produce its hypophagic effects by altering the synthesis and release of leptin—a peptide hormone produced by fat cells during the well-fed state—or by altering the leptin-receptor–mediated signaling cascade (17). Nicotinic acetylcholine receptors (nAChRs) are also found on autonomic, sensory, and enteric neurons which regulate feeding behavior by governing sympathetic and parasympathetic outflow.

Within the brain, nAChRs are found throughout the hypothalamus in important nuclei regulating appetite control and feeding behavior such as the arcuate, ventromedial, dorsomedial, paraventricular, and lateral hypothalamic nuclei. Because these nuclei are the sites for the production, detection and integration of anorexigenic [e.g., corticotropin releasing hormone and melanocortins such as α-melanocyte–stimulating hormone (α-MSH)] and orexigenic peptides [e.g., neuropeptide Y (NPY)], agouti-related peptide (AgRP)] along with neurotransmitters (i.e., GABA, glutamate, serotonin, and dopamine) known to be involved with appetite control, it is likely that nicotine's effects in these multiple hypothalamic nuclei play an important role in mediating postcessation weight gain.

As will be addressed in more detail later in this chapter, several lines of evidence also point to nicotine's effects on the endocannabinoid system (ECS) as a potential mediator of postcessation weight gain. While the precise mechanisms of action are not well understood, it appears that co-activation of α7 nAChRs and glutamate NMDA receptors elicits endocannabinoid (e.g., anandamide) formation in rat cortical neurons (18). Although the biosynthetic pathways for endocannabinoid production may differ between neural and nonneural tissues (18), the ubiquitous distribution of nAChRs in the brain and periphery described above make it seem plausible that nicotinic cholinergic receptors in various brain and peripheral tissues may trigger endocannabinoid release which is a known regulator of food intake and energy balance (19). There is also growing evidence that increasing endocannabinoid tone intensifies, while disrupting CB_1 receptor signaling diminishes, nicotine reward and possibly withdrawal (20), further implicating the ECS as a potential mediator of postcessation weight gain. However, as we will see later in this chapter, the most compelling evidence for a role of endocannabinoids in mediating weight gain after quitting smoking is the consistent evidence that CB_1 blockade attenuates postcessation weight gain in smokers with prolonged abstinence.

WHICH INTERVENTIONS ARE EFFECTIVE IN PREVENTING OR REDUCING POSTCESSATION WEIGHT GAIN?

Both pharmacological and behavioral methods of preventing or limiting postcessation weight gain have been investigated, with some studies examining the combination of these two types of treatment. In this section, we summarize the findings regarding the short- and long-term efficacy of extant therapeutic strategies to address postcessation weight gain. For a more comprehensive synthesis of this literature, we would refer the reader to the recent review by Heffner et al. (2006) (21).

Pharmacological Interventions

Currently, there are several choices of pharmacotherapies that have been approved by the U.S. Food and Drug Administration (FDA) as smoking cessation aids; these include nicotine replacement therapy (available in a variety of formulations, including nicotine patch, lozenge, gum, nasal spray, and inhaler), buproprion, and varenicline. Nicotine replacement therapy has received the most empirical attention to date in terms of its potential effects on postcessation weight gain. The results of this line of research suggest that nicotine replacement has the capacity to delay, but not to prevent, the weight gain that frequently accompanies smoking cessation. The weight-attenuating effect appears to be limited to the period of active use of the medication (22,23) and may not extend to all types of nicotine replacement. That is, the evidence seems to suggest that shorter-acting formulations, including nicotine gum and nasal spray (22–24), are more effective in delaying weight gain than the longer-acting nicotine patch (25,26).

Buproprion, another first-line agent for the treatment of nicotine dependence, has also been investigated in terms of its potential to reduce or prevent postcessation weight gain. The majority of extant studies point toward a weight-attenuating effect of buproprion (27,28). At this point, however, it is not clear whether the effects of buproprion on postcessation weight represent delayed gain, as appears to be the case with some nicotine replacement therapies, or sustained reduction in weight gain attributable to smoking cessation.

Varenicline has not been studied specifically in terms of its potential to limit postcessation weight gain, but reports from clinical trials of its efficacy as a smoking cessation aid suggest that its use is associated with modestly reduced weight gain as compared to placebo (29). Additionally, estimates of posttreatment weight gain in head-to-head comparisons of the efficacy of varenicline versus buproprion (29) and varenicline versus NRT (30) suggest that the average gain associated with varenicline is similar to that of buproprion and NRT.

Other pharmacotherapeutic agents that have been investigated as potential inhibitors of postcessation weight gain include topiramate (31), fluoxetine (32), and naltrexone as an augmentation to NRT (33). Although the efficacy of these agents has not been studied extensively, each has demonstrated short-term efficacy in at least one methodologically sound clinical trial. Notably, topiramate was actually associated with a decrease in the average body weight of successful quitters (31). Although replication and extension of these findings are necessary prior to drawing any strong conclusions, they are nonetheless provocative and warrant further study.

Behavioral Interventions

A number of studies have investigated the efficacy of behavioral and/or cognitive-behavioral approaches that address diet, physical activity, and/or weight concerns as a means of limiting or preventing postcessation weight gain. In general, the results of these studies are similar to those of the pharmacological intervention studies described above. Specifically, behavioral interventions have the potential to delay postcessation weight gain, but there is little evidence of long-term efficacy (34,35). Additionally, the empirical support for short-term efficacy is not unanimous (36). One of the significant challenges in terms of the long-term efficacy of dietary and exercise interventions is poor adherence (36), which tends to worsen over time (37). We are aware of only one study that has demonstrated a significant long-term benefit of a behavioral intervention in reducing postcessation weight gain. In this study (38), participants who received cognitive-behavioral therapy (CBT) for weight concerns maintained a lower average weight gain than those who received either nonspecific group support or a more structured dietary assistance at both 6- and 12-month follow-up. The perplexing aspect of these findings is that the CBT intervention was not found to actually reduce weight concerns, so the reasons for its observed efficacy are unclear.

Combined Pharmacological and Behavioral Interventions

Several investigations have been conducted to determine the efficacy of combined pharmacotherapy and behavioral therapy on postcessation weight gain. The vast majority of these studies, all of which involved some form of nicotine replacement, suggest that the addition of a behavioral and/or cognitive-behavioral weight control component does not improve the weight-attenuating effects of nicotine replacement alone (39–41). Again, however, adherence to exercise and dietary interventions has proven to be problematic (40), especially over the long term (37), and is arguably one of the primary challenges to the efficacy of behavioral methods of reducing postcessation weight gain.

CAN POSTCESSATION WEIGHT GAIN BE ATTENUATED THROUGH CANNABINOID CB_1 RECEPTOR BLOCKADE?

While CB_1 antagonists (e.g., rimonabant, taranabant, and others) have not yet been approved by the FDA for any indication, nor have they been approved for smoking cessation or mitigating postcessation weight gain by any regulatory agency including the European Medicines Agency (EMEA), there remains much interest in the use of such agents for this possible indication. This is a result of the consistent results found in a series of studies examining rimonabant as an aid to smoking cessation along with the clear evidence that this CB_1 blocker promotes weight loss and reduces several cardiometabolic risk factors as reviewed elsewhere in this text.

One Phase 2 study (42) and four Phase 3 studies (43,44) have tested rimonabant as a potential aid to smoking cessation in a program of development named by the drug's manufacturer as Studies of Rimonabant and Tobacco Use or STRATUS. Regarding the Phase 2 trial and the first of the STRATUS short-term trials (STRATUS-US) in which our group participated, there were remarkably consistent postcessation weight gain–attenuating effects observed despite the fact that the proof-of-concept study used a dosage double than that chosen subsequently for clinical development in the larger Phase 3 STRATUS and Rimonabant in Obesity (RIO) trials (i.e., 20 mg/day). Rimonabant-treated prolonged quitters gained 75% (19) and 84% (42) less weight, respectively, than sustained quitters treated with placebo. Similarly, consistent weight-attenuating effects were observed in the subsequent STRATUS-Europe and STRATUS-Meta short-term trials (44).

The STRATUS Worldwide study used a maintenance of abstinence design and was of 1-year duration. It was designed, in part, to determine whether a lengthier exposure to this CB_1 blocker would mitigate weight gain longer term. Indeed, those prolonged abstainers who were treated with the 20-mg dosage up to 1 year gained significantly less weight than those participants who quit but were re-randomized to 5 mg of rimonabant or placebo (43).

In addition to these placebo-controlled, randomized clinical trials, another trial conducted by Rigotti et al. compared rimonabant 20 mg/day and a placebo patch with rimonabant and transdermal nicotine replacement therapy (NRT) (45). This study, dubbed the CIRRUS trial, tested the hypothesis that combining rimonabant with the nicotine patch would improve cessation rates and maintain the medication's weight-gain–attenuating effects (45). Although the trial lacked adequate control groups (i.e., double dummy placebo and NRT-alone treatment arms) to fully place the results in context, of significance to this chapter is that prolonged abstainers in both the rimonabant and placebo patch, and rimonabant and NRT groups gained trivial amounts of weight (+0.1 kg vs. +0.5 kg, respectively) in this 10-week treatment trial (45). Taken together, and as reviewed in detail elsewhere (46), these studies provide consistent evidence that rimonabant 20 mg/day markedly reduces postcessation weight gain in patients achieving prolonged abstinence while taking the drug and may modulate weight gain in the long term.

CONCLUSIONS

Preclinical studies demonstrating crosstalk between the ECS and the nicotinic cholinergic system combined with consistent evidence that the CB_1 antagonist, rimonabant, diminishes postcessation weight gain provide powerful clues that dysregulation in these systems produced by chronic smoking or nicotine withdrawal may play an important role in mediating weight gain subsequent to smoking cessation. While this discovery adds yet another level of complexity to our understanding of why smokers usually gain weight after quitting, it also opens the door for the development of new treatment strategies to address this relatively common and presently intractable side effect of successful smoking cessation.

REFERENCES

1. Mathers CD, Loncar D. Projections of global mortality and burden of disease from 2002 to 2030. PLoS Med 2006; 3(11):e442.
2. Perkins KA. Issues in the prevention of weight gain after smoking cessation. Ann Behav Med 1994; 16(1):46–52.
3. Schiller JS, Nelson C, Hao C, et.al. Early release of selected estimates based on data from the January–June 2004 National Health Interview Survey. National Center for Health Statistics 2004. 2008.
4. U.S. Department of Health and Human Services. The Health Benefits of Smoking Cessation. U.S. Department of Health and Human Services, Public Health Service, Centers for Disease Control, Center for Chronic Disease Prevention and Health Promotion, Office on Smoking and Health. DHHS Publication No. (CDC) 90-8416, 1990.
5. Eisenberg D, Quinn BC. Estimating the effect of smoking cessation on weight gain: An instrumental variable approach. Health Serv Res 2006; 41(6):2255–2266.

6. Klesges RC, Meyers AW, Klesges LM, et al. Smoking, body weight, and their effects on smoking behavior: A comprehensive review of the literature. Psychol Bull 1989; 106(2):204–230.
7. Klesges RC, Winders SE, Meyers AW, et al. How much weight gain occurs following smoking cessation? A comparison of weight gain using both continuous and point prevalence abstinence. J Consult Clin Psychol 1997; 65(2):286–291.
8. Brouwer RJ, Pomerleau CS. "Prequit attrition" among weight-concerned women smokers. Eat Behav 2000; 1(2):145–151.
9. Copeland AL, Martin PD, Geiselman PJ, et al. Predictors of pretreatment attrition from smoking cessation among pre- and postmenopausal, weight-concerned women. Eat Behav 2006; 7(3):243–251.
10. Meyers AW, Klesges RC, Winders SE, et al. Are weight concerns predictive of smoking cessation? A prospective analysis. J Consult Clin Psychol 1997; 65(3):448–452.
11. Jeffery RW, Hennrikus DJ, Lando HA, et al. Reconciling conflicting findings regarding postcessation weight concerns and success in smoking cessation. Health Psychol 2000; 19(3):242–246.
12. O'Hara P, Connett JE, Lee WW, et al. Early and late weight gain following smoking cessation in the Lung Health Study. Am J Epidemiol 1998; 148(9):821–830.
13. Williamson DF, Madans J, Anda RF, et al. Smoking cessation and severity of weight gain in a national cohort. N Engl J Med 1991; 324(11):739–745.
14. Wise RA, Enright PL, Connett JE, et al. Effect of weight gain on pulmonary function after smoking cessation in the Lung Health Study. Am J Respir Crit Care Med 1998; 157(3 Pt 1):866–872.
15. Burnette MM, Meilahn E, Wing RR, et al. Smoking cessation, weight gain, and changes in cardiovascular risk factors during menopause: The Healthy Women Study. Am J Public Health 1998; 88(1):93–96.
16. Flegal KM, Troiano RP, Pamuk ER, et al. The influence of smoking cessation on the prevalence of overweight in the United States. N Engl J Med 1995; 333(18):1165–1170.
17. Jo YH, Talmage DA, Role LW. Nicotinic receptor-mediated effects on appetite and food intake. J Neurobiol 2002; 53(4):618–632.
18. Stella N, Piomelli D. Receptor-dependent formation of endogenous cannabinoids in cortical neurons. Eur J Pharmacol 2001; 425(3):189–196.
19. Anthenelli RM. Cannabinoid antagonists: CB1 receptors as a therapeutic target for nicotine dependence. In: George TP, ed. Medication Treatments for Nicotine Dependence, 1st ed. Boca Raton, FL: Taylor & Francis, 2006:187–198.
20. Merritt LL, Martin BR, Walters C, et al. The endogenous cannabinoid system modulates nicotine reward and dependence. J Pharmacol Exp Ther 2008.
21. Heffner JL, Winders-Barrett S, Anthenelli RM. Obesity and smoking. In: McElroy SL, Allison DB, Bray G, eds. Obesity and Mental Disorders. London, UK: Taylor & Francis Books, 2005:123–144.
22. Gross J, Stitzer ML, Maldonado J. Nicotine replacement: Effects of postcessation weight gain. J Consult Clin Psychol 1989; 57(1):87–92.
23. Sutherland G, Stapleton JA, Russell MA, et al. Randomised controlled trial of nasal nicotine spray in smoking cessation. Lancet 1992; 340(8815):324–329.
24. Doherty K, Militello FS, Kinnunen T, et al. Nicotine gum dose and weight gain after smoking cessation. J Consult Clin Psychol 1996; 64(4):799–807.
25. Hughes JR, Hatsukami DK. Effects of three doses of transdermal nicotine on post-cessation eating, hunger and weight. J Subst Abuse 1997; 9:151–159.
26. Transdermal Nicotine Study Group. Transdermal nicotine for smoking cessation. Six-month results from two multicenter controlled clinical trials. JAMA 1991; 266(22):3133–3138.
27. Hays JT, Hurt RD, Rigotti NA, et al. Sustained-release bupropion for pharmacologic relapse prevention after smoking cessation. A randomized, controlled trial. Ann Intern Med 2001; 135(6):423–433.
28. Hurt RD, Sachs DP, Glover ED, et al. A comparison of sustained-release bupropion and placebo for smoking cessation. N Engl J Med 1997; 337(17):1195–1202.
29. Nides M, Oncken C, Gonzales D, et al. Smoking cessation with varenicline, a selective alpha4beta2 nicotinic receptor partial agonist: Results from a 7-week, randomized, placebo- and bupropion-controlled trial with 1-year follow-up. Arch Intern Med 2006; 166(15):1561–1568.
30. Aubin HJ, Bobak A, Britton JR, et al. Varenicline versus transdermal nicotine patch for smoking cessation: Results from a randomised, open-label trial. Thorax 2008.
31. Anthenelli RM, Blom TJ, McElroy SL, et al. Preliminary evidence for gender-specific effects of topiramate as a potential aid to smoking cessation: Gender effects of topiramate in smoking cessation. Addiction 2008; 103:687–694.
32. Borrelli B, Spring B, Niaura R, et al. Weight suppression and weight rebound in ex-smokers treated with fluoxetine. J Consult Clin Psychol 1999; 67(1):124–131.
33. O'Malley SS, Cooney JL, Krishnan-Sarin S, et al. A controlled trial of naltrexone augmentation of nicotine replacement therapy for smoking cessation. Arch Intern Med 2006; 166(6):667–674.
34. Hall SM, Tunstall CD, Vila KL, et al. Weight gain prevention and smoking cessation: Cautionary findings. Am J Public Health 1992; 82(6):799–803.

35. Marcus BH, Albrecht AE, King TK, et al. The efficacy of exercise as an aid for smoking cessation in women: A randomized controlled trial. Arch Intern Med 1999; 159(11):1229–1234.
36. Marcus BH, Lewis BA, Hogan J, et al. The efficacy of moderate-intensity exercise as an aid for smoking cessation in women: A randomized controlled trial. Nicotine Tob Res 2005; 7(6):871–880.
37. Ussher M, West R, McEwen A, et al. Randomized controlled trial of physical activity counseling as an aid to smoking cessation: 12 month follow-up. Addict Behav 2007; 32(12):3060–3064.
38. Perkins KA, Marcus MD, Levine MD, et al. Cognitive-behavioral therapy to reduce weight concerns improves smoking cessation outcome in weight-concerned women. J Consult Clin Psychol 2001; 69(4):604–613.
39. Nides M, Rand C, Dolce J, et al. Weight gain as a function of smoking cessation and 2-mg nicotine gum use among middle-aged smokers with mild lung impairment in the first 2 years of the Lung Health Study. Health Psychol 1994; 13(4):354–361.
40. Pirie PL, McBride CM, Hellerstedt W, et al. Smoking cessation in women concerned about weight. Am J Public Health 1992; 82(9):1238–1243.
41. Ussher M, West R, McEwen A, et al. Efficacy of exercise counselling as an aid for smoking cessation: A randomized controlled trial. Addiction 2003; 98(4):523–532.
42. Dale LC, Anthenelli RM. Rimonabant as an aid to smoking cessation in smokers motivated to quit: Results from a U.S. multicenter study—STRATUS US Trial. Abstract Presented at the Annual Meeting of the American College of Cardiology, New Orleans, Louisiana, March 2004.
43. Niaura R, Dale L, Anthenelli R. Long-term treatment with rimonabant for smoking cessation and the maintenance of abstinence: Results from the STRATUS-Worldwide Trial. Poster Presented at the International Conference of the American Thoracic Society, San Diego, California, May 2005.
44. Cinciripini PM, Aubin HJ, Dale LC, et al. Pooled analysis of three short-term, randomized, double-blind, placebo-controlled trials with rimonabant 20 mg/d in smoking cessation. Poster Presented at the 8th Annual Conference of the Society for Research on Nicotine and Tobacco (SRNT) Europe, Kusadasi, Turkey, September 2006.
45. Rigotti NA, Gonzales D, Dale LC, et al. Efficacy and safety of adding a nicotine patch to rimonabant for smoking cessation: A randomized controlled trial. Paper Presented at the 13th Annual Meeting of the Society for Research on Nicotine and Tobacco. Austin, Texas, February 2007.
46. Cahill K, Ussher M. Cannabinoid type 1 receptor antagonists (rimonabant) for smoking cessation. Cochrane Database Syst Rev 2007; (3):CD005353.

33 Future Developments 2: Cannabinoid CB_1 Receptor Blockade in Weight Gain Subsequent to Psychiatric Disorder Treatment

Ester Fride, Shimon Rabichev, and Nikolai Gobshtis
Departments of Behavioral Sciences and Molecular Biology, Ariel University Center, Ariel, Israel

INTRODUCTION

Psychotropic medications were introduced in the 1950s. Despite their significant contribution to the management of psychiatric disease, they have been known from the onset of their usage as promotors of appetite and food intake, (1) and as a consequence of undesirable increase in body weight. More recently, the risk factors associated with weight gain and obesity have been delineated (1). These disease states include hypertension, type 2 diabetes, heart disease, stroke, and certain types of cancer (1–9).

The weight gain induced by psychotropic drugs may reach incidence rates of 44% with the antidepressant amitriptyline and 70% with nortriptyline (1), for body weights between 2 and 17 kg (2). In addition to the pathophysiologies associated with excessive body weight and obesity, psychiatric drug–induced weight increases frequently leading to noncompliance with the treatment, which in turn puts the patient at risk for relapse of mental disease (2,3,10).

Many second-generation antipsychotic medications, although having a much-improved side effects profile with regard to motor symptoms, increase weight gain to an even greater extent (1).

It seems that no class of psychotropic drugs is spared this side effect (2,11), although a few drugs seem to be devoid of weight gain induction. A few notable exceptions of such drugs include the antidepressant bupropion and two mood stabilizers (for use in bipolar disorder), carbamazepine and topiramate (2,12–13).

With respect to antischizophrenic drugs, the weight gain is severe and especially notable upon administration of widely used atypical antipsychotics, such as olanzepine and clozapine (1). Although antipsychotic drugs are associated with greater weight gain than antidepressants (2–3), antidepressant-induced weight increase carries a greater problem for the population at large, as antidepressant prescriptions are far more common (10–40% of the population) than antipsychotic medications (~1%) (2,8). Body weight increase upon administration of both antidepressant and (atypical) antipsychotic drugs is accompanied by glucose and lipid abnormalities, which are symptoms of the metabolic syndrome (1,14).

The major classes of antidepressant medications are the tricyclic antidepressants that prevent reuptake of norepinephrine and/or serotonin and the selective serotonin reuptake inhibitor (SSRI) drugs, which elevate levels of serotonin (7–8). Both types of drugs have been observed to initially induce weight loss (which was anticipated in view of the increase in serotonin levels), after which a "paradoxic" weight gain is often observed—after about 1 year of treatment (2,15)—for example, a 76-week study using combined fluoxetine/olanzepine therapy for major depressive disorder with or without treatment-resistant depression (16).

The psychiatric drug–induced weight gain is complex as depression and/or recovery by themselves may be associated with either weight gain or weight loss (15,17). The noncompliance, which often results from excessive weight gain, may amount to 48% (5,18).

Mood stabilizers, such as valproate and lithium used in the treatment of manic-depressive disease, may lead to a 6 to 10 kg weight gain (2,11). However, this review will focus on antidepressant and antipsychotic drugs.

MECHANISMS UNDERLYING PSYCHIATRIC DRUG–INDUCED BODY WEIGHT ELEVATION

The cause of weight gain as a result of antidepressant treatment is apparently multi-factorial, involving multiple-serotonin receptors in the case of SSRI-induced side effects and a number of additional systems including histamine-1 (H1R), opiate receptors, and/or the appetite suppressing hormone leptin in the case of tricyclic antidepressants (11). Many antipsychotics and SSRI antidepressants block 5-HT2 C receptors result in enhanced food intake (11,19). Additionally, the histamine-1 receptor is a mediator of food intake and carbohydrate craving, such that blocking these H1R receptors increases appetite and weight gain (11,14), while H1R knockout mice are obese (20). A recent study has shed new light on the mechanism of weight induction, at least in patients using atypical antipsychotic medication. Thus, Kim et al. demonstrated that antipsychotics, which are associated with severe weight gain, such as clozapine and olanzepine, activate the "fuel sensor" molecule AMPK (AMP protein kinase) through antagonism of the histamine H1R receptor (32).

PRESENT THERAPEUTIC AND/OR PREVENTIVE APPROACHES

A number of pharmacological agents have been proposed as a co-treatment along with long-term antidepressant medication with the aim to prevent weight gain. The drawback of at least some of these agents is their psychoactive and addictive potential and/or the absence of a known weight-loss mechanism (3–4). Included in such treatments are (1) topiramate, H2-antagonsists, naltrexone and serotonergic drugs, and leptin, as well as the peripherally acting orlistat and metformin. However, such combined treatment has been investigated only in open, short-term studies. For example, the anticonvulsant topiramate has been combined with the antipsychotic clozapine, resulting in dramatic weight loss, reported, however, as a single case study (21). Side effects with topiramate alone include sedation, dizziness, and impaired concentration (1). The opiate receptor antagonist naltrexone was used in a small clinical study with tricyclic antidepressants (1). However, in an animal study, naloxone was ineffective in reducing the antipsychotic sulpiride-induced weight gain (22). When the selective norepinephrine reuptake inhibitor reboxetine was combined with the antischizophrenic olanzepine in a 6-week study, weight gain was attenuated, although it was still present (23).

THE ECS, WEIGHT CONTROL, AND PSYCHIATRIC CONDITIONS

In recent years, appetite and body weight regulation by cannabinoid CB_1 receptors have been explored (24). In a series of phase III clinical trials involving over 13,000 subjects (25), the CB_1 receptor antagonist/inverse agonist SR141716 (rimonabant, acomplia), successfully reduced body weight and improved lipid profiles in obese subjects. In comparison to other current weight loss agents (orlistat and subitramine), the side effect profile of rimonabant was significantly more favorable than that of orlistat, while it was similar to that of subitramine—the latter drug, however, is contraindicated for patients with hypertension (26). Rimonabant did display significant rates of anxiety and depression, although afflicting less than 5% of the subjects (26). This will be discussed below in more detail. Importantly, the weight loss (4–5 kg) was at least as large as that upon adminstration of orlistat (2.85 kg) or subitramine (4.85 kg) (26–27).

Endocannabinoids and Obesity

This topic is extensively reviewed in other chapters of this book. It is sufficient to state here that the Endocannabinoid system (ECS) has been shown to interact with several major players in weight regulation and the metabolic syndrome. These include leptin (28), ghrelin, and perhaps NGF (nerve growth factor) (see Ref. 29) and more recently, mutual regulation of the ECS and histamine and AMPK have been demonstrated.

Thus, enhanced histamine release after local infusion of cannabinoids in the tuberomammillary nuclei of the hypothalamus was shown (30). However, an older study reported a decrease in brain histamine turnover upon the administration of Δ^9-tetrahydrocannabinol (Δ^9-THC) (31). Since these studies widely differ in methodologies, future research will have to determine the causal relationship and the dose dependence between the ECS and histamine in the regulation of food intake and obesity. However, it is of interest that the H1R receptor is being considered as a useful target for antiobesity pharmacotherapy (14,32). An additional adipokine, NGF, may be regulated by cannabinoid receptors, as shown, for example, by endocannabinoid stimulation of CB_1 and CB_2 receptors on peripheral nerves of NGF receptor tyrosine kinase A (TrkA) activation-induced inflammatory hyperalgesia (33).

Finally, the fuel sensing molecule AMPK is stimulated in the hypothalamus and inhibited in adipose tissue by Δ^9-THC (34), offering an additional explanation of the involvement of the ECS in appetite promotion and fat deposition.

The ECS, Mood Regulation, and Psychosis

The many (patho)physiological functions in which the ECS plays a regulatory role, include mood regulation, depression, and perhaps schizophrenia (8,35–37). Underlying such involvement may be ECS interactions with the serotonin system, such as activation of the serotonin receptors 5-HT_1, 5-HT_2, and 5-HT_3 (38) and enhanced firing of serotonergic and noradrenergic neurons as seen after application of URB597, an inhibitor of the endocannabinoid hydrolyzing enzyme "fatty acid amide hydroxylase" (39), or the rich interactions with the hypothalamic–pituitary–adrenal (HPA) stress axis (see Pagotto, this volume) and the dopamine system (40).

Depression

Cannabinoids may have antidepressant potential, whereas cannabis use may be motivated by self-medication for depression (41). Behavioral studies investigating the putative relationship between depression, the serotonin, and the ECSs, however, have yielded contradictory findings. Thus, antidepressant effects of cannabinoid CB_1 receptor antagonist/inverse agonists mouse behavioral assays (42–45) have been reported, while, in contrast, an antidepressant effect of the cannabinoid CB_1 receptor agonist (arachidonyl-2-chloroethylamide) was observed in the "Porsolt forced swimming" assay for mice (46). The latter finding is consistent with an antidepressant effect of the cannabinoid CB_1 receptor agonist HU-210 and the anandamide reuptake inhibitor AM404 in the forced swimming test in rats (47) and with an antidepressant-like effect induced by URB597 (see previous section) (39). Finally, in some studies cannabinoid CB_1 receptor antagonists (AM251 and rimonabant) were devoid of any activity in the forced swim test in rats (47) and mice (39,48), respectively. Since species, strain, and dose differences could underlie the varying outcomes, the involvement of the cannabinoid CB_1 receptor in the regulation of depressive behavior is clearly complex. Witkin and colleagues (49–50) have extensively reviewed the multiple roles of the cannabinoid CB_1 receptor in depression and anxiety disorders. Their overall impression is of an antidepressant potential for cannabinoid CB_1 receptor antagonist. As to the modulation of anxiety, these authors note that cannabinoid CB_1 receptor mediation is complex and often contradictory.

However, in previous studies it was demonstrated that biphasic effects of exocannabinoids (45,51) and endocannabinoids (52) on neurotransmitter release and behavioral parameters, may underlie at least some of the apparent contradictory outcomes when measuring cannabinoid-induced effects.

It is therefore interesting that in some of the clinical trials performed with rimonabant in overweight patients, a mild but significant increase in cases with anxiety or depression was reported (53). In our hands, rimonabant had no depressive-like effect in mice, whether it was administered acutely (Fig. 1), or chronically (Fig. 2). Interestingly, 30 days after the cessation of a 4-month treatment period, the rimonabant-treated group displayed a "rebound" depression-like behavior in the Porsolt forced swimming assay (Fig. 3).

Schizophrenia

The role of cannabis smoking as a risk factor for schizophrenia remains controversial (41), although a recent review of a number of longitudinal studies concludes that in vulnerable individuals, cannabis use may precipitate schizophrenia (54). Several lines of evidence are supportive of elevated endocannabinoid activity in schizophrenia-relevant behaviors or brain areas, such as the prefrontal cortex (see Ref. 55).

Based on such findings, it may be hypothesized that a CB_1 receptor antagonist and/or a CB_1 receptor inverse agonist may counteract symptoms of schizophrenia (56). Indeed in a recent animal study, rimonabant restored performance in the pre-pulse inhibition assay (PPI; a

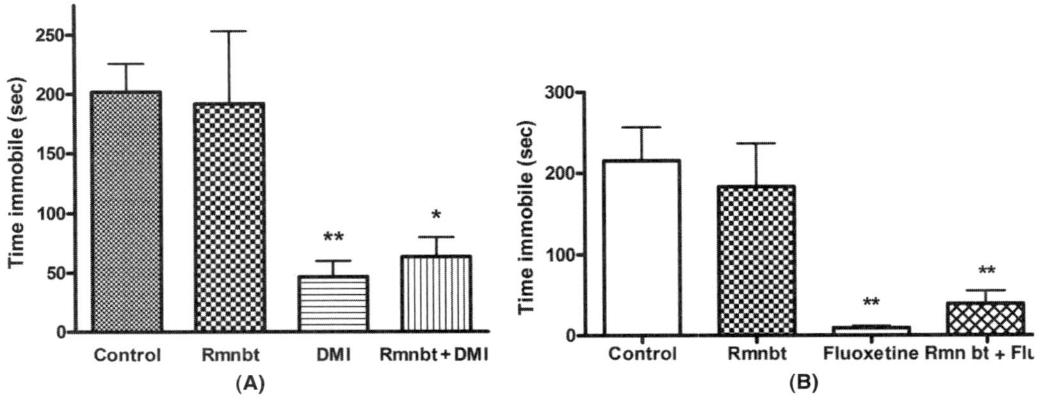

Figure 1 The antidepressant effects of an acute injection of desipramine (DMI) or fluoxetine; no effects of rimonabant. Female mice (Sabra strain), 2–3 months old, received two intraperitoneal injections of either control solution (ethanol:cremophor:saline = 1:1:18) or rimonabant (SR141716, 5 mg/kg, Rmnbt), 30 minutes before saline or **(A)** desipramine (DMI; 15 mg/kg) or **(B)** fluoxetine (20 mg/kg). Thirty minutes later, mice were observed in the "Porsolt forced swimming" test, which assesses antidepressant drug potential. The mice were scored for "immobility" (lack of movements except those necessary to stay afloat) by three independent observers, for 9 minutes. Data were analyzed with a one-way ANOVA, with Newman–Keuls post hoc analyses (Control, i.e., Vehicle + Saline). Values are presented as mean ± SEM. $^{*}p \leq 0.05$, compared to rimonabant; $^{**}p \leq 0.05$, compared to Control (for DMI and Fluoxetine) or compared to rimonabant (for Rmnbt+Fluox).

behavioral assay for sensorimotor gating, commonly used to diagnose schizophrenia in humans or schizophrenia-like symptoms in laboratory animals), after disruption by phencyclidine, apomorphine or dizocilpine (57). In another study, however, schizophrenia-like symptoms (D1 and D2 receptor agonist–induced stereotypy) were exacerbated by rimonabant (58). A third study found that rimonabant counteracted Δ^9-THC–induced impairment of PPI, but only in isolated rats (59). We have recenty confirmed a lack of rimonabant-induced impairment of PPI (Fig. 4). Finally, a clinical multi-center trial, which compared the antipsychotic potential of rimonabant to that of three other potential neuroleptic drugs and to that of the prototypical haloperidol over a 6-week period, found no antipsychotic activity for rimonabant (60).

INHIBITING THE ECS TO PREVENT PSYCHIATRIC DRUG–INDUCED WEIGHT GAIN

Despite the complex involvement of the cannabinoid CB_1 receptor in mood regulation and psychosis, the robust antiobesity effect of cannabinoid CB_1 receptor antagonists, and the theoretical plausibility that CB_1 receptor antagonism may be helpful or neutral in combating depression or psychosis (see above), suggests that combined treatment of a CB_1 receptor antagonist together with conventional psychiatric medication, may be a possible solution for psychiatric drug-induced overweight.

In a recent study (48), we investigated the effects of receptor antagonism/inverse agonism (using rimonabant) both on weight gain as well as on antidepressant-induced struggling behavior in the Porsolt forced swimming test. Thus, in this study, we showed for the first time that long-term treatment (daily injections for 4 months) with an antidepressant (the tricyclic desipramine, 5 mg/kg/day), induced a significant 7% increase in weight gain in mice, which in humans is defined as a clinically significant weight gain (61). Moreover, similarly to human patients, after initial reduction in weight gain, the excessive increase in body weight only started to become apparent after 2 months of treatment, which is equivalent to year long treatment in patients (6–7,48). Importantly, we showed that co-treatment with rimonabant (2 mg/kg/day) prevented the excessive weight gain, while, when periodically tested in the forced swimming test for anti-depressant activity (Fig. 2), the effectiveness of desipramine was preserved over the whole period of treatment.

In order to prevent the stress-induced inhibition of weight gain resulting from daily injections (48), we are now administering antidepressant or antipsychotic drugs, with the CB_1 receptor antagonist, via the drinking water.

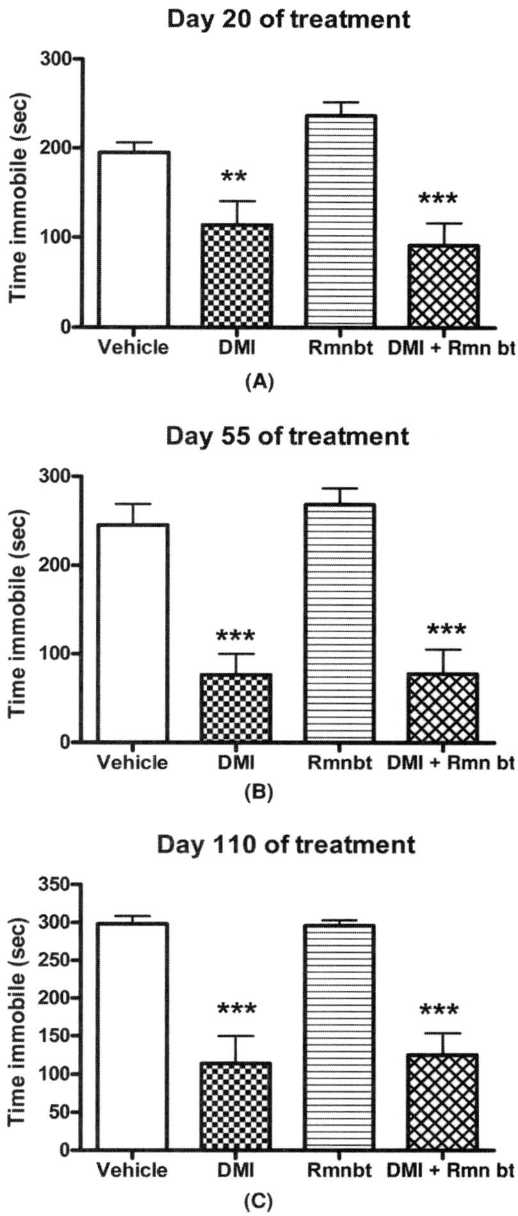

Figure 2 Chronic treatment with desiramine with or without rimonabant does not interfere with the antidepressant effect of desipramine. Long-term (116 days including an 14-day interruption) treatment (one daily intraperitoneal injection) with saline, desipramine (DMI; 5 mg/kg), rimonabant (Rmnbt; 2 mg/kg) or desipramine + rimonabant to female mice (Sabra strain), 2- to 3-month old. Mice were periodically tested in the forced swim test, that is, at 20, 55, and 110 days after the onset of treatment. Desipramine and desipramine+rimonabant significantly decreased immobility on days 20, 55, and 110. Rimonabant did not differ significantly from vehicle controls on any test day [see (A), (B), and (C)]. Values are presented as mean ± SEM. **Different from its control (desipramine vs. Vehicle; desipramine + rimonabant vs. rimonabant), $p \leq 0.01$; ***different from its control (desipramine vs. Vehicle; desipramine + rimonabant vs. rimonabant), $p \leq 0.001$.

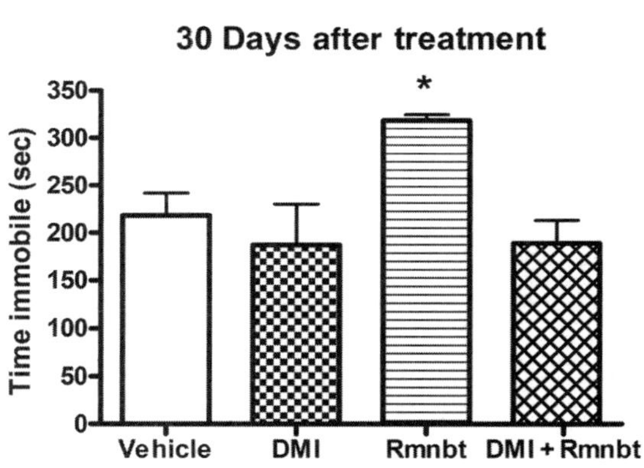

Figure 3 Rebound pro-depressive effect of rimonabant, 30 days after cessation of 4 months of treatment. Long-term treatment with saline, desipramine (DMI; 5 mg/kg), rimonabant (Rmnbt; 2 mg/kg) or desipramine + rimonabant to female mice (Sabra strain), 2- to 3-month old. Mice were tested in the forced swim test at 30 days after the cessation of treatment. Desipramine and desipramine + rimonabant did not differ significantly from vehicle controls; rimonabant displayed significantly elevated immobility. Values are presented as mean ± SEM. *Different from Vehicle, $p \leq 0.05$.

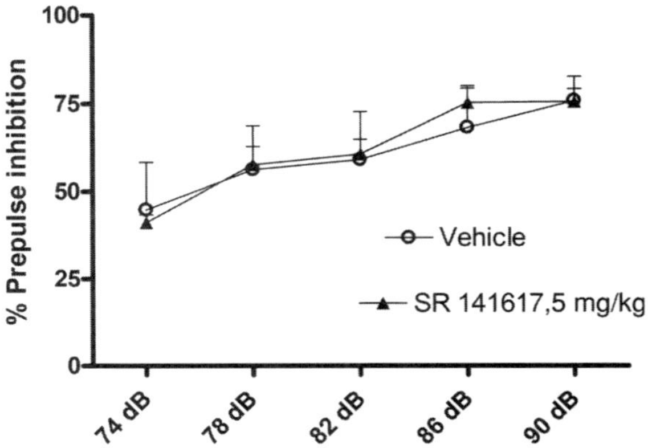

Figure 4 Rimonabant (5 mg/kg) does not affect prepulse inhibition female Sabra mice (2–3-month old) were tested for prepulse inibtion of the acoustic startle response (PPI) after peritoneal administration of vehicle (ethanol:cremophor:saline = 1:1:18) or rimonabant (5 mg/kg). One hour later they were tested for PPI—the sound level of the startle stimuli was 120 dB and that of the prepulse stimuli was 74, 78, 82, 86, and 90 dB (Kinder, CA, U.S.A.). Values are presented as mean ± SEM.

Similarly to the antidepressants, it is not clear whether rimonabant may improve, impair or be inactive with regard to ongoing antipsychotic pharmacotherapy (see section, "Schizophrenia"). Also here, no long-term studies have been performed to address the issue. Therefore, we are currently investigating whether rimonabant will effectively prevent antipsychotic-induced excessive weight gain, while preserving its antischizophrenic effectiveness.

CONCLUSIONS

In conclusion, in view of the involvement of the ECS in appetite, body weight regulation and metabolism, together with its profound yet complex influence on mood and cognition, manipulation of the CB_1 receptor may prevent excessive weight gain and obesity, which is a disturbing side effect of many psychiatric drugs. No optimal solution is available at this time (1). However, since it appears that the effect of blocking the CB_1 receptor on psychiatric functions may be dependent on many factors including the intrinsic activity of the CB_1 receptor antagonist, such therapeutic potential needs to be studied carefully for each psychiatric medication and each type of CB_1 receptor antagonist (neutral antagonist as well as inverse agonists).

ACKNOWLEDGMENTS

SR141716 was kindly supplied by RTI, North Carolina, U.S.A. and by Sanofi-Aventis, France. Financial support: Israel Ministry of Absorption (to N. G.) and Sanofi-Aventis, France, are also acknowledged for providing financial support.

REFERENCES

1. Zimmermann U, Kraus T, Himmerich H, et al. Epidemiology, implications and mechanisms underlying drug-induced weight gain in psychiatric patients. J Psychiatr Res 2003; 37(3):193–220.
2. Schwartz TL, Nihalani N, Jindal S, et al. Psychiatric medication-induced obesity: A review. Obes Rev 2004; 5(2):115–121.
3. Schwartz TL, Nihalani N, Virk S, et al. Psychiatric medication-induced obesity: Treatment options. Obes Rev 2004; 5(4):233–238.
4. Van Ameringen M, Mancini C, Pipe B, et al. Topiramate treatment for SSRI-induced weight gain in anxiety disorders. J Clin Psychiatry 2002; 63(11):981–984.
5. Himmerich H, Schuld A, Haack M, et al. Early prediction of changes in weight during six weeks of treatment with antidepressants. J Psychiatr Res 2004; 38(5):485–489.
6. Kachur SG, Hannan CL, Ward KE. Antidepressant-induced weight gain. Med Health R I 2005; 88(10):359–361.
7. Ferguson JM. SSRI antidepressant medications: Adverse effects and tolerability. Prim Care Companion J Clin Psychiatry 2001; 3(1):22–27.
8. Pacher P, Kecskemeti V. Trends in the development of new antidepressants. Is there a light at the end of the tunnel? Curr Med Chem 2004; 11(7):925–943.

9. Wirshing DA. Schizophrenia and obesity: Impact of antipsychotic medications. J Clin Psychiatry 2004; 65 (Suppl. 18):13–26.
10. Schwartz TL, Jindal S, Simionescu M, et al. Effectiveness of orlistat versus diet and exercise for weight gain associated with antidepressant use: A pilot study. J Clin Psychopharmacol 2004; 24(5):555–556.
11. Virk S, Schwartz TL, Jindal S, et al. Psychiatric medication induced obesity: An aetiologic review. Obes Rev 2004; 5(3):167–170.
12. Chengappa KN, Gershon S, Levine J. The evolving role of topiramate among other mood stabilizers in the management of bipolar disorder. Bipolar Disord 2001; 3(5):215–232.
13. Weisler RH, Johnston JA, Lineberry CG, et al. Comparison of bupropion and trazodone for the treatment of major depression. J Clin Psychopharmacol 1994; 14(3):170–179.
14. Meltzer HY. Illuminating the molecular basis for some antipsychotic drug-induced metabolic burden. Proc Natl Acad Sci U S A 2007; 104(9):3019–3020.
15. Harvey BH, Bouwer CD. Neuropharmacology of paradoxic weight gain with selective serotonin reuptake inhibitors. Clin Neuropharmacol 2000; 23(2):90–97.
16. Corya SA, Andersen SW, Detke HC, et al. Long-term antidepressant efficacy and safety of olanzapine/fluoxetine combination: A 76-week open-label study. J Clin Psychiatry 2003; 64(11):1349–1356.
17. Maina G, Albert U, Salvi V, et al. Weight gain during long-term treatment of obsessive–compulsive disorder: A prospective comparison between serotonin reuptake inhibitors. J Clin Psychiatry 2004; 65(10):1365–1371.
18. Pijl H, Meinders AE. Body weight change as an adverse effect of drug treatment. Mechanisms and management. Drug Saf 1996; 14(5):329–342.
19. Bickerdike MJ, Vickers SP, Dourish CT. 5-HT2 C receptor modulation and the treatment of obesity. Diabetes Obes Metab 1999; 1(4):207–214.
20. Masaki T, Chiba S, Yasuda T, et al. Involvement of hypothalamic histamine H1 receptor in the regulation of feeding rhythm and obesity. Diabetes 2004; 53(9):2250–2260.
21. Levy E, Margolese HC, Chouinard G. Topiramate produced weight loss following olanzapine-induced weight gain in schizophrenia. J Clin Psychiatry 2002; 63(11):1045.
22. Baptista T, Lacruz A, Acosta A, et al. Naltrexone does not prevent the weight gain and hyperphagia induced by the antipsychotic drug sulpiride in rats. Appetite 2000; 34(1):77–86.
23. Poyurovsky M, Pashinian A, Gil-Ad I, et al. Olanzapine-induced weight gain in patients with first-episode schizophrenia: A double-blind, placebo-controlled study of fluoxetine addition. Am J Psychiatry 2002; 159(6):1058–1060.
24. Fride E, Bregman T, Kirkham TC. Endocannabinoids and food intake: Newborn suckling and appetite regulation in adulthood. Exp Biol Med (Maywood) 2005; 230(4):225–234.
25. Wadman M. Appetite downer awaits approval. Nature 2005; 437(7059):618–619.
26. Wierzbicki AS. Rimonabant: Endocannabinoid inhibition for the metabolic syndrome. Int J Clin Pract 2006; 60(12):1697–1706.
27. Padwal RS, Majumdar SR. Drug treatments for obesity: Orlistat, sibutramine, and rimonabant. Lancet 2007; 369(9555):71–77.
28. Di Marzo V, Goparaju SK, Wang L, et al. Leptin-regulated endocannabinoids are involved in maintaining food intake. Nature 2001; 410(6830):822–825.
29. Fride E. The endocannabinoid-CB Receptor system: A new player in the brain–gut–adipose field. Biomedical Reviews 2006; 17, 1–20.
30. Cenni G, Blandina P, Mackie K, et al. Differential effect of cannabinoid agonists and endocannabinoids on histamine release from distinct regions of the rat brain. Eur J Neurosci 2006; 24(6):1633–1644.
31. Oishi R, Itoh Y, Nishibori M, et al. Delta9-Tetrahydrocannabinol decreases turnover of brain histamine. J Pharmacol Exp Ther 1985; 232(2):513–518.
32. Kim SF, Huang AS, Snowman AM, et al. From the cover: Antipsychotic drug-induced weight gain mediated by histamine H1 receptor-linked activation of hypothalamic AMP-kinase. Proc Natl Acad Sci U S A 2007; 104(9):3456–3459.
33. Farquhar-Smith WP, Jaggar SI, Rice AS. Attenuation of nerve growth factor-induced visceral hyperalgesia via cannabinoid CB(1) and CB(2)-like receptors. Pain 2002; 97(1–2):11–21.
34. Kola B, Hubina E, Tucci SA, et al. Cannabinoids and ghrelin have both central and peripheral metabolic and cardiac effects via AMP-activated protein kinase. J Biol Chem 2005; 280(26):25196–25201.
35. Hill MN, Gorzalka BB. Is there a role for the endocannabinoid system in the etiology and treatment of melancholic depression? Behav Pharmacol 2005; 16(5–6):333–352.
36. Fride E, Russo E. Neuropsychiatry: Schizophrenia, depression and anxiety. In: Onaivi E, Di Marzo V, eds. Endocannainoids: Marijuana of the Human Body, Brain And Testes. Boca Raton, FL: CRC Press, 2004.
37. Hainer V, Kunesova M, Bellisle F, et al. Psychobehavioral and nutritional predictors of weight loss in obese women treated with sibutramine. Int J Obes (Lond) 2005; 29(2):208–216.
38. Morales M. Cannabinoids and the central serotonergic system. In: Onaivi E, Sugiura T, Di Marzo V, eds. Endocannabinoids: The Brain and the Body's Marijuana and Beyond. Boca Raton: Taylor and Francis; 2006:249–260.

39. Gobbi G, Bambico FR, Mangieri R, et al. Antidepressant-like activity and modulation of brain monoaminergic transmission by blockade of anandamide hydrolysis. Proc Natl Acad Sci USA 2005; 102(51):18620–18625.
40. Martin AB, Fernandez-Espejo E, Ferrer B, et al. Expression and function of CB(1) receptor in the rat striatum: Localization and effects on D(1) and D(2) dopamine receptor-mediated motor behaviors. Neuropsychopharmacology 2008; 33(7):1667–1679.
41. Fride E, Russo E. Neuropsychiatry: Schizophrenia, depression and anxiety. In: Onaivi E, Sugiura T, Di Marzo V, eds. The brain and body's marijuana. Boca Raton: CRC Press, 2006:371–382.
42. Shearman LP, Rosko KM, Fleischer R, et al. Antidepressant-like and anorectic effects of the cannabinoid CB1 receptor inverse agonist AM251 in mice. Behav Pharmacol 2003; 14(8):573–582.
43. Petit-Demouliere B, Chenu F, Bourin M. Forced swimming test in mice: A review of antidepressant activity. Psychopharmacology (Berl) 2005; 177(3):245–255.
44. Griebel G, Stemmelin J, Scatton B. Effects of the cannabinoid CB1 receptor antagonist rimonabant in models of emotional reactivity in rodents. Biol Psychiatry 2005; 57(3):261–267.
45. Tzavara ET, Davis RJ, Perry KW, et al. The CB1 receptor antagonist SR141716A selectively increases monoaminergic neurotransmission in the medial prefrontal cortex: Implications for therapeutic actions. Br J Pharmacol 2003; 138(4):544–553.
46. Rutkowska M, Jachimczuk O. Antidepressant-like properties of ACEA (arachidonyl-2-chloroethylamide), the selective agonist of CB1 receptors. Acta Pol Pharm 2004; 61(2):165–167.
47. Hill MN, Gorzalka BB. Pharmacological enhancement of cannabinoid CB1 receptor activity elicits an antidepressant-like response in the rat forced swim test. Eur Neuropsychopharmacol 2005; 15(6):593–599.
48. Gobshtis N, Ben-Shabat S, Fride E. Antidepressant-induced undesirable weight gain: Prevention with rimonabant without interference with behavioral effectiveness. Eur J Pharmacol 2007; 554(2–3):155–163.
49. Witkin JM, Tzavara ET, Davis RJ, et al. A therapeutic role for cannabinoid CB1 receptor antagonists in major depressive disorders. Trends Pharmacol Sci 2005; 26(12):609–617.
50. Witkin JM, Tzavara ET, Nomikos GG. A role for cannabinoid CB1 receptors in mood and anxiety disorders. Behav Pharmacol 2005; 16(5–6):315–331.
51. Tzavara ET, Wade M, Nomikos GG. Biphasic effects of cannabinoids on acetylcholine release in the hippocampus: Site and mechanism of action. J Neurosci 2003; 23(28):9374–9384.
52. Sulcova E, Mechoulam R, Fride E. Biphasic effects of anandamide. Pharmacol Biochem Behav 1998; 59(2):347–352.
53. Pi-Sunyer FX, Aronne LJ, Heshmati HM, et al. Effect of rimonabant, a cannabinoid-1 receptor blocker, on weight and cardiometabolic risk factors in overweight or obese patients: RIO-North America: a randomized controlled trial. JAMA 2006; 295(7):761–775.
54. Degenhardt L, Hall W. Is cannabis use a contributory cause of psychosis? Can J Psychiatry 2006; 51(9):556–565.
55. Linszen D, van Amelsvoort T. Cannabis and psychosis: An update on course and biological plausible mechanisms. Curr Opin Psychiatry 2007; 20(2):116–120.
56. Scatton B, Sanger DJ. Pharmacological and molecular targets in the search for novel antipsychotics. Behav Pharmacol 2000; 11(3–4):243–256.
57. Ballmaier M, Bortolato M, Rizzetti C, et al. Cannabinoid receptor antagonists counteract sensorimotor gating deficits in the phencyclidine model of psychosis. Neuropsychopharmacology 2007; 32(10):2098–2107.
58. Ferrer B, Gorriti MA, Palomino A, et al. Cannabinoid CB1 receptor antagonism markedly increases dopamine receptor-mediated stereotypies. Eur J Pharmacol 2007; 559(2–3):180–183.
59. Malone DT, Taylor DA. The effect of Delta9-tetrahydrocannabinol on sensorimotor gating in socially isolated rats. Behav Brain Res 2006; 166(1):101–109.
60. Meltzer HY, Arvanitis L, Bauer D, et al. Placebo-controlled evaluation of four novel compounds for the treatment of schizophrenia and schizoaffective disorder. Am J Psychiatry 2004; 161(6):975–984.
61. Fava M, Judge R, Hoog SL, et al. Fluoxetine versus sertraline and paroxetine in major depressive disorder: Changes in weight with long-term treatment. J Clin Psychiatry 2000; 61(11):863–867.

Index